MENTAL HEALTH CONCEPTS APPLIED TO NURSING

Mental Health Concepts Applied to Nursing

LOIS CRAFT DUNLAP, R.N., M.S.

Editor

Assistant Professor
University of San Francisco
School of Nursing
San Francisco, California

A WILEY MEDICAL PUBLICATION
John Wiley & Sons
New York • Chichester • Brisbane • Toronto

Library of Congress Cataloging in Publication Data
Main entry under title:

Mental health concepts applied to nursing.

  Bibliography: p.
  Includes index.
  1. Psychiatric nursing. 2. Sick-Psychology. I. Dunlap,
Lois Craft. [DNLM: 1. Mental disorders — Therapy — Nursing
texts. 2. Psychiatric nursing. WY160 M547]
RC440.M35   610.73'68   77-22962
ISBN 0-471-04360-5

Manufactured in the United States of America
10 9 8 7 6 5 4 3 2 1

Composed and printed at the
Waverly Press, Inc.
Mt. Royal and Guilford Aves.
Baltimore, Md. 21202, U.S.A.

Dedicated to:
Marion E. Kalkman,
*Teacher, friend, and source of
immeasurable inspiration*

CONTRIBUTORS

MILDRED ANDREINI, R.N., M.S.
Coordinator, Anchorage Child Abuse Board, Inc.
Anchorage, Alaska 99502

SR. PATRICE BURNS, O.C., M.A.
(As told to Lois C. Dunlap)
Counselor, West Coast Cancer Foundation
San Francisco, California

SHERRLYN CARPENTER, R.N., M.S.
Outreach Nurse
Sonoma County Mental Health Department
Sonoma, California

DIANA COHEN, M.A.
Licensed Family Therapist
Former Director of Education
Walnut Creek Hospital
Walnut Creek, California

DANA L. CONNELL, M.S.W.
Social Worker
Norwalk Hospital
Norwalk, Connecticut

ALICE DEMI, R.N., M.S.
Former Nursing Coordinator
Hospice of Marin
Marin County, California
D.N.S.
University of California
San Francisco, California

JANNE DUNHAM, M.S.
Continuing Education
University of Michigan
Ann Arbor, Michigan

BARBARA R. DUNLAP, B.S.
Counselor, Mt. St. Joseph's Group Home
San Francisco, California

LOIS CRAFT DUNLAP, R.N., M.S.
Assistant Professor, School of Nursing
Doctoral Student, School of Education
University of San Francisco
San Francisco, California

CAROL FINK, R.N., B.S.
Psychiatric Liaison Consultant with
Trauma and Burn Units
San Francisco General Hospital
San Francisco, California

BEVERLY J. HENDLER, R.N., M.S.
Psychiatric Nurse Specialist
Walnut Creek, California

DORIS HOUSER, R.N., M.A.
Clinical Nurse Specialist, Cardiovascular Disease
University Hospital
Iowa City, Iowa

DARRYL S. INABA, PHARM.D.
Director of Pharmaceutical Services,
Drug Detoxification
Haight-Ashbury Free Medical Clinic
San Francisco, California

JEANETTE JUSTICE, R.N., M.S.
University of Nevada
School of Nursing
Reno, Nevada

SR. M. MARTHA KIENING, S.M., R.N., M.S.
Professor Emeritus, School of Nursing
University of San Francisco
San Francisco, California

D. ALLAN LEVY, M.D.
San Mateo, California

ELEANOR L. METZ, R.N., M.N.
Assistant Professor
University of San Francisco
School of Nursing
San Francisco, California

CAROL EDGERTON MITCHELL, R.N., M.N.
Assistant Professor, Mental Health and
Community Nursing
University of California at San Francisco
School of Nursing
San Francisco, California

JOHN H. QUINN, M.A., M.A.
Art Psychotherapist
Walnut Creek Hospital
Walnut Creek, California

RICHARD REUBIN, DR.P.H.
Director, Marin Suicide Prevention Center
San Anselmo, California

SUSAN PHELPS RHINEBERGER, B.S.
Registered Recreational Therapist
Director of Patient Activities
Walnut Creek Hospital
Walnut Creek, California

JERI E. RYAN, R.N., M.S.
Clinical Nurse Specialist
Mission Mental Health Center
San Francisco, California

LYNN SAVEDRA, R.N., D.N.S.
Assistant Professor, Department of
Family Health Nursing
University of California at San Francisco
School of Nursing
San Francisco, California

HARVEY J. WIDROE, M.D.
Medical Director
Walnut Creek Hospital
Walnut Creek, California

REV. LARS F. WILLIAMSON, M.A.
Co-Founder, Open Doors Ministries, Inc.
Sausalito, California

D. JEAN WOOD, R.N., M.S., PH.D.
Associate Professor
University of Michigan
School of Nursing
Ann Arbor, Michigan

Preface

SOME BOOKS OF READINGS develop out of formal studies conducted by an organization or group of educators or clinicians. Some present the various known theories on a particular topic. Still others bring together in one volume current articles which have appeared in many sources of professional literature in order to make available easy access to them.

This collection of all new readings dealing with the application of mental health concepts in both traditional and not so traditional settings for the nurse, evolved mainly in response to the knowledge of the fact that thousands of registered nurses from diploma and associate degree programs are returning to the educational scene each year. Some have been away from nursing for a period of time, others come from a variety of nursing specialties other than the care of the emotionally disordered. Only a relatively few are either skilled in psychiatric nursing, aware of current developments in the field or plan to specialize in that area. Most of these nurses will continue to work in a wide assortment of community and experimental agencies other than psychiatric facilities. It is necessary for them to become aware of trends and issues in today's care of the emotionally disordered, both in the hospital and the community, but the chief objective of concerned educators in the field of psychiatric nursing should be to better prepare these nurses to apply mental health concepts and principles in their own nursing specialty regardless of the setting. It is in many of these areas that the work of primary prevention can take place. The nurse must be aware of both the obvious and the unspoken needs of the patient or client and be able to respond to them in a therapeutic way. Much time has been wasted in the past putting these nurses through routine learning experiences aimed toward general objectives for all nursing students. This book is intended to meet the more specific needs of the student who is a registered nurse and to hasten the educational process for her. It brings together in one volume a vast wealth of material showing application of important concepts in the care of patients and clients. Perhaps such an overview of the reality of psychosocial nursing will also help to reduce some of the anxiety associated with the reentry into a dynamically changing professional education. It should be noted that this collection is inclusive and broad enough to be of tremendous value to the basic nursing student or to anyone who works with those who at this point in time have difficulty in dealing with the emotional problems of living.

This book also grew out of a long felt need to make available to the reader some examples of creative work being done by many dynamic and innovative clinicians. We can all learn from sharing the experiences of these committed persons, some of whom serve in out of the way places. This need has grown over the years as I have, in my professional life, become aware of these people, and others like them, and developed a deep sense of appreciation and respect for their contributions to the mental health field. Gradually, over my 30 years of professional experience in mental health nursing, I have become increasingly more aware of the role of the nurse in primary prevention, especially in the areas of critical care nursing. I have expanded my teaching in nursing education to include wholism and early intervention as vital to the prevention of emotional disturbances. Psychosocial concepts must be integrated into all patient care. The responsibility for providing assistance in meeting the psychosocial needs of any client rests on all of us who are engaged in helping professions or who are in any way involved in the delivery of such services.

This is not primarily a textbook but a sourcebook containing examples of the "how to do" from actual clinical experience. It is intended for the practitioner in any setting who is interested in the role of the nurse in effecting primary prevention of psychological and social maladjustment. There are many theories of mental health nursing represented "operationally" in these pages. The reader will find multiple points of view and approaches demonstrating examples of group and individual attempts to apply basic mental health concepts into a variety of settings.

This book has two main themes — the reality of working with the emotional aspect of the individual and the existential awareness of one's own humanness. Its credo is an approach to life as a whole wherein the helping person is a human being first and a scientist second. It is a recognition that the nurse and the patient share more than anything else in the commonality of their humanity, which means both the acceptance of human potential and the acceptance of individual limitations. Perhaps the deepest bond of the nurse-patient/client relationship emerges out of this unspoken recognition. Nurses who have truly incorporated this humanistic ethic are united in seeking growth-facilitating experiences for their patients and themselves. Therefore, this is not an attempt to present "identified" or rigid content around a framework of ordered concepts and constructs appropriate to many basic psychiatric nursing textbooks, but rather to explore the existential reality of psychosocial nursing today. However, the theory and application of such concepts are there, but incorporated into the presentation. Each author draws on practical experience to tell how it really is, the theory qualifying and verifying what is seen and felt.

Another theme the authors bring to the reader is the stress on the individual uniqueness of the patient or client. Each intervention or response from the nurse should in turn be as unique as the individual himself if it is to have the necessary potential for facilitating mutual growth.

In Part 1 the readings deal mainly with patients in the hospital setting in which are found those people who suffer from emotional distress sufficiently severe to produce symptoms that interfere with their functioning in society.

I attempt to set the tone of the book in the first reading by emphasizing the importance of love in the nurse-patient relationship, with all of its inherent elements necessary for a growth experience. The theme of humanistic ethic is integrated into each reading as some of the innovative approaches to treatment are discussed. Part 2 speaks to the need in the community for skilled practitioners in the mental health field by presenting readings which deal with certain groups of identified clients. Again, the above theme continues, and the importance of the therapeutic alliance is stressed. In Part 3 the reader will find examples of the application of mental health concepts and principles to specific specialty areas. There are many other clinical areas which could be appropriately discussed but the very practical aspect of size limits their inclusion herein. However, it is hoped that the reader who works with those other identified groups will be able to make the application on his/her own.

I would like to express my gratitude to all of those who have helped me to bring to fruition this book, which originated first in the form of a beautiful dream, an expression of an ideal. Speaking as a nurse, I wish to thank all of my patients of the past, and as a teacher, all of my wonderful students whom I have had the privilege of knowing. In sharing their lives and experiences with me, they have taught me the most. I thank God for my life experiences, both positive and negative, which have been for me a source of insight and understanding. Without the support of family and friends who have put up with some insanely "mad" behavior as the stresses of such an undertaking grew, this book would never have been completed. And to the many contributors, who cooperated so well in this project, I express my appreciation for both their faith in me and their willingness to share in this dream long enough to get the job done. It is my hope that those who read this book, because of their care and concern for the emotionally troubled, will find in the presentation of actual clinical experiences, suggestions for helping others to find comfort and more purpose to their lives.

L.C.D.

Contents

PART 3: THE APPLICATION OF PSYCHIATRIC NURSING CONCEPTS

PART 1

The Psychiatric Patient in the Hospital Setting

Chapter 1

the therapeutic process in the nurse-patient relationship

LOIS CRAFT DUNLAP

The process that takes place in therapy is described as one of ego strengthening, growth, adjustment and expansion. Nurses speak of the therapeutic process as a successful meeting of the patient's needs, a time of mutual growth. These statements are quite valid, but one must look closer to see what lies at the core of this intricate interaction.

Erich Fromm so accurately wrote of man's deepest need as being one of overcoming his separateness, his aloneness, and he logically concluded that the desire for interpersonal fusing had to be the most powerful striving in man. And love, Fromm felt, was the active power in man that accomplished this unity with others, that helps him to retain his own integrity. "In love the paradox occurs that two beings become one and yet remain two." (Fromm, 1956, p. 21)

It is this love or active process of giving (more accurately, of sharing) which is actually at the heart of the therapeutic process in the nurse-patient relationship. Its importance lies in the human element of giving oneself, of ones life, of that which is alive in oneself, thereby enriching the other person. As the patient grows and becomes more complete, what has been given is thereby returned to the giver. Rather than giving up or losing something the nurse also receives and is enriched. This is similar to what happens in any teaching-learning process. It has been correctly stated that no greater lessons are learned than those the teacher learns from her students if she remains open and receptive in the process.

Not only does love imply giving but also care and concern. (Fromm, 1956, p. 27) Nurses, however, in attempting to meet the needs of patients, get more concerned with the results that caring can produce instead of the necessary commitment to a *philosophy* of caring. Crucial to such a philosophy is the art of empathy. (Pendleton, 1976, p. 52) Somehow, in her relationship with the patient, this message of care and concern must get across to the patient, not necessarily by being said in so many words but conveyed in her actions toward him. The greatest asset the nurse can have toward accomplishing this is the ability to be herself, to be relaxed and natural. There is an element here of Carl Rogers' "congruence," a condition he states as necessary for learning to take place in therapy. (Rogers, 1969)

It is when this congruence exists that the nurse's genuineness will be conveyed to the patient. It is this humanness that is so vital in the therapeutic relationship. The nurse, in her acceptance of her own uniqueness, accepts the individual unique qualities of her patient. In order to accept one's own uniqueness it is necessary to listen to oneself. It means being real, being close to whatever is going on within oneself at the time that it is happening. This is very often a difficult task and one which goes on throughout one's entire life. To be real says that one is not basically afraid of whatever lies within oneself, and therefore is nondefensive and totally willing to be vulnerable. Realness such as this on the part of the nurse brings out much more real feeling from those other people around her and allows a closer, more caring relationship. Communicating this realness to another is far from easy because of the complexity of feelings and because one must push aside the security of any facade, instead speaking from deep within oneself. When the nurse is basically frightened or threatened in the relationship she cannot get close to what she is experiencing and consequently is not genuine or congruent. In turn, neither the care nor the concern, necessary elements of love, are communicated to the patient. In accepting the patient's unique qualities the nurse is also allowing the patient to be his own realness and to be separate from her with his own ideas and values which may be totally different from hers. Here again is the paradox. Kahlil Gibran speaks of this separateness yet oneness in *The Prophet*:

Let there be spaces in your togetherness,
And let the wind of the heavens dance between you.
Love one another, but make not a bond of love:
Let it rather be a moving sea between the shores of your souls . . .
Give your hearts, but not into each others keeping.
For only the hand of Life can contain your hearts.
And stand together yet not too near together:
For the pillars of the temple stand apart,
And the oak tree and the cypress grow not in each others shadow. (Gibran, 1923, pp. 19–20)

Nurses need to overcome their anxiety in approaching this kind of closeness. One way of viewing such hesitation is that it represents a fear of being "swallowed up" or of being pulled out of one's role and merged with that of the patient who has been identified as "sick." This is a role of much less status and authority and one certainly not desired.

Fromm also emphasized the element of responsibility in love. (Fromm, 1956, p. 28) To the loving person the life of his brother is not only his brother's concern but also his. He feels as responsible for others as for himself. This accounts for the nurse becoming professionally involved with the patient in the therapeutic relationship as in the form of taking direct and specific actions. For years educators have taught students that getting involved with patients was to be avoided and that involvement would make the nurse less effective if allowed to take place. Pendleton believes, however, that getting involved does not decrease one's effectiveness. In fact, it is "the fear of getting involved" that decreases a nurse's effectiveness. She actually advocates encouraging students to get involved, to be a participant in "active empathic envolvement rather than falling into passive, sympathetic immobility." (Pendleton, 1976, p. 53) This responsibility also accounts for her recognition of the necessity for limit-setting with the patient and for definite preventive measures when acting out behavior seems probable. When the nurse establishes the therapeutic alliance and/or a verbal contract with her patient she is exercising this responsibility. It is in the felt need for physical and verbal confrontation in the relationship that the nurse expresses her feeling of responsibility for the patient. These active interventions initiated by the nurse express also the care and concern she feels for the patient.

There is also the third of Fromm's components of love present in the nurse-patient relationship, namely, respect. "Respect is not fear and awe; it denotes, in accordance with the root of the word (respicere-to look at), the ability to see a person as he is. Respect, thus implies the absence of exploitation." (Fromm, 1956, p. 28) Respect also implies Rogers' genuineness. The patient must be allowed to grow and enfold for his own sake and in his own way. It becomes obvious that the nurse cannot respect the patient in this sense of the word if she herself has not achieved independence, for respect exists only where freedom exists also. This returns us again to the necessary acceptance of one's unique qualities, whatever they may be, and a continual awareness of what is being experienced at the time, moment to moment. With respect for the patient comes also a greater appreciation of the patient in a growth-promoting way.

When the nurse respects the patient she acknowledges his identity as a distinct and separate individual, as a human being important to himself and to others. She gives the necessary recognition which maintains and confirms whatever semblance of a self-concept he may have. The sick individual, especially one with an emotional disturbance, has a tremendous need to be recognized as a person. So frequently, his ego boundaries are vague and poorly developed or shattered by emotional turmoil, and he is not really sure who he is in relation to others. It is through this respect, a vital element in love, that the nurse recognizes a patient's behavior, whatever it may be, to be a manifestation of his illness. Her acceptance is based on an understanding of its meaning and does not reflect a value judgement against the behavior. And most important, respect for the patient also includes the necessary recognition of the patient's inherent capacity to change. I am totally convinced that many patients have regressed and lived out a vegetative existence on the back wards of state mental hospitals because no one conveyed to them their belief in this capacity which exists within all persons. We tend to stereotype patients, putting them in catagories and expecting certain behavior according to whatever diagnostic "pile" they fall into. The withdrawn schizophrenic patient does not have to remain that way, always apart from others, and the delusional patient need not always be ruled by his suspicions of those around him. The depressed and self-destructive can indeed learn to see the value in living and the possibility for happiness and self-enjoyment. The young seclusive patient can only learn to see himself as

something other than that if those around him, through their respect, recognize him as an individual capable of change, treat him and refer to him as such, and give him the necessary "space" to change and to grow. The concept of the "I" emerging from the "Thou" as the infant develops, as presented by Arieti comes to mind. (Arieti, 1974 pp. 551–587) If the "Thou", or the significant others within the patient's environment (as the nurse), see him as unable to change, the positive "I" or self will not form. Without a positive "Thou" there can be no positive "I."

The fourth basic element common to all forms of love, Fromm identifies as knowledge. (Fromm, 1956, p. 29) He states clearly that it is impossible to respect a person without knowing him. All four elements are tied very closely together. Care and responsibility would lead nowhere if they were not guided by knowledge of the person. Likewise, Fromm points out that knowledge would be useless if it is not motivated by care and concern. Knowledge also facilitates respect. This knowledge that the nurse must have about the patient tells her more than the fact that he is angry, for example, whether it is blatantly out in the open or is hidden. It tells her that beyond that he is basically lonely, frightened, hurt and feeling guilty. She not only transcends her own problems and feelings, whatever they may be, but sees a suffering insecure human being seeking her understanding and acceptance rather than the angry person attempting to shove her away. The shouting and obscenities are seen as manifestations of a more basic need.

Fromm also tells us that not only does love help man to overcome his sense of isolation by "fusing" with another but that it also fills man's need and desire to know or to penetrate into the secret of man's soul, to have full knowledge of the innermost part of him, of life as it really is, way down deep. . . . (Fromm, 1956, p. 29) So it is through the act of loving that one gives of oneself, discovering both oneself and one's fellow man, and reaches out toward full knowledge. As the nurse, through her love for the patient, grows in knowledge not only of herself and of him as a unique and separate individual, she also grows in knowledge of man in general and of life itself. This she passes back to the patient and both grow and benefit from the process. All of the elements discussed—care, concern, responsibility, respect, knowledge— are mutually interdependent.

The love, which exists between the patient and the nurse and which is the vital element operating within the therapeutic process, is of the most fundamental kind, identical with brotherly love as described by Fromm. (Fromm, 1956, p. 47) It is not as all exclusive as is sexual love—it is a love for all human beings, a desire to help and enhance the life of another who is more like you than not and a recognition of a general sense of brotherhood. It is the kind of love referred to in the Bible where man is told to love his brother and where another element inherent within it is spoken to. "In love there is no fear." (The first letter of John, Ch. 4, Verse 18) Fear is cast out because of the presence of all those vital interdependent elements of love which are in full operation—the warmth and acceptance, care and concern, respect, depth of knowledge, absence of judgement or criticism, and a sense of responsibility. There is no ambivalence, only consistency. It is in the absence of fear that the patient feels safe and secure and risks can be taken. It is only in such a milieu that a patient is given the opportunity to grow and the growth will take place. We do not create growth in our patients anymore than a man and woman create a new life in sexual union. They merely bring together living cells into the necessary environment for fusion, nurturing and growth to take place. We provide for our patients in the nurse-patient relationship an emotional environment conducive to growth by giving and sharing of ourselves through the love demonstrated in the therapeutic process. This love says to the patient, "Hold on to my hand and share the strength I feel. Use my eyes in your moment of blindness to see the light of hope and the beauty of the world around you. Hear through my ears the words of encouragement and expressions of tenderness and concern which you need and desperately desire. Feel in me a safeness necessary in order to shed the tears of grief you feel. Allow me to tend your wounds so that they might heal with little scarring. Accept from me that which was freely given to me from another and which I wish to pass on to you." These words may not be spoken to the patient as such but must be accurately perceived by the patient before the risk taking, the working through, the ego growth and the insight will take place, because only then will there be enough trust felt in the relationship. When the patient turns to the nurse and asks a personal question, such as, "Are you married?" or "Do you have any children?", she is advised to turn the question back to the patient, "Why do you ask?" Most nursing educators teach students this kind of behavior. The truth of the matter is that, handled in such a manner, the nurse loses a valuable opportunity to share of herself with her patient without focusing the interview of the nurse's life and problems—the fear of which seems to be at the base of such teaching. The nurse cannot always *take* in the relationship, she must also *give*.

We speak of giving and the expression of warmth as though it did not include any element of tenderness. Yet, in order to be human we need to be tender—and to be tender implies to give, because it is in giving that tenderness is expressed. It is through tenderness that one's kinship with other human beings can be felt and one's being is affirmed. The therapeutic process is more than an educative process—it is also a meaningful feeling-relationship. The following has been cited as a case in point:

A father brought his son to Plato and enrolled him in Plato's classes. The boy worked with Plato for a year. At the end of that time, the father came to Plato quite angry. He said to the Great Master, "My boy knows nothing." Plato replied, "Of course not, he doesn't love me."

(Leland, 1960, p. 21)

Students ask, "How do I do these things? What do I say to the patient? What do I do for him?" Theory serves a purpose but so often authors speak in global terms. What does it mean to be sensitive, to care, to have empathy, patience and persistence? How do we respect the patient and show that he is accepted? How do we create a warm and safe environment? How does the nurse help the patient to be less frightened by the emotions and feelings he sees in himself and others so that he might look at them, identify them, and gain satisfactory control over them? How does she convey understanding so that the patient no longer feels alone? Students best receive the answers to these questions by observing a skillful clinician actually interacting with a patient or by observing the role-play of a simulated situation.

Roland, age 18, has been lying on his bed motionless and mute, his eyes closed since his admission the previous afternoon. He would maintain a position he was placed in for long periods of time. The rather sudden onset of this behavior followed his witnessing the brutal murder of his father. When the doctors, on their morning rounds about the unit asked, "Good morning, Roland. How are you?", he gave no answer. "Are you frightened, Roland?" Roland opened his eyes and slowly said, "No." — his first words since his arrival. The doctor replied, "You look frightened." Roland closed his eyes saying no more.

A nurse, having witnessed this, pulled a chair up to Roland's bed after the doctors had left. Now is the time to establish an alliance with this young man whom she was observing for the first time, she thought. She knew Roland was unable at this moment to take the risk involved in saying, "Yes, I am frightened." Instead of expecting this, looking directly at his unopened eyes, she introduced herself and began to express for him those feelings which her many years of working with patients told her he was experiencing. It would be much easier for him to give, at first, nonverbal affirmation if he felt truly understood and if it were expressed for him. She began, "I know how you are feeling, Roland. It is a scary thing to be here in this hospital, especially when it is the first time anything like this has happened to you. You are sick. We want to do everything we can to help you get well — to help you to feel better and to understand what this is all about. Let me help you feel less frightened." Speaking very slowly she began to orient Roland to the reality of time and place, acknowledging for him his felt confusion. He responded only with his eyes which closely followed

her lips. Again she stated as sensitively as she knew how, "I know how frightened you are feeling." Roland opened his eyes and nodded his head. "The other young men here in this room have also been sick and understand the difficult time you are having," she said. Then introducing him to John, also 18, as he approached, she said, "John sleeps in the bed next to yours. He is feeling much better now than he did when he arrived here a week ago." Expressing concern the nurse asked, "Have you had breakfast, Roland? It is especially important that you drink enough fluids." She attempted to convey to Roland by tone and modulation of voice, — it is safe to speak. I know you are able to do this. He than replied, softly but clearly, "Yes." With a well formulated plan in mind the nurse began, "Have you ever been in a psychiatric hospital before, Roland?" Out it came, the first sentence. "No, this is the first time." "Well", she replied, "it is better for you to be up and around as much as possible rather than to remain in bed. We can even go out on the patio — it's a beautiful sunny day." Slowly she helped him to get up, encouraging him with each step that she knew he was able to do it with little physical assistance from her. Holding his hand they walked up and down the corridor, at first silently. Then he looked at her and with an attempt to smile said, "Gee, thanks for helping me out."

Here we see the beginning of the therapeutic process in the nurse-patient relationship, with the communication in actions to the patient of the love described by Fromm with its elements of care and concern, respect, responsibility and knowledge, and of all the other therapeutic attitudes necessary for the expression and working through of conflictual feelings by the patient. Here we see the beginning of trust and the risky business of expressing meaningful feelings. The process of reality testing begins and the patient slowly allows the nurse to enter his safer but more isolated world. In the future work which lies ahead there will be many ups and downs, pitfalls and times of progress. There will also be times when it seems certain that both patient and nurse are on a downhill course. However, with early evidence of warning and the awareness of corrective measures applicable to the situation, the correct action will again further the therapeutic process toward the desired goal. Much can be learned from these periods of little progress—they can be anticipated and utilized in a positive way.

MacKinnon and Michels define the therapeutic alliance as the relationship between the doctor's analyzing ego and the healthy, observing rational component of the patient's ego. (MacKinnon and Michels, 1971, p. 11) This realistic therapeutic alliance has its origin in infancy and is based on the bond of real trust between the child and his mother. These authors go on to say that in all interviewing aimed at uncovering deep feelings is the fundamental technique of attempting to stimulate the patient's curiosity. The therapist starts early in the relationship to use "his own genuine curiosity to awaken the patient's interest in himself." (MacKinnon and Michels, 1971, p. 57) This curiosity is directed to the most superficial aspects of the patient's conflict rather than at deeply repressed issues—which are defended at a great cost. Thus, the nurse working with Roland dealt with the here and now, the confusing aspects of his present reality. She did not deal with the traumatic experience of his father's murder and the feelings surrounding it.

And what is involved in one's being able to give love in the nurse-patient relationship? Again we turn to Fromm. The nurse must be objective, overcoming her own narcissism, the concern with only that which exists within oneself as being real. People and things in the outside world must be seen as they are, apart from internal fears and desires. The nurse must be reasonable and have an attitude of humility. She must practice rational faith, a quality of firmness and certainty in her own convictions. This faith is "rooted in an independent convic-

tion based upon one's on productive observing and thinking." (Fromm, 1956, p. 123) Faith implies courage, the ability to take risks and complete commitment. Part of the nurse's faith is her belief in the patient's potentialities, his ability to grow and to change. Fromm accurately states that "love is an act of faith, and whoever is of little faith is also of little love." (Fromm, 1956, p. 128) Likewise, the nurse-patient relationship void of love and all of its vital elements will never provide the growth experience necessary for the patient to learn a more effective and satisfying way of life.

BIBLIOGRAPHY

Arieti, S. Schizophrenia: the psychodynamic mechanisms and psychostructural forms. In Arieti, S. (Ed.), *American Handbook of Psychiatry*, Vol. III. New York: Basic Books, Inc., 1974, pp. 551–587.

Baumgartner, M. Empathy. In Carlson, C. (Ed.), *Behavoral Concepts in Nursing*. Philadelphia: J. B. Lippincott Co., 1970, pp. 29–37.

Burgess, A. W., and Lazare, A. *Psychiatric Nursing in The Hospital and Community*, 2nd ed. Englewood Cliffs, New Jersey: Prentice-Hall Inc., 1976, pp. 85–174.

Carter, F. M. *Psychosocial Nursing*, 2nd ed. New York: MacMillan Co., Inc., 1976, pp. 135–178.

Fromm, E. *The Art of Loving: An Enquiry into the Natury of Love*. New York: Harper and Row, 1956.

Gibran, K. *The Prophet*. New York: Alfred A. Knopf, 1923, pp. 19–20.

Leland, T. Tenderness: a haven in a hurricane. *Voices* 2: 21, 1960.

MacKinnon, R. A., and Michels, R. *The Psychiatric Interview in Clinical Practice*. Philadelphia: W. B. Saunders Co., 1971.

Pendleton, M. K. When the need to be human conflicts with the need to be professional. In *Current Perspectives in Psychiatric Nursing—Trends & Issues*, Vol. I. St. Louis: The C. V. Mosby Co., 1976.

Robinson, L. *Psychiatric Nursing As A Human Experience*. Philadelphia: W. B. Saunders Co., 1972, pp. 11–39.

Rogers, C. *Freedom to Learn*. Columbus, Ohio: Charles Merrill & Co., 1969.

Sullivan, H. S. *The Psychiatric Interview*. New York: W. W. Norton & Co., 1954.

The New Testament

Chapter 2

conducting a therapeutic community

JANNE DUNHAM

Nurses, because of their continuous observation and interaction with patients, are an indispensable part of a therapeutic community. They are present in the unit environment more than any other staff members. Therapeutic community principles are based on the belief that the way a person interacts outside the hospital will be reflected in the way this person relates to others in the day to day activities and relationships on the unit. The staff member who has 24-hour, day to day responsibility on the unit is the nurse. Thus, the nurse, more than any other staff member, is going to be observing how a patient is relating to others on the unit and is going to be constantly interacting with the patients. (*Note:* While a therapeutic community is used most often on psychiatric units, its principles can also be applied to other hospital units, such as rehabilitation, surgical or obstetrical units. — Williams, 1970, pp. 957–962.)

DEFINITION OF A THERAPEUTIC COMMUNITY

The term "therapeutic community" originated with Maxwell Jones in the early 1950's. He described it as follows:

It would seem that in some, if not all, psychiatric conditions there is much to be learned from observing the patient in a relatively ordinary and familiar social environment so that his usual ways of relating to other people, reaction to stress, etc., can be observed. If at the same time he can be made aware of the effect of his behavior on other people and helped to understand some of the motivation underlying his actions, the situation is potentially therapeutic. This is believed to be the distinctive quality of a therapeutic community. Clearly there is the possibility of any interpersonal relationship being therapeutic or antitherapeutic. It is the introduction of trained staff personnel into the group situation together with planned collaboration of patients and staff in most, if not all, aspects of the unit life which heightens the possibility of the social experience being therapeutic. (Jones quoted in Wilmer, 1958)

In a therapeutic community, every hour and each interaction on the unit is significant and can be used effectively in the treatment of a patient. This is in contrast to the more traditional psychotherapeutic belief that the patient's hour with his therapist is the "therapy" while the other 23 hours of the day just serve to maintain the patient.

Therapeutic community applies the democratic process to the treatment realm. Each person must accept the responsibility of his actions and make his own decisions. The goals of a therapeutic community include honestly sharing information with patients, followed by involving them in the decision making process. These goals are accomplished through the environment, or milieu, as it is called in psychiatric literature. Any aspect of this milieu, or environment, will affect the patient. In order that this have a therapeutic effect, the total milieu must be carefully examined and everyone present involved in its support. This includes the patients, members of the health team (nurses, psychiatrists, psychologists, social workers, occupational and recreational therapists, etc.), and even the personnel from housekeeping and food service. After all, the way the janitor copes with mopping the cluttered floor of a patient's room, or answers a patient's questions about why he (the patient) can't have a pass, can significantly affect the patient's perception of the unit, as well as affect the patient's treatment process.

Clarification of feelings and discussion of events assist in the decision making process, also. The people involved have more data to use when making a decision. They find other ways of dealing with situations within a more protected environment. More options are available and hopefully their sense of self-esteem is increased at the same time. After having some successes on the unit, the patients can, hopefully, begin to try some of these new alternatives in their life situations.

Patients may not like participating in decision making because it also means they have responsibility. Their expectation of hospitalization may be that they get a well deserved rest—or that someone will magically make them better with no effort on their part. A therapeutic community structure expects them to be active, be responsible for their actions, to give as well as receive. It can be painful for the patients to verbalize feelings, give or receive feedback or take responsibility for their actions. Because this is different from the traditional medical model, patients have a right to know about this community structure before they come to the hospital unit.

Patients may have inaccurate perceptions about others when they come to the unit. The clarification of events and people's feelings can help the patients identify their distortions and begin to be more realistic in their outlook.

Sharing information in decision making has another purpose. Often, patients are not accustomed to verbalizing their feelings or even recognizing them. For instance, they may not verbalize their anger, holding it bottled up inside. The open communication taking place on the unit may help them verbalize this anger for the first time. Or maybe they seem angry in everything that they do. They will probably get feedback about this. Others may find themselves responding in anger. All are sources of discussion on the unit. This can lead not only to recognition of feelings but also can lead to a resolution of the original problems of several patients. As they are discussing one person's problem they may be resolving some of their own.

Sometimes the most effective therapists on the unit are the patients themselves. Seeing another patient who has gone through a similar crisis and who seems to be successfully resolving it can have a great impact. At times, patient A might be really looking up to patient B when patient B experiences a failure or has a relapse of illness. This has an impact and needs some discussion time. Sometimes, it never occurred to patient A that he could help patient B. It also is frightening to patient A because he begins to wonder if this could happen to him. Such a possibility is also open to discussion for we all have failures as well as successes, and the hospital or treatment does not guarantee success.

No two units that have therapeutic communities are alike, and likewise, within a unit the culture is constantly changing. As staff and patient populations change, the structure and culture change. Sometimes it is a very dynamic community and at other times very dull. The composition of any therapeutic community is dependent upon the personalities of the people within it. It tends to be more dynamic if the group are working together, are able to be honest with each other, and fill a mutual trust and respect.

TREATMENT PROGRAM

A wide range of behaviors is usually accepted in a therapeutic community with limits also being defined. This is accomplished through group support and group pressure. Community meetings are a formal example of this. Everyone (patients and staff) attends community meetings where the current happenings on the unit are discussed. Problems are brought up and, hopefully, clarified and resolved. Decisions are made about privileges or passes, anticipated changes are discussed, new people are introduced, etc. Everyone is a part of this process. If a group of patients is upset with a staff member's actions, that is just as relevant as the staff's perception that a patient is having a problem which is affecting the unit. Anything can be brought up by anyone. Group support and group pressure can be a very strong influence in these meetings. Support or pressure can be on a patient-patient, patient-staff, or staff-staff basis.

Emergency community meetings are called whenever a serious matter arises that needs to be discussed immediately. For example, if a patient has made a suicide attempt, this fact is shared with the total staff and patient group. The person who made the suicide attempt is present, if possible, and is a part of this process with other people expressing their feelings directly with this patient. Ways that others can help are discussed. Emergency community meetings are often very emotionally charged meetings. Patients and staff are both experiencing feelings about the incident involved. Usually anger and sadness are both expressed. Several people may be crying.

Since the patients are to have responsibility for decision making, a structure is decided upon for patient government. The definition of their duties depends on individual units and should be drawn up and changed as necessary by the patients and staff on the unit. Staff may or may not be present at the official patient government meetings. Patients' tasks are defined and often include such common unit concerns as bathrooms being dirty (this may be a patient or housekeeping problem), changing the food menus, getting the record player fixed, or asking someone to turn down the volume of his radio at night. Patients often have concerns that they discuss directly with hospital administration. Maybe they want permission to extend the hours that they can be gone on a pass, or maybe they feel the recreational facilities are inadequate. They may contribute remodeling ideas to the unit. Their focus may vary from patient or staff problems to administrative ones. The process of working these out is the important goal of therapy. Some problems aren't resolved so that patients have to consider other alternatives or decide that it's a matter that can't be changed. This is all part of the learning process that needs to occur on a unit.

Individual and group therapies are both found in therapeutic communities. Careful consideration should be given as to how these will intermesh with the rest of the milieu program. Periodic evaluation should follow. Individual and group therapies need to be conducted by staff who support the therapeutic community philosophy.

Occupational and recreational therapy often become a unit event with several staff members participating with the patients. This promotes a mutual sharing and respect that is also carried into other activities on the unit. If a patient does not play volleyball well, he may find that a staff member he looks up to doesn't play well either. Yet, that staff member is a part of the group and seems to be enjoying himself, or a couple of members of the community may discover a mutual interest which they can share. New skills are learned here by staff as well as patients. Special unit events may be planned by the community for everyone, i.e., a picnic, a softball game or a party.

Daily activities are also shared. Staff eat with patients and both groups help with preparation and clean-up. Patients may have some housekeeping responsibilities. This varies from hospital to hospital, but patients should have the responsibility of keeping their rooms in an acceptable condition. The "acceptable condition" needs to be defined by the community realizing that there will be some public health codes that must be maintained.

The patient's family or significant friends should be included in the treatment program. The family or friends may have a special group with patients and staff where they work on problems concerning this current hospitalization. If no group is available, much can be accomplished by staff members meeting with patients and their families individually or on an informal basis. The structure for including families varies from unit to unit but must be considered and reevaluated periodically. Families will affect the unit community and need to be included in its structure.

PHYSICAL ENVIRONMENT

The physical environment is another important aspect of a therapeutic community. An environment that is as homelike as possible is most conducive to the treatment program. Bars on windows, locked doors, and seclusion rooms do not tell the patient that he is a responsible individual. If doors are open and the physical environment resembles a home, an open feeling is gained simply by looking about the unit. The effect of an unlocked entry door on the unit atmosphere can be very great. As soon as this door is locked, the unit seems smaller and one feels more closed in. The tension level increases with both staff and patients. Other physical factors are important although they may seem like small things that are taken for granted in a home. Telephones need to be available to patients. A full length mirror, clocks and calendars, and grooming equipment are all found in a home. It is most therapeutic if these are available to patients.

Each patient also needs a space of his own. A bed, dresser or locker, bedside table or ledge, even a bulletin board gives the patient a place that belongs to just him. Some patients enjoy decorating this space. Many patients bring in their own stereo sets or put up posters. The way a patient uses his space can become an important treatment issue. This space and the opportunity to individualize it are important aspects of a patient's hosptial stay.

OTHER FACTORS AFFECTING THE THERAPEUTIC COMMUNITY STRUCTURE

Other things may be happening with staff and patients in the milieu that will effect the therapeutic community structure. These situations may be difficult to work through but can be resolved in support of this philosophy.

A very simple factor concerns the patients' right to choose their own roommates. This can become an excellent learning process. They may choose another patient on the unit or have the next new patient assigned to their room. If they are not getting along with their roommate, this needs to be worked out. The way this is dealt with is important. It is tempting for a staff member involved in these situations to take over and help make these decisions for the patient. However, for the patient, this will not be the most helpful method of handling the problem. In these situations, staff should supply additional data or options that the patients haven't thought of, and/or encourage the patients to express their feelings with each other, but the decisions should be left up to the patients involved.

Unit life can become disrupted by a patient in an acute stage of psychiatric illness. This presents an unresolved problem for the therapeutic community. Sometimes the community will help special the patient and assist in his care. However, this patient might require a more secure space than the overall unit provides. If an intensive care area is available, this can be an excellent solution, although involvement in the community should take place as soon as possible. If secure space isn't available, the community may be faced with many problems. Other patients may have belongings destroyed or taken, the unit may be locked, and patients may be frightened or angry. The acutely disturbed patient may not be able to assume responsibility for himself right away. The community must deal with these difficulties as they arise. For example, the unit may be locked because of one person when the rest of the patients are responsible enough to have the unit open. The patients may have to wait for staff to unlock doors, causing them to feel caged. This adds to the tension in the community. The community may resolve this by applying group pressure on the patient involved. This is effective at times but the situation might have to continue until medications or treatments have taken effect. These issues are discussed in community meetings and informally around the unit.

Another factor affecting the therapeutic community structure is length of stay. In a unit with an acutely ill population the patients may have an average hospital stay of 3 to 4 weeks. The patients who have been there longer help to orient new patients to the unit. If the patient turnover is too rapid, this orientation may not take place adequately. More responsibility for orienting new patients, then, must rest with the staff. Therapeutic community is most effective when the patients are there long enough to experience its benefits and be able to pass this along to newer patients. Perhaps a 1- to 2-month stay would achieve this effect.

Another problem occurs within this structure. Some patients will like the unit so much that they won't want to leave. This also must be dealt with in the community. Remaining on the unit is not an available alternative. As patients progress, they are able to have more privileges and leave the unit more often. The unit life might be far more supportive than their home life. They still must leave but feelings need to be discussed. They may be able to come back to the unit for part of a day or evening and thus grow away from the unit gradually. A referral to an outpatient clinic or therapist is also helpful at this point. It may be that some patients will come back to see a specific staff member on an outpatient basis. This depends on what the hospital administration allows.

If unit staff members can be involved in pre- and postdischarge care, this can be very helpful for both patients and staff. Patients must become acquainted with a lot of people on the unit. Friendships and meaningful relationships are started. Continuing these relationships can be therapeutic. (This is not to negate the importance of saying goodbye. In the community they may have been able to express, for the first time in their lives, the anger and sadness of ending a relationship.) Staff experience the same thing and may wonder what has happened to a certain patient they worked with. Having the opportunity to continue to see this patient, using the relationship they already have established, can facilitate a patient's progress and add to a staff member's job satisfaction.

Another problem occurs when patients are distrustful of the therapeutic community structure. They do not believe that the unit really functions that way, but that it is just a facade or a trick. When this happens, it is a topic for discussion both informally with others on the unit and also in the community meeting.

Staff may experience personal difficulties. They may not be accustomed to talking openly about feelings, or they may have distortions about events, just as the patients do. Other staff and patients may be giving them feedback about this. It is not always a comfortable time for either staff or patients.

Staff may be having problems among themselves. Several authors have discussed this problem as it has an effect on the patient population (Cumming and Cumming, 1970; Stanton and Schwartz, 1954). In a therapeutic community, the staff problems are also discussed with the patients. For example, if a nursing staff member has been counseled several times and finally is fired, this is an important topic of discussion in the community. Maybe this staff member has been involved with a couple of patients who think this person is doing a better job than the rest of the staff. When the staff member is fired early one evening, an emergency community meeting should be called so this can be discussed. Staff who are not working that shift may be called in for the meeting. The reasons for the staff member's leaving would be discussed. Rumors about this will have been circulating and these issues need to be clarified and feelings expressed.

Lastly, hospital administration's support can be very important. The usual hospital administrative structure does not allow sharing confidential information about one patient with another patient. If a therapeutic community is started, it is very important to have the hospital administration's support and understanding of what this involves. It is also important that the administration support and delegate more staff decision making on a unit level. A therapeutic community cannot be achieved without the formal authority granted by hosptial administration.

PROGRAM EVALUATION

When evaluating a situation that arises on the unit, a decision that has been made, or a program to be started, think about the basic principles of the therapeutic community. Have these principles been supported? Is the patient being treated as a responsible human being? Is the patient given the chance to do any task he is capable of doing? Is the patient the initiator and manager of his own affairs with the staff assisting him? Is the patient being taught how to problem solve and is he being given the opportunities to practice these skills? Is the patient learning more adaptive behaviors? (Dunham and Krone, 1975, p. 15)

Staff behavior must also be evaluated. Are the staff who will carry out decisions regarding patient care actively involved in making those decisions? Are the staff responsible for evaluating their performance in patient care and seeking to improve their performances? Are they willing to share experiences in patient care and willing to accept or give feedback on their own and others' performance? Is there constant and effective communication flowing freely amongst the disciplines? (Dunham and Krone, 1975, p. 15)

If a therapeutic community is not functioning effectively, there will be many signs and symptoms to indicate this. The climate of the unit may be laden with tension or be very quiet with the feeling that nothing is happening. Staff may be dissatisfied and staff turnover may increase. There may be actual suicides and destructive behavior on the part of the patients. Staff may be constantly staying in the nursing office and not spending time with patients. Dichotomies among staff (and/or patients) may be taking place and allowed to continue festering unresolved. Tempers may be flaring. All of these signs and symptoms are significant and must be discussed and resolved. This can be a very painful process. If the problems are allowed to continue, the result can be devastating.

A note is in order here if one is evaluating a unit and comparing it with what the literature defines as therapeutic community. There are many good books and articles written about therapeutic milieu that also apply to the therapeutic community. Cumming and Cumming (1970) is an excellent reference. Therapeutic milieu happenings should be taking place in a therapeutic community. Therapeutic community expands these milieu definitions and adds the democratic ingredient. It states that patients are responsible for their own actions and should be involved in the decision making process.

SUMMARY

In summary, a therapeutic community is based on the belief that most casual, everyday activities of living offer opportunities for patient growth in areas such as social interaction, problem solving, and enhancing self-confidence. Interchange, debate, self-assertion and adjustment to others are necessary skills, and opportunities to develop these skills are found in an active and flexible milieu. The planning of activities as a group, the discussion of the effect of one person's behavior on another and all of the many routine activities of daily living faced by people in a social milieu become the instrument of treatment.

Staff within a therapeutic community need to be asking, what it is that patients cannot do for themselves and how staff can provide growth experiences for them so that they can learn to do for themselves. The staff uses any situation that might arise in order to help patients become more aware of their feelings, thoughts and behaviors, and the effects these behaviors have on others. The patients then need the opportunity to try out new skills and make decisions in a safe environment. This opportunity will enhance the patients' feelings of self-worth. It will also assist them in dealing more effectively with problems that arise in everyday living. Nurses, because of their continuous observation and interaction with patients, are an indispensable part of the therapeutic community structure.

BIBLIOGRAPHY

Abroms, G. M. Defining milieu therapy. *Arch. Gen. Psychiatry* 21: 533–560, 1969.
Barker, P., and Ward, P. Milieu therapy in a child psychiatric unit. *Nurs. Times* 68: 1579–1581, 1972.
Bonn, E. A therapeutic community in an open state hospital – administrative and therapeutic links. *Hosp. Community Psychiatry* 20 (9), 1969.
Chappell, C. I. Participation training – an instrument for milieu change. *Hosp. Community Psychiatry* 20: 355–357, 1969.
Cumming, E. Therapeutic community and milieu ther-

apy strategies can be distinguished. *Int. J. Psychiatry* 7: 204–208, 1969.

Cumming, J., and Cumming, E. *Ego and Milieu*. New York: Atherton Press, 1970.

Dunham, J., and Krone, C. *A Study to Identify How the University Hospital Psychiatric Nursing Staff Define Therapeutic Milieu*. Master's thesis, University of Michigan School of Nursing, 1975.

Ellsworth, R., Maroney, R., Klett, W., Gordon, H., and Gunn, R. Milieu characteristics of successful psychiatric treatment programs. *Am. J. Orthopsychiatry* 41: 427–441, 1971.

Gottlieb, B. M. Modifications of a therapeutic community on a brief stay ward. *Hosp. Community Psychiatry* 22: 23–24, 1971.

Herz, M. I. The therapeutic milieu – a necessity. *Int. J. Psychiatry* 7: 209–212, 1969.

Holmes, M., and Werner, J. *Psychiatric Nursing in a Therapeutic Community*. New York: The Macmillan Co., 1966.

Jones, M. *The Therapeutic Community*. New York: Basic Books, Inc., 1953, p. 1053.

Jones, M. In Wilmer, H. A., *Social Psychiatry in Action*. Springfield, Ill: Charles C Thomas, 1958.

Kish, G. B. Evaluation of a ward atmosphere. *Hosp. Community Psychiatry* 22: 159–161, 1971.

Kraft, A. M. The therapeutic community. In *American Handbook of Psychiatry*, Vol. 3. New York: Basic Books, Inc., 1966.

Kramer, M. *Reality Shock*. St. Louis: The C. V. Mosby Co., 1974.

Leedy, P. D. *Practical Research: Planning and Design*. New York: The Macmillan Co., 1974.

Lewis, A. B., Jr., and Selzer, M. Some neglected issues in milieu therapy. *Hosp. Community Psychiatry* 23: 293–298, 1972.

Litwin, G. H., and Stringer, R. A. *Motivation and Organization Climate*. Division of Research, Graduate School of Business Administration, Harvard University, Boston, 1968.

Neff, S. *Work and Human Behavior*. New York: Atherton Press, 1968.

Robinson, J. P., and Shaver, P. R. *Measures of Social Psychological Attitudes*. Survey Research Center, ISR, Ann Arbor, 1973.

Rossi, J., and Filstead, W. *The Therapeutic Community: A Source Book of Reading*. New York: Behavioral Publications, 1973.

Schiff, S. A therapeutic community in an open state hospital – administrative framework for social psychiatry. *Hosp. Community Psychiatry* 20 (9), 1969.

Stanton, A. H., and Schwartz, M. S. *The Mental Hospital: A Study of Institutional Participation in Psychiatric Illness and Treatment*. New York: Basic Books, Inc., 1954.

Stauble, N. J. Milieu therapy and the therapeutic community. *Can. Psychiatric Assoc. J.* 16: 197–202, 1971.

Tollinton, H. J. The organization of a therapeutic community. *Br. J. Med. Psychol.* 42: 271–275, 1969.

VanPutten, T. Milieu therapy: Contraindications. *Arch. Gen. Psychiatry* 29: 640–643, 1973.

White, N. F. The descent of milieu therapy. *Can. Psychiatric Assoc. J.* 17: 41, 1972.

White, N. F. Reappraising the inpatient unit: Obit milieu. *Can. Psychiatric Assoc. J.* 17: 51–53, 1972.

Williams, R. B., Jr. The use of a therapeutic milieu on a continuing care unit of a general hospital. *Ann. Intern. Med.* 73: 957–962, 1970.

Yalom, I. *The Theory and Practice of Group Psychotherapy*. New York: Basic Books, Inc., 1970.

Zeitlyn, B. B. The therapeutic community – fact or fantasy. *Int. J. Psychiatry* 7: 195–199, 1969.

Chapter 3

current uses of psychiatric drugs

HARVEY J. WIDROE

More than any other factor, the development of psychopharmacological agents over the last 25 years has dramatically increased our ability to reduce or eliminate serious psychopathology. Psychopathological behavior and suffering from mental illness can now be effectively treated with a far greater likelihood of a patient's returning to normal living than ever before. In recent years the discovery of still other psychopharmacological agents and the development of greater skills in using those psychopharmacological agents already available have bettered the prognosis for any given patient with a serious mental illness or another form of severe behavioral disturbance. No mental health professional of today can afford to be without a basic knowledge of concepts and facts concerning contemporary psychopharmacology.

OBJECTIONS TO THE USE OF PSYCHIATRIC DRUGS

Many objections to the use of psychiatric drugs have been raised not only by fearful patients but even by a number of unenlightened or misguided mental health professionals. Because all mental health professionals meet these objections in day to day work with patients, it is necessary to examine them in order to determine how best to overcome them.

Therapists' objections to psychiatric drugs usually stem from a lack of familiarity with psychoactive medications and consequent inability to use them with optimal results. This lack of knowledge may lead the therapist to use drugs only when he feels that his patient cannot benefit from psychotherapy or that psychotherapy alone has been a failure. Thus, the use of medications is conceived as an alternative to psychotherapy. In reality the effects of medication do not solve the problems of the patient's life. What we actually observe is that psychiatric medications are an adjunct to psychotherapy rather than an alternative to it. Patients who distort reality, have scattered thinking, are impulse-driven, or are overwhelmed by strong affects, cannot solve problems effectively and find great difficulty in using psychotherapy constructively. It follows that 1) if a patient is hallucinating less and his reality testing is more intact, 2) if his thought processes can follow along the usual lines of syntax and logic, 3) if he has greater impulse control and greater tolerance to tension, and 4) if his affects are more stable and not of overwhelming intensity, only then will he be in a position to learn from those around him about the origins and consequences of his behavior and problems. It is this type of problem solving which, when effectively achieved, contributes to personality growth and self-actualization.

Other therapists' objections to psychiatric drugs may arise from a commitment to the philosophy of a particular school of psychology which postulates that drugs mask psychopathology, suppress the expression of a patient's true self, decrease or increase the intensity of the regressive transference, etc. This division of the field of psychiatry into schools of psychology or cults marked a phase in the early history of psychiatry when little scientific information had been collected. Fortunately, this cultism is giving way, albeit grudgingly, to a respectable eclecticism, the pronouncements of which stand less on declarations of faith and dogma and more on the dialectical progression of organization and explication of fact.

Patients' objections to the use of psychiatric drugs are based on 1) the meanings they attach to the act of taking medication, and 2) the meanings they attach to the feelings produced by the medication, whether therapeutic effects or side effects. The meanings the patient attaches to the act of taking medication or to the feelings produced by taking the medications are a product of fantasies which have dynamic significance for a given patient.

1. Patients whose oral level conflicts are most prominent are those with diagnoses such as schizophrenia, borderline schizophrenia and character disorders. The fantasies of these patients lead them to object to the use of psychiatric drugs; the fantasies reflect fears of helplessness, submission, dissolution, annihilation, bodily distortion, mutilation, decay, poisoning, loss of reality testing, loss of control of thought, or destruction of possessions or loved ones. For example, a fantasy commonly encountered in the acute schizophrenic patient—that of being poisoned by the medication—may lead to the patient's increased anxiety or outright refusal to take the medication.

2. Patients with neurotic character, anxiety states, and psychoneurotic depressions, may interpret taking medication as a confirmation of feelings of helplessness, a state which threatens still further regression.

3. Patients' objections to taking psychiatric drugs may also be related to phallic level fantasies which vary with the sex of the patient. For example, homosexuality and castration are the prominent themes of fantasies of men who object to taking psychiatric drugs, whereas fantasies of women center on confirmation of castration or oral impregnation. An example of male phallic level fantasy regarding drugs is that of a man who interpreted taking the medication the doctor prescribed as being forced into a condition of homosexual submission. An example of a female phallic level fantasy is that of a woman who interpreted taking medication as a sexual assault which confirmed her castration and sense of worthlessness.

Even though the therapist might understand a patient's motivation for objecting to the use of psychiatric drugs, it is extremely unlikely that at the time the patient is psychologically prepared for examination of the motives behind his objections. Insofar as the patient's fantasies about medication are detrimental to the effects of the drug or may interfere with the patient's taking the drug, the therapist must do all that can be done to dispel the fantasies. Most important in overcoming the patient's objections is the presentation of explicit information about the medications and their side effects by the doctor and the nursing staff at the onset of administration and as a patient's objections arise. Patients should be told the names of the medications they are taking, the intended effect of the medications, and the more frequently encountered side effects of medications. For example, the psychotic patient with defective reality testing is less likely to become frightened if he has been told that his blurred vision is due to the use of his medication rather than to an exacerbation of his mental illness. Side effects which may appear secondary to suggestion are more readily dispelled than a patient's reaction to the appearance of unexpected or unexplained symptoms.

Another means of dispelling fantasies about taking drugs is to clearly indicate to the patient that the medication he will take is "weak." The importance of this approach is apparent if one considers that one of the goals in treatment is to foster a patient's autonomy. He may ask for medication of tremendous strength while he feels helpless, but at a later date he will be concerned about solving problems with no external assistance. By emphasizing the lack of potency of the medication, the physician and nursing staff may assist the patient in diminishing the effects of fantasies related to submission and castration and hasten the growth of self-confident feelings.

A patient's questions and objections concerning medication often reflect the patient's fantasies. These statements give the physician and nursing staff an opportunity to explore the fantasies with the patient or to assist the patient in suppressing or repressing his fantasies by providing accurate information. For example:

Patient: "Is it a tranquilizer?"
Staff: "Yes, it is a kind of tranquilizer. You may have read about them. Have you? What have you read?"
Patient: "I feel ill at ease about taking medication. I want to solve my problems all by myself. Shouldn't I?"
Staff: "You feel you should do it yourself? You will. You sell your own abilities short, and you think this medication can perform wonders. The fact is that the medication can help you have a little more control over your feelings, but the problem solving falls completely on your shoulders."
Patient: "Is it a sugar pill?"
Staff: "No, it is not a sugar pill. I doubt that you could place much trust in us if we were to give you sugar pills."
Patient: "I don't need any medication. I can control myself any time I want to."
Staff: "The fact is that recently you haven't had the kind of control that you would like to have. For the time being the medication will help you to maintain that control until you can handle the whole thing by yourself."

Psychotic patients may present a somewhat different set of objections. Replies should assist the patient to test the reality of his perceptions and ideas:

Patient: "I won't take it. You are trying to poison me!"
Staff: "No, we are not trying to poison you, and the medication is not poison. The medication is to help you feel better. I can understand how confused you must feel about things and how hard it is for you to know whom to trust, but we are all here to help you, and this medication will be good for you. It will help you to feel better."

In replies to patients' objections to the use of psychiatric drugs the staff assists the patient in suppressing and repressing fantasies about medication by 1) identifying the medication, 2) explaining its effects and side effects, and 3) discussing the fantasies in whatever form they are presented.

PATIENTS WHO DEMAND PSYCHIATRIC DRUGS

Patients who demand psychiatric drugs often have fantasies about magical help. As a rule the patient feels in great distress and sees himself as helpless in the face of forces he cannot control. It is best for the physician and/or nursing staff to honor such requests for medication. If the patient seeks pills to make him more comfortable and has little awareness of his psychological problems or cannot tolerate such an awareness, then even the most tactful suggestion that the patient examine his difficulties instead of receiving medication will result in his seeing the staff as punitive rather than benign as intended. The doctor's prescribing the medication and the nursing staff's providing medication may be the only basis on which a therapeutic alliance can be established. This rapport may enable the patient to come to deal with his problems in psychotherapy. At worst the patient will see the staff as his ally, trying to determine the most effective schedule of the medications prescribed. At best the patient may begin to discuss his psychological problems after a short time. Thus, the administration of psychiatric medications to the patient who demands them need not reinforce the patient's denial of his problems. When prn medication is demanded, the nursing staff, after granting the request, may then be in an optimal position to discuss with the patient those circumstnaces which led to the increase in the patient's symptoms.

Another function of administration of drugs to the patient who demands them may be the strengthening of obsessive defenses by the taking of medication at regular intervals. For example, a patient, who was frightened of suicidal impulses, was advised to take a mild sedative at hourly intervals until she felt she had control of her thoughts and feelings.

HOW DO PSYCHIATRIC DRUGS WORK?

Psychiatric drugs affect human behavior by affecting parts of the brain in a differential manner. Thus, if the activity of one functional area of the brain is enhanced or decreased, the net effect may be the realignment of a neurological subsystem which accounts for a particular area of human behavior. A psychiatric drug is useful if its effect is to realign a subsystem which in a state of imbalance has led to pathological behavior, feelings, or thoughts. The subsystem concept can be envisioned at a number of different levels. For example, at a biochemical level we might envision certain depressed states as a product of a relative norepinephrine deficiency. The use of antidepressant medications may increase the amount of norepinephrine available for synaptic transmission leading to an improvement in mood. An example of the subsystem concept at an anatomical level would be excessive activity of the amygdaloid nucleus contributing to raging behavior. The effect of haloperidol (Haldol) in reducing electrical activity of the amygdaloid nucleus subsequently leads to a reduction in rage behavior.

DRUGS USED FOR ANXIETY IN NONPSYCHOTIC PATIENTS

Anxiety in the nonpsychotic patient can be diminished in most instances by the judicious use of so-called minor tranquilizers. Those drugs included in the minor tranquilizer class and which are most commonly employed are phenobarbital, meprobamate, chlordiazepoxide hydrochloride (Librium), diazepam (Valium), oxazepam (Serax) and clorazepate dipotassium (Tranxene).

Minor tranquilizers act on the brain by sedating the cerebral cortex. These drugs tend to provide rapid relief of anxiety — often within 15 to 30 minutes. Because patients have a conscious appreciation of the sense of relief these drugs provide, they tend to be prescribed frequently by physicians. Unfortunately, they are readily abused by patients who seek instant relief from discomfort. Patients who use cortical acting sedatives for any period of time may develop both a psychological dependence and a physiological tolerance with significant withdrawal symptoms if dosages are withheld. Because they do suppress activity of the cerebral cortex, minor tranquilizers impair patients' judgement, thus making them more subject to affective outbursts. For example, patients who use diazepam (Valium) are more prone to crying or to

rage. Barbiturate addicts are characterized by affective volatility, minimal tension tolerance and poor judgement. Cortical acting sedatives all tend to intensify depression to the point of increasing suicidal thinking and feelings. The most commonly occurring side effects of cortical acting sedatives are manifestations of cerebellar ataxia, including slurred speech, poor coordination and ataxic gait. Commonly employed dosages are: meprobamate, 400 to 800 mg. q.i.d.; phenobarbital, $1/4$ to 1 grain q.i.d.; chlordiazepoxide hydrochloride (Librium), 10 to 50 mg. q.i.d.; diazepam (Valium), 5 to 15 mg. q.i.d.; oxazepam (Serax), 15 to 30 mg. q.i.d.; and clorazepate dipotassium (Tranxene), 7.5 to 15 mg. q.i.d.

DRUGS USED FOR ALCOHOLISM, BARBITURATE ADDICTION, OR ADDICTION TO OTHER CORTICAL ACTING SEDATIVES

In the treatment of addiction to cortical acting sedatives the function of medication is to prevent the emergence of withdrawal symptoms in the absence of the substance to which the patient is addicted. Withdrawal symptoms may include sweating, nausea and vomiting, diarrhea, tremulousness, hyperirritability, agitation, grand mal seizures or florid psychosis. For safe and relatively comfortable detoxification of addicted patients, the physician substitutes another cortical acting sedative for the substance to which the patient is addicted. The substituted drug is then gradually reduced as a function of the patient's improvement. For example, a patient who is addicted to alcohol may be given diazepam (Valium) and diphenylhydantoin sodium (Dilantin) instead. Or a patient addicted to meprobamate might be given chlordiazepoxide hydrochloride (Librium) and diphenylhydantoin sodium (Dilantin). The exception to the premise of substituting one cortical acting sedative for another is ethchlorvynol (Placidyl) addiction which can be treated only by - gradual reduction of the drug itself. Chlordiazepoxide hydrochloride (Librium) and diazepam (Valium) are most commonly employed as substitute cortical acting sedatives because they are excellent anticonvulsants when used alone and yet, even at relatively high dosages, have minimal effects on depressing respiration. For example, a patient undergoing delirium tremens as a result of alcohol withdrawal could safely be given chlordiazepoxide (Librium) 50 mg. IM q. 1 to 2 hours until his agitation, visual hallucinations and tremulousness have diminished. For alcoholics in particular, vitamins by injection or by mouth are helpful in treating the nutritionally depleted cerebral enzymes and coenzymes.

Medications can be prescribed which produce alcohol intolerance. Disulfiram or metronidazole (Flagyl) when taken daily can produce an alcohol intolerance. If a patient ingests alcohol while taking disulfiram or metronidazole (Flagyl), he experiences an intense toxic reaction. He will feel hot and flushed all over and experience nausea and vomiting, diffuse myalgia and even cardiovascular collapse and death. The reaction of alcohol plus disulfiram is quite severe whereas the reaction to metronidazole (Flagyl) and alcohol is less marked. To avoid a toxic reaction a patient ought *not* to start taking disulfiram or metronidazole (Flagyl) for at least 72 hours after alcohol usage. Patients should be cautioned not to drink for at least 72 hours after their last dosage of disulfiram or metronidazole (Flagyl). Disulfiram in itself, even at therapeutic levels, can produce serious psychopathology, including depression, paranoia and depersonalization. A safe maintenance dosage of disulfiram is .125 to .25 gm. daily. Metronidazole (Flagyl) is used at 250 mg. b.i.d. with no serious psychopathology discerned to date.

DRUG USE FOR THE TREATMENT OF SCHIZOPHRENIC PSYCHOSES, SCHIZOAFFECTIVE DISORDERS AND PSYCHOTIC DEPRESSION

Phenothiazines and phenothiazine-like drugs are the medications of choice in the treatment of schizophrenic psychoses, schizoaffective disorders and psychotic depression. These medications may be divided into three groups according to the degree of sedation they produce. Thus, a medication is often chosen by the degree of sedation a given patient may require. Maximally sedating phenothiazines include thioridazine (Mellaril), chlorpromazine (Thorazine), and mesoridazine (Serentil). Moderately sedating phenothiazines include perphenazine (Trilafon) and prochlorperazine (Compazine). The latter is relatively ineffectual in the treatment of major psychoses. Loxapine succinate (Loxitane) is a nonphenothiazine which has a moderately sedating action. The nonsedating group includes phenothiazines such as trifluoperazine hydrochloride (Stelazine) and fluphenazine hydrochloride (Prolixin) and phenothiazine-like medications including haloperidol (Haldol), thiothixene (Navane), and molindone hydrochloride (Moban).

Frequently encountered side effects of these medications include dry mouth, blurred vision, photosensitivity, postural hypotension, along with extrapyramidal symptoms such as parkinsonism, dystonic reactions, and akathisia responses. Extrapyramidal symptoms can almost always be avoided by the prophylactic use of antiparkinsonian agents such as benztropine mesylate (Cogentin), trihexyphenidyl hydrochloride (Artane), procyclidine hydrochloride (Kemadrin), and amantadine hydrochloride (Symmetrel). Parkinsonism and dystonic symptoms will respond to benztropine mesylate (Cogentin) 2 mg. IM on an acute basis, whereas akathisia symptoms may require both an antiparkinsonian medication plus Benadryl for symptomatic relief. Dermatitis, liver function changes, and blood dyscrasias are rarely occurring toxic effects of the phenothiazines and phenothiazine-like drugs. Commonly employed dosages are: chlorpromazine (Thorazine), 100 to 500 mg. q.i.d.; thioridazine (Mellaril), 50 to 150 mg. q.i.d.; mesoridazine (Serentil), 50 to 150 mg. q.i.d.; perphenazine (Trilafon), 4 to 16 mg. q.i.d.; prochlorperazine (Compazine), 10 to 25 mg. q.i.d.; loxipine succinate (Loxitane), 10 to 50 mg. q.i.d.; trifluoperazine hydrochloride (Stelazine), 5 to 20 mg. q.i.d.; fluphenazine hydrochloride (Prolixin), 5 to 20 mg. q.i.d.; molindone hydrochloride (Moban), 10 to 25 mg. q.i.d.; haloperidol (Haldol), 2 to 25 mg. q.i.d.; thiothixene (Navane), 2 to 15 mg. q.i.d.

Many psychotic patients demonstrate suspiciousness along with paranoid delusions concerning taking medication. Consequently they may "cheek" and discard medications given in tablet form. To insure the likelihood that the floridly psychotic patient will receive the medication he needs, he should be given medication in oral concentrate forms if possible. Injectable medication may be necessary early in the patient's treatment.

Many psychotic patients recover in a hospital setting and then decompensate once again because of failure to continue the prescribed use of antipsychotic medications. Once such a propensity is clear, these patients are candidates for regular injections of depot drugs, such as fluphenazine enanthate or decanoate. Dosages may vary from 25 mg. IM q. 2 weeks to 50 mg. IM q. 2 days. Occasional psychotic patients may not respond to medications given in the prescribed dosage ranges. A certain number of these patients will achieve remissions from psychotic episodes only if so-called megadosages are employed. Fluphenazine hydrochloride (Prolixin) may be used in dosages up to 500 mg. daily. Perphenazine (Trilafon) has been used in dosages up to 500 mg. daily. Haloperidol (Haldol) is effective in dosages up to 150 mg. daily. Other medications are used in megadosages less frequently. At times a combination of phenothiazines or a phenothiazine plus a phenothiazine-like drug may bring about a remission in a psychotic patient who has previously been refractory to treatment. After a remission has been achieved, antipsychotic medications should be continued in lower dosages for approximately 6 months or more in order to increase the likelihood that a patient will not experience an exacerbation of his psychosis. Patients who have had multiple psychotic episodes may need to take small doses of phenothiazines for an indefinite period in order to prevent additional psychotic episodes.

Occasionally lithium plus a phenothiazine will bring about a successful remission from a psychotic episode which has been refractory to the use of phenothiazines alone. This combination is most successful when the patient's psychosis includes a marked affective component; however, at times patients without an affective component to their schizophrenic psychoses may respond to the lithium-phenothiazine combination.

DRUG USE IN THE TREATMENT OF MANIC PSYCHOSES OR RECURRENT UNIPOLAR DEPRESSION

While lithium is most dramatic in its effect on patients with manic psychoses, it may be of value in the treatment of many patients with conditions featuring affective instability. It is also helpful in the treatment and prophylaxis of patients with endogenous recurrent unipolar depression. The effectiveness of lithium is measured by clinical response related to serum-lithium levels. A given drug dosage will produce a particular lithium level within 2 to 3 days, whereas the clinical effect of the lithium dosage may not be apparent for 6 to 10 days. Because of this delay in effect, maximally sedating phenothiazines are indicated early in the treatment of the manic patient concurrent with the use of lithium. A safe dosage that is unlikely to produce toxic effects is: lithium, 300 mg. t.i.d. Frequently, physicians will employ dosages as high as 600 mg. q.i.d. for several days in order to achieve a rapid buildup of the serum-lithium level. If such large dosages are used, then daily serum-lithium levels need to be measured. The therapeutic range of lithium is 0.5 to 1.5 mEq. Toxic symptoms usually begin to appear at serum-lithium levels of 2.0 or above, but may appear at levels less than 1.5. These symptoms include nausea, vomiting, diarrhea, hand tremor, ataxia, confusion and bone marrow depression. Concomitant use of diuretics must be avoided where lithium is used in order to prevent the retention of lithium to toxic levels.

DRUGS USED IN THE TREATMENT OF DEPRESSION

Drugs used in the treatment of depression are: the amphetamines and amphetamine-like drugs, the tricyclic antidepressants and the monoamine oxidase inhibitors. Medications in the amphetamine group include dextroamphetamine sulfate (Dexedrine), dextroamphetamine sulfate and amobarbitol (Dexamyl), methylphenidate hydrochloride (Ritalin), and methamphetamine hydrochloride (Desoxyn). Tricyclic antidepressants are divided into the nonsedating group consisting of imipramine hydrochloride (Tofranil), desipramine hydrochloride (Norpramin or Pertofrane) and protriptyline hydrochloride (Vivactil), and the sedating group consisting of amitriptyline hydrochloride (Elavil), nortriptyline hydrochloride (Aventyl), and doxepin hydrochloride (Sinequan). Currently available monoamine oxidase inhibitors include isocarboxazid (Marplan), phenelzine sulfate (Nardil) and tranylcypromine sulfate (Parnate). Side effects of the amphetamine group include nervousness, anorexia, sleeplessness, palpitation and anxiety. The amphetamine group are rapid acting with an antidepressant effect noted on the 1st day of use. Patients using the amphetamine group acquire a partial tolerance to drug use after the 2nd day. Prospects for addiction and abuse exist but are infrequent. Fears of addiction to prescribed amphetamines are highly exaggerated. Amphetamines can be used with tricyclic antidepressants if necessary. Antidepressants in the amphetamine group are relatively safe, even in the presence of cardiovascular disease. A shift of antidepressants from the amphetamine group to the tricyclic group is safe without any time interval between the cessation of the amphetamine and the prescription of the tricyclic. When a patient stops using an amphetamine, he commonly experiences 48 to 72 hours of apathy and hyperirritability and should be cautioned that these symptoms may appear.

Dosages for the amphetamine group include: dextroamphetamine sulfate (Dexedrine), 5- to 15-mg. Spansule each morning; dextroamphetamine sulfate and amobarbitol (Dexamyl), 10- to 15-mg. Spansule each morning; methylphenidate hydrochloride (Ritalin) 5 to 20 mg. b.i.d.; and methamphetamine hydrochloride (Desoxyn), 2.5 mg. t.i.d.

Tricyclic antidepressants have many side effects including tachycardia, sweating, constipation, urinary retention, agitation, cardiac arrhythmias, blurred vision, edema, tremor, insomnia, impotence, vertigo, hypotension and dry mouth. Tricyclic antidepressants are slower acting with the antidepressant effect noted about 1 week from the time the drug is begun. Tricyclic antidepressants exhibit no tolerance or addiction, but the antidepressant effect may decrease in about a month, and higher doses may be necessary. Small doses of thyroid may enhance the antidepressant effect of tricyclic antidepressants in women. Ordinarily tricyclics may not be used with monoamine oxidase inhibitors. If the physician intends to substitute a monoamine oxidase inhibitor for a tricyclic antidepressant, he must wait at least 72 hours after the last dose of the tricylcic antidepressant. Tricyclic antidepressants are contraindicated in patients with cardiovascular disease. If used with cortical acting sedatives, tricyclic antidepressants produce a high incidence of acute brain syndrome. Combinations of tricyclic antidepressants with moderately sedating phenothiazines (Etrafon or Triavil) are very useful in the treatment of agitated depression. Thus, perphenazine (Trilafon) plus amitriptyline hydrochloride (Elavil) are very effective. Commonly employed dosages of the tricyclic antidepressants vary from 50 to 200 mg. daily except protriptyline hydrochloride (Vivactil) which is prescribed at a dosage of 10 to 30 mg. daily.

Patients taking monoamine oxidase inhibitors may experience side effects such as hypotension, sweating and constipation. If particular dietary restrictions are not observed, patients may experience hypertensive crises. Thus, patients who are taking monoamine oxidase inhibitors must adhere to a monoamine oxidase inhibitor diet which *excludes* pickled herring, chicken livers, red wine, aged cheese, raisins, lima beans and chocolate. These foods all contain tyramine, an amino acid which combines with the biological monoamines to produce pressor amines with subsequent blood pressure elevation. Monoamine oxidase inhibitors are slower acting with an antidepressant effect noted in about 1 week. Monoamine oxidase inhibitors produce no tolerance or addiction. The antidepressant effect of these medications continues over prolonged periods. Monoamine oxidase inhibitors are relatively safe even for patients with cardiovascular disease. The incidence of side effects secondary to administration of monoamine oxidase inhibitors is lower than the incidence of side effects in patients using tricyclic antidepressants. Commonly employed dosages of monoamine oxidase inhibitors are isocarboxazid (Marplan) 10 to 30 mg. daily, phenelzine sulfate (Nardil) 15 to 60 mg. daily, and tranylcypromine (Parnate) 10 to 60 mg. daily.

PSYCHIATRIC DRUGS OF THE FUTURE

Development of new psychiatric drugs must answer two needs:

1. Drugs must be developed which can be administered more effectively.

2. Drugs must be developed which are more effective for some groups of patients than those currently available.

Many patients do not achieve functional recovery because they fail to continue using psychiatric drugs after discharge from a hospital. The use of fluphenazine hydrochloride (Prolixin), fluphenazine enanthate (Prolixin Enanthate) and fluphenazine decanoate (Prolixin Decanoate) as long-lasting injectables usually administered at 1- to 2-week intervals has drastically improved the prognosis for many of these patients. Penfluridol, a medication currently being tested, exemplifies a long-lasting oral medication which can be given at weekly intervals for the treatment of schizophrenic psychosis. Research is currently underway regarding phenothiazines or phenothiazine-like drugs which can be inserted subcutaneously in pellet form at 6-month intervals. It must be cautioned that long-acting forms of psychoactive medications ought *not* to be used early in a patient's treatment in order to avoid the persistence of serious side effects or toxic effects should they occur.

Other drugs currently under development are quadricyclic antidepressants, and new families of phenothiazine-like antipsychotic agents.

Although many of these new medications may serve only to parallel drugs already in use, some patients will respond to the new agents despite these patients having been unresponsive to other drugs previously employed. Each new medication is a welcome addition to our rapidly growing armamentarium of psychoactive drugs.

BIBLIOGRAPHY

Ayd, F. J., Jr. Long acting injectable neuroleptics. *Int. Drug Therapy Newsletter* 7: 1–7, 1972.

Fieve, R. Overview of therapeutic and prophylactic trials with Lithium in psychiatric patients. In Gershon, S., and Shopsin, B. (Eds.), *Lithium: Its Role in Psychiatric Research and Treatment.* New York: Plenum Press, 1973, pp. 329–332.

Jarvik, M. Drugs used in the treatment of psychiatric disorders. In Goodman, and Gilman (Eds.), *The Pharmacological Basis of Therapeutics.* New York: MacMillan, 1970, pp. 181–193.

Prien, R., Levine, J., and Cole, J. O. High dose trifluoperazine therapy in chronic schizophrenia. *Am. J. Psychiatry* 126: 305–313, 1969.

Quitlar, F. Lithium in other psychiatric disorders. In Gershon, S., and Shopsin, B. (Eds.), *Lithium: Its Role in Psychiatric Research and Treatment.* New York: Plenum Press, 1973.

Voltolina, E., and Widroe, H. Brain subsystems in the genesis of schizophrenia. In Widroe, H. (Ed.), *Human Behavior and Brain Function.* Springfield: Charles C Thomas, 1975, pp. 93–96.

Widroe, H. Understanding the use of psychiatric drugs. In *Ego Psychology and Psychiatric Treatment Planning.* New York: Appleton-Century-Crofts, 1968, pp. 129–139.

Chapter 4

the nurse as a group therapist

BEVERLY J. HENDLER

The care and treatment of patients with psychiatric or emotional problems usually involves the utilization of a variety of treatment modalities. One method of treatment that is well-favored and that is frequently recommended and employed in outpatient and inpatient psychiatric treatment is group therapy. Group therapy has become increasingly popular as a psychiatric treatment modality primarily because of its overall therapeutic effectiveness in the management and care of patients.

The continued popularity and acceptance of group therapy as an integral part of a patient's treatment has created a demand for more qualified, skilled, and theoretically prepared individuals to assume the role of group therapists. The demand for increased numbers of qualified group therapists has been an important, contributing factor to the registered nurses' advancement to that role. Another element that has influenced the nurses' progression to the position of group therapist relates to the continued expansion of the role of the nurse.

Over the past 8 to 10 years nurses have begun to function more actively as group therapists. Prior to that time nurses were not considered for that role because of the inadequate clinical and theoretical preparation (or in some instances, a total lack of preparation) given in a basic or graduate nursing program. The involvement of more nurses as group therapists has required nursing educators in basic and graduate nursing programs to carefully evaluate and revise the kind of theoretical and clinical experience the student receives in preparation for functioning therapeutically in a group. Consequently, many schools of nursing now offer a more well-rounded clinical and theoretical experience in group therapy courses for the basic and graduate nursing student. However, a complaint that is often voiced by students is that many of the available courses tend to focus excessively on group theory and place less emphasis on the clinical component of group therapy. A course in group therapy that presents an effective and appropriate balance between the theoretical and clinical elements is far more meaningful and practically useful to the student.

The statement has been made regarding the increased popularity of group therapy for patients with emotional or psychiatric problems. It must be remembered that group therapy is not limited to the psychiatric patient. During recent years, groups have been established for patients with various physical problems for the purpose of helping the patient learn to cope with a particular disability. Examples of these kinds of groups include groups for the psoriasis patient, the cancer patient, the cardiac patient, and the mastectomy patient.

The beginning student in group therapy is usually frightened, anxious, insecure, and confused about participating in group sessions with patients. The questions most frequently asked usually relate to specific clinical and interpersonal situations that affect the student's ability to function as a participant and/or therapist in the group.

The purpose of this chapter is to explore some of the more salient issues and situations with which the group leader/therapist is confronted. The material that is presented focuses on specific theoretical concepts and opinions that are related to group therapy and offers relevant clinical examples to demonstrate the practical application of the theory. The scope of this chapter will be limited to the discussion of group therapy for patients with psychiatric or emotional problems.

For the purpose of this chapter the terms group leader and group therapist will be used synonymously.

THE THERAPEUTIC EXPERIENCE

It should be understood that group therapy is not appropriate for all psychiatric patients in terms of being therapeutically beneficial. The rationale for referring a patient for group psychotherapy must be clearly defined after careful evaluation and assessment of the client. The goals for treatment in group therapy must be thoroughly outlined in the client's treatment plan. It is imperative that the group therapist be aware of and follow the patient's treatment plan and revise the plan as necessary.

Group Structure and Group Goals

The goals and structure of a therapy group may be described or labeled as an exploratory or confrontive group or as a supportive or nonconfrontive type of treatment approach. Careful consideration must be given to the type of group to which a client is referred. For example, a patient in need of a supportive type of group should not be a member of an exploratory or confrontive group whose goal is to explore intrapsychic conflicts in clients' lives. Members of an exploratory group usually have healthier egos which enable them to more easily engage in introspection.

The goals of a supportive group are to strengthen ego defenses and to assist the client in the suppression and repression of unconscious conflicts. Therefore, the exploration of conflictual issues in a patient's life is avoided. The floridly psychotic patient who exhibits a reality testing defect and a thought process disorder is an example of a candidate who can profit most from a supportive group.

Case Illustration

A 40-year-old, hospitalized patient with a manic-depressive illness, manic-type, was referred to an exploratory psychotherapy group. During his first session he became extremely agitated after being in the group for about 15 minutes. He left his chair several times and began to discuss topics that were entirely unrelated to the group. He became quite argumentative and attempted to challenge the group therapist to "a game of words." He expressed his displeasure with the group and made a number of provocative, uncomplimentary statements to several members of the group. It was obvious that the patient was losing control and could not function in the session at that time. The nurse therapist intervened and, in a supportive manner, pointed out to the patient that he seemed anxious and told him that he should leave the group. The patient appeared greatly relieved and promptly left the session.

Some therapists might argue the point that the patient should have remained in the group and have been allowed to "vent" his ideas and feelings. However, the nurse realized that the patient's anxiety continued to increase and this made it difficult for the patient to maintain control over his feelings and behavior. The patient's positive response to the nurse's recommendation that he leave the group demonstrated that the nurse had exercised good clinical judgment.

The clinical example illustrated that the patient was not a candidate for exploratory group therapy. He would have benefited more from a supportive group approach.

Some of the ways the group therapist best meets the goals of a supportive type of group include the following: 1) avoiding conflictual issues/material in a patient's life; 2) focusing on reality testing when indicated or necessary; 3) helping a patient organize his thoughts if he appears to be confused or if he is unable to follow logical speech sequences; 4) allowing the client to leave the group, or requesting that he leave the session, if he is unable to cope with the events in the group; 5) placing limits on the amount of time spent in a session—e.g., a supportive group might meet for $1/2$ hour to 45 minutes, whereas an exploratory group might meet for 1 or $1^1/2$ hours; and 6) involving the group members in a structured, nonconflictual activity that has a clear, concise, uncomplicated directive. Examples of structured activities include having the patients in the group discuss their favorite vacation or a favorite pet, involving the clients in an exercise period, or having the patients participate in an art project. To reiterate, the objective is to avoid areas or issues around which there is conflict for the client which, consequently, could create increased anxiety for the patient and impede his ability to cope.

Group Relationships: Establishing a Therapeutic Alliance

Group therapy, like all other types of psychotherapy, involves the establishment of a therapeutic alliance between the patient and the therapist for the purpose of facilitating effective psychiatric treatment. DeWald (1971, pp. 99–100) states that the therapeutic alliance is "where the healthy aspects of the patients ego form a partnership with the therapist in which they, as a pair, pit themselves against the neurotic or the sick elements in the patient's mental life, in an attempt to influence or change the latter. The healthy ego processes include such things as capacities for communication, self-awareness, intelligence, motivation, object relationships and overall capacity for integration and synthesis."

Case Illustration

A 35-year-old woman was referred to a supportive, outpatient therapy group after experiencing an acute psychotic episode which had required hospitalization. The patient expressed a great deal of fear about attending the group sessions. She failed to attend four consecutive sessions after the referral was made. The group leader called the client each week to discuss her reluctance to participate in the group. The patient was given an opportunity to relate her concerns and fears to the therapist. She had the fantasy that she might be verbally and/or physically attacked by members of the group. She also expressed the concern that she would "be forced" to talk. The group therapist reassured the patient that she would not be attacked or forced to talk in the sessions. The therapist was careful to explain the structure—e.g., group rules, standards, and norms—of the group. The therapist was quite supportive of the client. The nurse made a deliberate effort to let the patient know that group therapy was a crucial part of her treatment. The patient concurred with the leader and began attending the group sessions.

The first two sessions that she attended seemed to evoke tremendous anxiety in the patient. She arrived 20 to 30 minutes early and asked to see the therapist for "a few minutes" before the other members of the group arrived. The therapist reminded the patient that she realized that the client was anxious about participating in the group but that, in the therapist's judgment, the patient was able to cope with the situation. The therapist also pointed out to the patient that the fact that she managed to get to the session for two consecutive meetings was evidence that she could deal effectively with her fears and concerns about group therapy. The client agreed with the group leader and appeared to be less anxious. The patient made it a point to sit next to the leader during the first two or three meetings.

Analysis of the case example demonstrates the way in which the therapeutic alliance developed between the patient and the therapist. The nurse therapist was therapeutically responsive to the patient in several ways: 1) she offered adequate support to the client; 2) she set firm and meaningful limits for her; 3) she reinforced, as well as appealed to, the healthier parts of the patient's ego, particularly as it relates to her capacity to communicate, her capacity for integration, her level of motivation, and the degree of self-awareness; 4) she maintained clear communication with the patient.

The development of the therapeutic alliance occurs when the client and the therapist can establish some sense of rapport. Establishing a rapport can be easily accomplished with some patients, and yet it can be a very difficult task to achieve with others. The case presentation illustrates that the establishment of a rapport between the therapist and the client requires careful work on the part of the therapist to enable the patient to enter into a therapeutic relationship with the therapist and the group. The relationship between the therapist and the patient is essential to the successful treatment of clients.

Group Relationships: Transference and Counter-Transference

Transference, as discussed by Widroe (1968, p. 108), "generally refers to an irrational repetition of behavior patterns that have their genesis in the patient's modes of relating to important objects of his childhood. These behavior patterns have not adjusted to conform with the realities of the patient's present situation. Thus transference behavior stands in contrast to reality adjusted behavior." Obviously, transference phenomenon is a crucial element of the therapeutic process in group as well as in individual psychotherapy. Therefore, it is of utmost importance that the group therapist have a clear understanding of the significance of the transference principle and tool in the treatment of patients.

Transferences occur among members of the group as well as with the therapist. Patients inherently develop transferences to those individuals who best represent their infantile subjects. It must be pointed out, however, that the therapist is the single most dominant transference figure in the group (Durkin, 1964, p. 148).

A student sometimes fails to appreciate and treat seriously the way in which he influences the group as a participant or as a group therapist.

Singer (1965, p. 290) defines counter-transference as an unconsciously determined set of attitudes that are held by the therapist and that can interfere with his work with a patient. (This definition is not universally accepted, however). Counter-transference is generally understood to be a development that is quite similar to transference. The need for the therapist to understand and appreciate the counter-transference concept is just as important as the need to understand the phenomenon of transference.

Transference and counter-transference can be described as either positive or negative.

Case Illustration

A 28-year-old, depressed, single woman was referred for outpatient exploratory group therapy following her discharge from a psychiatric hospital. She had been hospitalized because of a suicide attempt.

During the first several sessions she appeared to be withdrawn and participated minimally with the members of the group. Her physical appearance was characteristic of a fragile, helpless child who needed to be taken care of completely by others. Most of the time that she was in group she sat staring blankly at the group therapist. When questioned by someone she spoke very softly and had to be asked several times to speak louder. There were a number of attempts to try to engage her in the interactive process in the group.

At one point in her therapy, she began telephoning the group therapist several times daily to talk about her problems and her feelings of helplessness. She became upset and tearful if the therapist would not spend time with her. The therapist tried to set firm limits with her but most of the attempts at limit-setting were, for the most part, ineffective. The therapist became increasingly angry with the patient and during a group therapy session she sternly confronted and admonished the patient regarding her clinging, demanding behavior. The patient fled the group in tears.

The therapist soon realized that her negative counter-transference feelings were, indeed, interfering with her ability to work with the patient. The group leader also recognized that she had failed to identify the character of the transference—e.g., a regressive, maternal transference—which, subsequently, created problems in the patient's management and care in the group as well as outside the group.

After careful exploration of the situation, the nurse therapist acknowledged that her angry reaction to the patient related to her difficulty in dealing with manipulative, demanding, and excessively dependent, clinging people. She was able to recall that her mother and sister frequently behaved in a fashion similar to the patient and that she, the therapist, usually responded with anger and/or disgust.

In evaluating the case more closely, several points must be considered. They include: 1) the character of the transference must be identified very early in treatment; 2) the therapist should maintain an appropriate level of awareness as well as keeping a perspective about the character of the transference; 3) the therapist needs to explore counter-transference issues with colleagues or in supervision sessions; 4) the therapist must recognize that she will not like all patients with whom she works, nor will all clients like her. The beginning group therapist generally has some difficulty accepting this idea.

Functioning as a Group Therapist

Leadership in a group involves a multitude of responsibilities and expectations. Leadership in group therapy requires the willingness on the part of the nurse to function as a role model for the patient members of the group.

The qualified, effective, and competent group therapist is one who is prepared to deal with almost any situation or activity in the group. Naturally this implies an enormous amount of risk-taking on the part of the therapist. Obviously this is extremely difficult for some nurses since assertiveness, or risk-taking, is an attribute that has not always been inherent in the practice of nursing.

Another important component of effective group leadership is the nurse's ability to utilize the nursing process and to be prepared to exercise her clinical judgment and decision-making ability. In making decisions regarding the care and treatment of patients in the therapy group the nurse must keep in mind the need for treating all clients as individuals.

The nurse's use of herself in group therapy (or functioning as a role model) is therapeutically valuable in terms of facilitating change in patients. For example, a nurse therapist, who is willing to confront and set limits on an acting-out adolescent who is disrupting the group process, sets an example for other group members. Furthermore, she communicates the message that it is all right to confront people and that members of the group have permission to deal with issues that are disturbing or that affect the therapeutic process in the group.

A question that is often raised by the beginning group therapist is whether or not it is appropriate to share with the members of the group information about herself. Years ago the philosophy was to maintain a distinctly distant relationship with the patient and to always "behave in a professional manner." The interpretation of this latter statement usually meant that the nurse was not, under any circumstances, to disclose any information about herself. The rationale for this is still unclear. That aside, it has been demonstrated in a patient's response to treatment that the therapist can, indeed, share certain kinds of information about herself with the patient. It should be emphasized that the nurse should avoid disclosing the more personal parts of her life.

Case Illustration-1

During a group therapy session a patient asked the nurse therapist if she ever became depressed and, if so, how she coped with the depression. The therapist answered the patient honestly and offered the client information about the coping mechanisms that she, the therapist, utilized in handling the feelings of depression.

Case Illustration-2

During a therapy session in a supportive type of group a confused patient asked the nurse therapist several questions regarding the therapist's sexual life. The group therapist responded to the patient's questions by pointing out to the client that his questions were quite inappropriate and were regarded as unacceptable social behavior and that the patient must discontinue that particular line of questioning. The nurse's attitude toward the patient was not punitive but, instead, her attitude was realistically and supportively firm. By reality testing for the patient the therapist was able to give clear feedback about his behavior.

The two contrasting case examples illustrate how the nurse therapist must exercise her judgment and discretion about self-disclosure.

SUPERVISION

Supervision is a crucial element of any type of nursing practice. Supervision promotes continued professional and personal growth of the individual as well as offering a tremendous support system for the therapist. As in the case of the nurse in private practice, the nurse group therapist needs to establish and maintain adequate and ongoing resources for the supervision of her work with patients.

In inpatient settings, supervision of the nurse's work as a group therapist is accomplished in "feedback" or "rehash" sessions in which other members of the staff are usually present. This method of group supervision is generally quite meaningful and practically useful if the focus is on the thorough analysis and evaluation of all aspects of the events that transpired in the therapy meeting.

In order to facilitate a useful feedback session the therapist should share, in a sequential order, as much information about the group as possible. Examples of the information that should be discussed with other staff members include: 1) whether the group began on time or not (which is quite important), 2) the names of the individuals who were tardy or who did not show up for the meeting, 3) whether the group began in an orderly or a chaotic manner, 4) the seating arrangements of the members of the group, 5) the member(s) who initiated the interactive process, 6) all unusual verbal and nonverbal interactions in the group, 7) the level of participation of the members of the group, 8) the group process — e.g., the way in which all members of the group interacted during the entire meeting, 9) the level and degree of participation of the therapist, 10) any techniques that were utilized and the rationale for utilizing them, 11) the theme of the group — e.g., rejection, separation, etc., 12) the overall affect of the group — e.g., depressed, flat, and 13) amy other information that affects, in any way, the functioning of the group. Obviously, this is not an exhaustive list.

The feedback session should be a teaching/learning session for all staff members involved in the treatment and care of the psychiatric patient. A problem that sometimes occurs in the rehash meeting is the staff's tendency to relate what happened in the group on a verbal level and omit the nonverbal component of the group meeting. Also, the inclination at times is to fail to use the feedback or rehash period as a teaching/learning experience so that input is given from a number of sources about the way in which the group functioned.

Obviously, effective supervision in the feedback session is facilitated by the availability of a skilled, qualified and competent supervisor who is adequately prepared clinically and theoretically in the theory and practice of group therapy.

Supervision of a therapist's work in outpatient group therapy is often done on an individual basis. With this type of supervision the therapist does not have the advantage of receiving input from several sources, a method of supervision which is usually quite beneficial to the therapist.

SUMMARY

This paper has offered a discussion of some of the most prominent issues that relate to group therapy with exploration of the nurse's role as a group therapist. The nurse who assumes a group therapist role must be prepared personally and professionally to meet the demands and responsibilities that relate to that position. Participation in therapy groups is a challenging experience and requires that the group leader be adequately prepared educationally for the experience.

BIBLIOGRAPHY

Bross, R. The 'deserter' in group psychotherapy. *Int. J. Group Psychother.* 6: 419–427, 1956.

Cartwright, D., and Zander, A. *Group Dynamics, Research and Theory,* New York: Harper and Row, 1968.

DeWald, P. A. *Psychotherapy: A Dynamic Approach.* New York: Basic Books, Inc., Publishers, 1971.

Durkin, H. Transference in group psychotherapy revisited. *Int. Group Psychother.* 21: 11–21, 1971.

Durkin, H. *The Group in Depth.* New York: International Universities Press, Inc., 1964.

Fried, E. Some aspects of group dynamics and the analysis of transference and defenses. *Int. J. Group Psychother.* 15: 44–56, 1965.

Guttmacher, J. A., and Birk, L. Group therapy: What specific therapeutic advantages? *Compr. Psychiatry* 12: 546–556, 1971.

Hare, P. *Handbook of Small Group Research.* New York: The Free Press, 1962.

Jacobs, M. and Christ, J. Structuring and limit setting as techniques in the group treatment of adolescent delinquents. *Community Ment. Health J.* 3: 237–244, 1967.

Kotkov, B. Favorable clinical indications for group attendance. *Int. J. Group Psychother.* 8: 419–427, 1958.

Luft, J. *Group Processes: An Introduction to Group Dynamics.* Palo Alto: National Press Books, 1970.

Martin, J. T. Regressed patient in group therapy. *Perspect. Psychiatr. Care* 8: 131-135, 1970.

Model, Y. Adolescent group psychotherapy in a hospital setting. *Am. J. Psychoanal.* 30: 68-72, 1970.

Munzer, J. Acting out: Communication or resistance? *Int. J. Group Psychother.* 16: 434-441, 1966.

Newman, G., and Hall, R. Acting out: An indication for psychodrama. *Group Psychother. Psychodrama* 24: 87-96, 1971.

Singer, E., *Key concepts in Psychotherapy.* New York: Basic Books, Inc., Publishers, 1965.

Stotsky, B., and Zolick, E. Group psychotherapy with psychotics: 1921-1963 – A review. *Int. J. Group Psychother.* 15: 321-344, 1965.

Swanson, M. A check list for group leaders. *Perspect. Psychiatr. Care* 7: 120-126, 1969.

Weisselberger, D. Acting-out behavior in group psychotherapy: A re-appraisal. *Groups: J. Group Dynam. Psychother.* 5: 57-61, 1973-1974.

Whitaker, D., and Lickerman, M. *Psychotherapy Through the Group Process.* Chicago: Aldine Publishing Co., 1972.

Widroe, H. J. *Ego Psychology and Psychiatric Treatment Planning.* New York: Appleton. Century-Crofts, 1968.

Wolstein, B. Transference: Historical roots and current concepts in psychoanalytic theory and practice. *Psychiatry* 23: 159-172, 1960.

Yalom, I. D. A study of group therapy drop-outs. *Arch. Gen. Psychiatry* 14: 4, 1966.

Yalom, I. D. Problems of the neophyte group therapists. *Int. J. Soc. Psychiatry* 12: 52-59, 1966.

Yalom, I. D. *The Theory and Practice of Group Psychotherapy.* New York: Basic Books, Inc., 1970.

Zeligs, M. A. The psychology of silence. *J. Am. Psychoanal. Assoc.* 9: 7-13, 1961.

Chapter **5**

teaching the unreachable: psychotherapy in the classroom

DIANA COHEN

Classrooms can be chaos. Occasionally that chaos is the excitement of learning in progress, of a heated discussion of generating ideas and of students and teachers exchanging roles and learning from each other. More often, however, the chaos is that confusion which results when students who would much rather be anywhere other than the classroom confront the teachers who must perforce become jailer and task-master in order to deal with distracted, uninvolved youngsters. Picture for a moment a classroom full of severely disturbed adolescents who are inpatients in a psychiatric hospital. The variety, complexity and seriousness of the problems in this situation increase in geometric proportion; however, the level of chaos need not do the same. On the contrary, meeting adolescents on some of their own turf in the classroom may prove to be one of the most effective modalities of psychotherapy for working with this most difficult of age groups.

Of the few psychiatric institutions which have programs designed for the treatment of adolescents, only a small percentage have begun to explore the possibilities of includ-ing an academic component. The most frequently taken first step in this direction is the addition of community based tutors who help keep the youngsters from getting irreparably behind in their school work. Most traditional psychiatric institutions (as well as most educational institutions) seem to subscribe to the notion that one must choose to teach *either* the student or the subject. Consequently, for the most part, academics has remained the domain of the teachers and therapy the responsibility of the therapists.

In a 4-year project started in a 60-bed, private psychiatric hospital, integration of a secondary school into the overall treatment program was explored. The patients involved ranged in age from 12 to 20 years and represented the entire span of psychiatric diagnoses, including both psychotic and nonpsychotic illnesses, drug-related problems, behavior disorders and adjustment reactions of adolescence. The school was fully accredited and could therefore provide academic credit to the students, while at the same time it served as another modality of psychotherapy. The instructors in the school were involved on a daily basis in diagnostic and treatment planning sessions with the medical staff and in group and family therapy as well. The results of this project were, and continue to be, extremely exciting. It became apparent that psychotherapy can indeed be accomplished at the same time schooling takes place, oftentimes more efficiently than through other approaches.

This chapter attempts to isolate some of the most common objectives in working with disturbed and severely disturbed adolescents. These are: structuring, confrontation of character pathology and experimenting with learned behavior, socialization, developing communication skills, experiencing success, dealing with conflictual material and reality testing. In a general way, comments have been made on the role of a psychotherapeutic school in meeting these objectives. In addition, vignettes from actual cases and brief examples of the academic tasks that are commonly used have been provided in order to further illuminate the concept of the psychotherapeutic school.

STRUCTURING

Institutionalized adolescents, whether the location be in a juvenile hall or a psychiatric hospital, regardless of their respective diagnoses, have many past experiences in common. Many youngsters who find themselves in a hospital situation of some sort have come from troubled families, families not strong enough to supply a constructive environment in which to grow. In the vast majority of cases involving troubled adolescents, the parental relationships have been less than ideal. Constant fighting, total lack of communication between the parents, threats of separation or actual dissolution lie behind many. In the midst of such familial turbulence, children learn to push their limits to the extreme, encountering only sporadically the moderating force of a rational and caring parent figure. This experience translates, of course, when the adolescent is out in the world, involved in cutting class, breaking laws, and generally defying authority. The mere existence of a school in a hospital setting, with its clearly defined sets of rules, time schedules and expecta-

tions, can be used constructively in beginning to teach children where socially acceptable and functional limits lie. School can be seen as the "work" of an adolescent. It might be considered one of the most important responsibilities an adolescent has on the ward. A therapeutic school can provide the structure around which the adolescent must organize the rest of his activities.

The emphasis in recent years on "free schools" and "open classrooms" in certain areas of the country offers adolescents a wide variety of choice and extreme flexibility in scheduling. As exciting and broadening as these programs may be for some well-organized adolescents, the programs are easily manipulated and abused by those who have learned to test and stretch their limits at home. It is not rare for a youngster to relate having spent no more than 3 days per week at school, taking anywhere from one to three real courses and using the remainder of his time to smoke pot with friends just outside the boundaries of the school, all with seemingly few if any repercussions from the school authorities. In a therapeutic school, although a good deal of choice can and ought to exist within the curriculum for students who can benefit from it, assignments, hours of attendance and classroom regulations must be clearly stated and firmly adhered to.

Example

An obese, 15-year-old girl was admitted from the emergency room of a local hospital following an overdose of Dexamyl which she said had been prescribed for her for weight control. She stated that her weight was 267 pounds. She had become increasingly depressed following the recent death of a long-time family physician. She was the youngest of seven children in a family in which both parents worked up to 16 hours a day, spending virtually no time at home with her and letting her know that they were tired of raising children. Although she was quite a bright and artistically talented student, her school performance had begun to suffer terribly. She had no friends, as she invariably offended acquaintances with her crass and cruel statements and foul language. It was clear that the girl had never been asked to abide by household rules and that her parents were never around her to control her behavior. Thus, an important function of school in the hospital for her was to set firm limits and provide a structure within which she might learn more productive and acceptable behavior.

There are many academic techniques and tasks which can be used to supply guidance and structure to those adolescents who have, for either behavioral or psychiatric reasons, been unable to address themselves to school work. By the time they reach the point of institutionalization, many youngsters are simply out of practice with school. Others' internal processes are so chaotic that to ask them to impose their own structure is futile.

One of the richest tools for use in this type of school is the daily journal. Students know that if nothing else is assigned, a journal entry must be written every day. This, of course, can easily be integrated into the English curriculum. Even before an adolescent is ready to attend school sessions in the classroom, he is given a journal, a pen and a very specific assignment, in order for him to become familiar with one of the fundamentals of the school he will soon be joining. For youngsters who have been out of touch with academics in general for a while, writing "just anything" is a terrible task. Setting up some kinds of structure for them is very important in the beginning, regardless of the nature of the assignment. They might be asked to complete a full page, even if they must fill the remaining space with penmanship practice. In other instances, setting a time limit for writing, say 10 minutes, without stopping, provides a similar sort of structure which makes the early stages of journal writing somehow easier.

The journal can be used quite well in helping psychotic patients begin to organize their thoughts. They might be asked to use the journal as a diary of sorts, keeping track of their activities in list form. They might be asked to write very concrete and simple descriptions of objects or of other people. As their psychoses begin to clear, of course, any number of assignments can be created which can allow for increasingly more flexibility but at the same time supply a good amount of structure.

CONFRONTATION OF CHARACTER PATHOLOGY AND EXPERIMENTING WITH LEARNED BEHAVIOR

In a sense, a hospital classroom can become a microcosm of the worlds of the adolescents. It is often possible to generalize about the overall behavior of a student from his behavior in or concerning school. Frequently, school has been a source of stress, either socially or academically, for hospitalized adolescents.

Consequently, the classroom provides a natural setting for the confrontation of failure-oriented behavior. Problem areas become quite visible in a situation which puts demands on patients who are not accustomed to responding in an acceptable way to the demands of a responsible life. Failure to meet these demands, whether it be arriving at class late, not completing an assignment or interacting in inappropriate ways with teachers and other students, is firmly confronted and clearly interpreted.

As patients progress in their hospital treatment, they learn new behavior patterns, or become more comfortable expressing their true feelings. They are encouraged to experiment with their new skills in the classroom. The teacher/therapist can act as a referee when necessary, sometimes "protecting" newly vulnerable students (having come out from behind tough facades) from the potentially cruel reactions of peers. Discussion of this new behavior is encouraged, giving the patient a glimpse of the kinds of reactions he can expect after discharge and resumption of life in the real world.

Example

The 19-year-old son of a retired military man and a neurotic woman was admitted for severe depression following a 2-month spree during which he carelessly spent a $7000 inheritance. He had not finished the 10th grade, had never held a job for more than 3 months and had never really attempted to support himself. He had great difficulty attending to and completing the tasks which led the way to independence and autonomy. He was assigned to school, having expressed some desire to complete his high school education, perhaps by taking the high school equivalency examination, the GED. After 10 minutes of the first class, he began to make up excuses for not participating in the program, protesting that "It is just not for me." His resistance and desire to "cop out" were interpreted as representative of his basic problem, which, after having had it repeated to him hundreds of times, he could not avoid understanding. Small academic tasks were set up for him and he was asked to try to complete something, anything, to see how it felt. He gradually progressed over a period to larger assignments, and experienced the feeling of pride which comes with completing a new and difficult task.

It is possible, with an understanding of the dynamics operative in an individual or group, and a familiarity with English literature, both prose and poetry, to select works with which patients can identify enough to gain some often very powerful insight. I have found numerous short stories written at the junior high and high school levels which lend themselves well to first, a discussion of the behavior patterns of the protagonist and second, to the identification of similar patterns which exist in one or more of the adolescents participating.

Example

One 16-year-old girl who had been hospitalized for severe depression, excessive drug use, trouble with the legal authorities and other characterological problems was in the habit of "editing" what she heard. Her hearing "failed her" when things were said that she did not want to hear and occasionally created things that had never been said at all. Reading and discussing Richard Wright's story "The Kitten," an excerpt from "Black Boy," proved to be very helpful with her. In the story a young boy "hears" his father order him to kill a kitten, and in an effort at getting even with his father for his lack of attention, the boy "obeys," realizing the consequences of his action only long after the deed has been done. Through a discussion of this boy's "hearing problem" it was possible for the teacher/therapist and the other adolescents in class to confront the girl and help her begin to develop and practice her new hearing skills.

SOCIALIZATION

In hospitals where all age groups are integrated in the general ward program, a school can provide the opportunity for adolescents and other young adults to interact with people of similar ages. It almost need not be stated that many youngsters in this age group have problems relating to older people and authority figures. Many, however, have problems in dealing with peers as well; it is not unusual that hospitalized adolescents report having few, if any, friends.

There are few secrets kept in the classroom; students are encouraged to relate with openness and honesty, qualities which are considered foremost in the overall school atmosphere. The result is often the development of strong ties which have become friendships between hospitalized kids, continuing even after discharge.

Introverted patients, whose lack of real socialization with other people has reached the point where life is at a standstill, are encouraged to use the classroom setting for this purpose.

Example

A 24-year-old young man who had completed 1 year of college and part of a 2nd year, was admitted for depression and multiple somatic symptoms which had no discoverable physiological origin. He became unbearably anxious when talking to people, and this caused him a great deal of abdominal pain. This patient's authoritarian father had cowed him into virtual silence since childhood, instilling in him a deep feeling of inferiority. These feelings were accompanied by an increasingly powerful hatred of his father, who was at that time dying. The young man was asked to come to a couple of classes a day in order to experiment with peer interaction. In the classroom he was given the role of "assistant to the teacher" to help him recognize his better than average intellectual capability, and to encourage him to relate on a peer level with the young teacher/therapist as well as the older students.

Use of the psychotherapeutic journal, which was introduced earlier, is one of the most effective tools for encouraging socialization in the classroom setting. Reading journals aloud in class, whether it be a homework assignment or a special classroom exercise, is strongly encouraged, but not required of the patients. Frequently new students are reluctant to share their personal thoughts or to expose what they consider to be poor writing to the group. Gradually, though, with encouragement from the writings of more experienced class members, and with the proddings of other students, most patients eventually become quite comfortable with reading aloud, some to the point of quibbling about who gets to read first. As in group therapy, patients who are not speaking are responsible for listening actively to the reader, and are directed to respond if possible to that which is being read. All listeners are encouraged to ask questions and make interpretations when appropriate, suggestions which provide the impetus for verbal interaction and identification among the adolescents. Journal entries, when read aloud, are rarely subject to academic judgement or evaluation so that the patients are never discouraged in that manner from sharing their feelings with their peers. The following is an example of the sort of in-class writing assignment which might be used to stimulate social interaction.

Example

The teacher/therapist writes on the blackboard, "I think_____thinks I am. . . ." Students are asked to pair off randomly. Each person is asked to write a paragraph about how he thinks his partner perceives him; in other words, how he thinks he comes across to the other person. When this is finished, the teacher writes on the blackboard, "I think_____is . . .," and asks the students to reverse the process, writing how they perceive their partners. When everyone is finished writing, both sets of paragraphs are read aloud and the discrepancies are discussed openly. Frequently, students are quite surprised at the impressions they give others, both negative and positive, and often find that they have responded to other students based on inaccurate assumptions. Invariably, patients come away from this assignment with fresh feelings about themselves and all the other members of the group.

DEVELOPING COMMUNICATION SKILLS

Faulty communication and total lack of communication can be viewed as both cause and effect in the realm of psychopathology. Many psychological disturbances in adolescents appear to be the result of living for many years in environments where parents cannot communicate with each other in effective ways and therefore cannot impart communication skills to their children. The children are then unable to express their needs well enough to have them fulfilled, and they find living in a society which cannot clairvoyantly respond to them extremely difficult.

Discussion is the key to virtually all of the academic work selected for psychotherapeutic classes. These discussions, although to some degree structured, are allowed to evolve in the direction which best satisfies the needs of the participating students. As the patients feel more comfortable and able to open up in the classroom, common problems and common concerns begin to appear and these provide relevant material with which to experiment in communication, that is, just how accurately one can get a message across to another person. Clarity of speech is stressed, and ambiguities are immediately pointed out.

The theme of communication (or the lack thereof) is one which constantly appears in the literature selected for use in psychotherapeutic classes. A carefully chosen poem or piece of prose dealing with this (or any other conflictual topic) can serve as a springboard for the discussion of the individual subjective experiences of the students. There are a number of poems which have been used with significant success in getting adolescents to see how their patterns of communication do them a disservice. Often they can begin to understand that is is not just their words, but their facial and bodily movements, their tones of voice, and the contexts in which they say things which determine the actual messages they transmit. The following is an example of the sort of poem, actually written by a hospitalized 13-year-old, through which there has been very insightful discussion of the feelings underlying the tough facades which many adolescents sport.

I put on other people
to escape from being me
from seeing me
so I can look happy
look sexy, tough
look unafraid

look like I've got
peace of mind
everything I don't have
and wish I did
I'm not happy
not sexy, or tough
I'm afraid to look at myself
for what I really am
I have no peace of mind
just confusion and depression
maybe I should put on me.

It is possible, through discussions of this sort, to teach kids to communicate on a feeling level and to begin to cut through the garbage which clutters their communications and keeps them from "making contact" with other people.

EXPERIENCING SUCCESS

The vast majority of adolescents who are enrolled in psychotherapeutic schools have histories of chronic academic failure. Many of them describe themselves as having always been the "dummy" of their classes. Part of the teacher/therapist's responsibility here is to try to distinguish where intellective deficit, secondary to psychiatric disturbance, and poor study habits begin and end. Because of the unusual makeup of a hospital school, many of these low self-esteem patients can experience, if only briefly, a feeling of success and superiority in a schoolroom setting. The great diversity of ages and grade levels in a typical class provides the opportunity for almost every student at one time or another to be an instructor of sorts. Although a 12th grade student may have been at the bottom of his history class in public school, he is bound to be more familiar with the concept, or at least the term, the Cold War than an 8th grader who is now in the same class. The fact that some patients stay in the school program longer than others allows for a similar experience when they are asked to orient new patients to class procedures or recently covered material. It is always striking how much more interested and involved these patients become in the class immediately following the experience of feeling the slightest bit of academic success. For some patients it provides a much more long-lasting incentive to be prepared for and active in classes.

Example

A 17-year-old girl was admitted for an acute schizophrenic episode following the unexpected death of her mother. Her history indicated longstanding bizarre behavior, with a gradual decline in interest and success in school. She, had dropped out of continuation high school just one course away from graduation and indicated to the staff that she had no desire at all to try to make up the course credit while in the hospital. Nevertheless, her doctor assigned her to some of the classes as part of her therapeutic course when her acute symptoms were no longer evident. She turned out to be a basically intelligent girl with some background in academic subjects. When she relaxed into the noncompetitive atmosphere of school and realized that she actually knew more than a number of the other students, her classroom involvement and participation increased three-fold. She later committed herself to the course designed by the instructors to assure her of high school graduation.

The small size of the classes provides great potential for individual attention. The supportive atmosphere allows embarrassingly simplistic questions to be asked, questions which a patient would not have been able to bring himself to ask in a public school classroom for fear of ridicule. Adolescents are encouraged to take advantage of the hospital school to understand some of the basic concepts which they have pretended to know all along and without which it was impossible to comprehend new material which presupposed mastery of the former.

An interesting and effective technique which was developed in order to help patients experience some of these feelings of success is what I call the "each one teach one" class. The group of students sits in a circle and each person is asked to "teach" a subject for about 5 minutes. The subjects can be absolutely anything, but preferably something about which the rest of the group knows very little. In my experience, patients have spoken on such topics as gymnastics, horses and carpentry. The "teachers" have been astounded that the rest of the class was not only interested in what they had to say, but in reality knew next to nothing about the subject before the lesson was taught.

DEALING WITH CONFLICTUAL MATERIAL

The conflictual situations which underlie all mental illnesses must be dealt with very carefully. The how's and when's of working with this material vary drastically with each individual case. For those adolescents who have not been able to deal in a direct way with the situations which precipitated their hospitalization, academic material can serve a very useful purpose. When the teacher/therapist understands that the adolescent is indeed capable of beginning this exploration without suffering any exacerbation of his symptoms, materials which in some way relate to the inner dynamics of a particular student are carefully selected. Reading and writing projects, if selected with extreme care, can provide a smooth transition from the discussion of an objectified situation that exists only on paper, to a subtle and increasingly more personalized exploration of an adolescent's life situation. Quite often, more than one student can identify with the particular conflicts in discussion, an occurrence which lends support to the individual for whom the assignment was designed.

The following is a capsulization of one of the short stories which on numerous occasions has opened the door for patients to talk about some of the difficult areas of their lives. Following the resumé is a list of the kinds of questions which might be used to make the transition from talking about the fictional character to a more personal discussion.

Example

"The Kid Nobody Could Handle,"
by Kurt Vonnegut, Jr.

In this story, the central character, Jim Donnini, is a teenage boy whose life has been a series of unsuccessful foster home placements, each resulting in yet another rejection. He has never experienced love or stability or really any kind of warm, human interaction. Consequently, he appears in the story as a full-fledged juvenile delinquent, sporting shiny black boots (his prized possession), chains and a ballooning police record. He has recently changed homes again in the story and begins attending another new school. The music instructor of his new school, Helmholtz, who believes above all in the powers of music and love, tries valiantly to reach out to Jim, but to no avail. Jim, instead, vandalizes the music room one night and is caught, expecting anything but the response he gets from Helmholtz. The music instructor, out of despair for the miseries of humanity which could have created such destructiveness in a human being, smashes his own treasured trumpet, once played by John Philip Sousa. The final scene shows Jim playing Helmholtz' repaired trumpet in the last chair of the school's third level band.

1. What is your response to this story? What did you like or dislike?

2. Why do you think Jim was the way he was?

3. Jim was called "a bundle of scar tissue" in the story. What does that mean to you?

4. What were Jim's boots and tough clothing trying to say?

5. Everyone needs attention. How did Jim get his and what kind of attention did he get?

6. What is the difference between positive and negative attention? Describe a situation in which you might get one or the other.

Many patients have seen bits of their lives in Jim Donnini. Many hospitalized adolescents are the victims of loveless or disturbed families, or unsatisfactory foster homes. Others have spent their lives moving from one institution to another, creating, as Jim had, an array of well developed defenses in order to cope with the harshness of the world and the endless disappointments they experience. Never having been given much attention, they often resort to acting out, running away, and creating trouble as a means of getting that attention. In the context of this story, adolescents can begin to glimpse not only the qualitative but the quantitative difference between positive and negative attention. An adolescent who is used to getting negative attention, which usually comes in large and loud dosages, has a difficult time understanding that a positive stroke might consist of merely a couple of words.

The hopeful ending of this story provides food for thought and discussion also. Jim eventually drops his hostile pride and bravely grabs onto the hand that has reached out to help him. In doing that he has made a very difficult, but active, decision to try to change the direction of his life. He has begun to take responsibility for himself and his future.

REALITY TESTING

Reality testing refers to a person's ability to appropriately appraise the reality of a situation. A defect in reality testing can include such gross manifestations as auditory and visual hallucinations or merely misinterpretation of situations. The psychotherapeutic classroom provides many opportunities to help a patient restore that ego function which keeps his sense of reality congruent with that of most people. Adolescents whose reality testing is grossly defective are often not assigned to school until they seem to be able enough to cope with the large amount of external stimuli created by a room full of students.

Written materials of a factual nature provide a solid, irrefutable point of reference for students whose reality testing needs repair. If the adolescent begins to interpret material in an unrealistic way the teacher/therapist merely refers to the written words and points out any discrepancies. Newspapers, magazines and many other kinds of written materials serve this purpose well. In addition, the teachers are very careful to keep discussions on a strictly realistic plane, indicating if and when a patient exhibits loose associations or loses track of the conversation.

Other patients, though, often provide more effective reality testing than the teacher/therapist does. A confused adolescent is often reluctant to admit that his thoughts are unclear or that his statements and perceptions make no sense to other people. When confronted by authority figures, the adolescent is less likely to accept the observations as valid than when confronted by peers. Groups of patients have often displayed a profound understanding of and a genuine sympathy for the student having difficulty.

Example

A 15-year-old boy who was originally admitted to the hospital in a floridly psychotic and violently assaultive state, was enrolled in school as his acute symptoms began to sub-

side. He was asked to keep a journal and began bringing written material to class. When he read aloud, the material was not only full of violence and sex, but rambled so broadly that the teacher/therapist had to intervene at almost every sentence. The boy eventually became very defensive, suggesting that the therapist alone could not follow. The three other patients in that particular class jumped to the fore, letting the confused boy know very directly that they also found his writing very difficult to follow, and that they understood that his mental illness was causing him to be that way.

CONCLUSION

In this chapter eight of the numerous possible objectives in the psychiatric treatment of hospitalized adolescents and the way the therapeutic school can help meet those ends have been discussed. The mere existence of a well organized school with clearly stated parameters helps provide the structure which is mandatory for work with adolescents. Firm and consistent leadership by the person who is both instructor and therapist sets distinct limits. Invariably, failure-oriented behavior surfaces in the classroom and can be confronted by the teacher/therapist. The classroom also provides an arena for adolescents to experiment with new behavior patterns. Carefully selected literature frequently supplies patients with insights necessary for these behavioral changes. A group of adolescents with a common task, for example, an in-class writing assignment, with the guidance of a leader who is familiar with group process and intervention techniques, can be a perfect situation for encouraging socialization. The daily use of the psychotherapeutic journal and extensive group discussions offer a wealth of possibilities for peer interaction and the development of communication skills. The unusual makeup of a hospital class with its variety of age groups and grade levels and extensive individualized attention allow even chronically failing youngsters to experience some academic success. Dealing with conflictual material is often more easily accomplished through increasingly more personalized discussion of both poetry and prose, while more factual materials can be used in reality testing with psychotic patients.

None of this discussion is in any way mysterious; indeed, much of it may lean more toward the obvious. However, the fact that so few programs utilizing this particular modality of therapy exist indicates that many institutions which purport to treat adolescents could greatly benefit by exploring and expanding upon some of the ideas set forth here. It is my hope that readers of this text will in their own ways make attempts at implementing parts of what has proven to be a most valuable method of working with emotionally disturbed adolescents.

BIBLIOGRAPHY

Bandura, A., and Walters, R. H. *Adolescent Aggression*. New York: Ronald Press, 1959.

Erikson, E. H. *Childhood and Society*. New York: W. W. Norton and Co., Inc., 1963.

Furth, H. G. *Piaget for Teachers*. Englewood Cliffs, N. J.: Prentice-Hall, Inc., 1970.

Ginsburg, H. and Opper, S. *Piaget's Theory of Intellectual Development: An Introduction*. Englewood Cliffs, N. J.: Prentice-Hall, Inc., 1969.

Glasser, W. *Reality Therapy*. New York: Harper and Row, 1965.

Glasser, W. *Schools Without Failure*. New York: Harper and Row, 1969.

Glueck, S., and Glueck, E. *Unraveling Juvenile Delinquency*. New York: Commonwealth Fund, 1950.

Gordon, T. *P.E.T. Parent Effectiveness Training*. New York: Peter H. Wyden, Inc., 1970.

Havighurst, R. J., and Taba, H. *Adolescent Character and Personality*. New York: Wiley, 1949.

James, W. *Talks to Teachers on Psychology and to Students on Some of Life's Ideals*. New York: W. W. Norton and Co., Inc., 1958.

Mowrer, O. H. Identification: a link between learning theory and psychotherapy. In *Learning Theory and Personality Dynamics*. New York: Ronald Press, 1952, pp. 573–616.

Simon, S. B., Howe, L. W., and Kirschenbaum, H. *Values Clarification; A Handbook of Practical Strategies for Teachers and Students*. New York: Hart Publishing Co., Inc., 1972.

Smith, J. and Donald, E. P. *Child Management: A Program for Parents and Teachers*. Ann Arbor: Ann Arbor Publishers, 1970.

Stevens, J. O. *Awareness: Exploring, Experimenting, Experiencing*. New York: Bantam Books, 1972.

Vonnegut, K., Jr.: The kid nobody could handle. In *Welcome to the Monkey House*. New York: Dell Publishing Co., 1968.

Widroe, H. J. *Ego Psychology and Psychiatric Treatment Planning*. New York: Appleton-Century-Crofts, 1968.

Wright, R. *Black Boy*. New York: Harper and Row, 1945.

Chapter 6

poetry therapy

DIANA COHEN

In recent years, the trend in many psychiatric institutions has been one toward flexibility of technique and multiplicity of approach. This trend has allowed for the inclusion of many new modalities of therapy in overall treatment designs. Most mental health professionals arc at least superficially acquainted with the concepts and techniques associated with the art therapies, drawing and ceramics, music, dance and drama. Another medium, however, much less frequently used, and about which very little has been written, deserves some serious consideration—poetry therapy.

If one harkens back to high school days for a moment and recalls some of the standard definitions set forth by teachers of literature, i.e., "literature is a mirror image or reflection of human emotions, conflicts, and experiences, set down in words" one can begin to sense a parallel to the psychotherapeutic process. Literature in general, but specifically poetry combines the search for a deeper understanding of one's innermost emotional experiences with a verbal mode which the other art therapies do not supply. Poetry gives us a very special language with which to communicate the most deeply seated of human hopes, fears and needs. In addition, the nonverbal aspect of poetry, that is rhythm or meter, combines the rarely disputed advantages of music and dance therapies with immediately available words with which to discuss the sensations and experiences.

Poetry is a language, a form of communication, that is inherent in the nature of man. It is the artistic use and blending of words and sounds that are derived from human need and experience (Barron, 1974, p. 87).

The paucity of directive or suggestive writing about the use of poetry as a therapeutic medium allows us the freedom to try and to err in various contexts. It is feasible that poetry be used in individual, one-to-one psychotherapy, in groups of small to moderate size, or within the curriculum of the therapeutic classroom. Poetry may be used spontaneously or in a more structured and directive manner. The larger part of the following discussion is based on my experience in groups of adolescents and groups of mixed ages using poetry in a moderately directive way, aiming at both individual self-discovery and group process. It is difficult to plan too specifically or to predict the exact effect a particular poem will have in a given situation, but very likely, poetry chosen with a good amount of care and understanding will precipitate something of value.

Communication of the poetic mode which is syntonic with inner and primary process in elementary form is more able to penetrate the layers of sophistication and defensive structures, and reach a responsive recipient (Barron, 1974, p. 89).

What is it about the particular literary genre that causes such significant and emotionally charged responses? It has been suggested that the movement of poetry resembles the many natural rhythms of the universe: the flow of the tides and their relationship to the moon, the birth-do-death cycle which never stops, the perennial return of the seasons. Perhaps it is in part through movement that poetry can touch the deepest, most undefinable experiences of man. Some people are anxious to explore these sensations and to use poetry as a means of catharsis; others, however, fear the unraveling of what lies beneath their surface actions and thoughts. All poetic inspiration and imagination seem to spring from profound, universal emotions which provide the groundwork for the use of poetry as a therapeutic medium. Poetry which reflects the core emotions, experiences and hopes of man, becomes a perfect tool for the discussion of very personalized experiences within a group. As a session gets going and patient interaction increases, individuals observe other group members responding in similarly strong ways to the same poems. Much comfort comes from the realization that one patient is not alone in his misery; through the poems he often finds that the entire family of man has suffered similar distresses. It is very common that a patient has seen his problems as unique to himself, has felt that no one can empathize with him, and that he is therefore abnormal and sick. Through the process of ventilation that open discussion provides, the intensity of these feelings can be diminished. The interaction among patients concerning personal reactions to a certain poem creates a bond of understanding and compassion.

The language of the poetry itself, in its soothing, nonpsychiatric nature, is extremely helpful in encouraging patients to relax and interact in an open and honest fashion. Poetry provides a less direct and therefore less frightening medium for the discussion of problems than other kinds of therapy offer. As in discussing other kinds of literature, patients may first, if they like, discuss the subject through the third person of the author before beginning to get in touch with how their own lives might be applied.

Poetry is the epitome of the perfect synthesis of form and meaning; subject matter, movement and style become one. A short poem which exemplifies the totality of purpose of the poetic mode is Eve Merriam's "How to Eat a Poem." It is this quality which often produces for a patient a flash of insight that might have been more difficult coming through other modalities of therapy.

How to Eat a Poem

Don't be polite.
Bite in.
Pick it up with four fingers and lick the juice
   that may run down your chin.
It is ready and ripe now, whenever you are.

You do not need a knife or fork or spoon or
   plate or napkin, or tablecloth,

For there is no core
or stem
or pit
or seed
or skin
to throw away.

In other words, there is absolutely no waste. Every word, every pause, every beat in the rhythm contributes to the overall impact that most selections used in poetry groups have.

GENERAL RULES FOR SELECTION OF POEMS TO BE USED IN POETRY THERAPY

Almost any poem may spontaneously provoke the kinds of thoughts and discussion that become a mode of therapy in themselves. When using poetry in a group of people who meet regularly for therapeutic purposes, however, much care must go into choosing the right poems. In planning for a maximally effective session, certain rules are best adhered to for selecting poetry that will provide both stimultion and structure.

The first consideration must be, of course, the literary level of the group as a whole. Poetry can be used remarkably well with patients of all intellectual capabilities, from those with postgraduate degrees to those who have been deemed minimally retarded by school authorities. The important thing is choosing a poem which will be comprehensible to the majority of people in the group. Poetry which is complex or excessively symbolic or abstract is usually contraindicated except for occasional individuals, for whom such poems might be useful. Relatively simple verse serves the group's interests best for the most part, though, especially when many divergent abilities are represented in one group.

Poems which are developed with detail and specificity but which refer to or examine concerns of a generalized nature are the most workable. Part of the therapist's job is to choose poetry whose subject matter is particularly applicable to a few group members and will be of general interest, at least, to the rest of the group. Subject matter may naturally vary widely, but certain topics are best avoided. Poems which glorify death or suicide are very rarely constructive. Once, when a poem with the mere mention of the word "suicide" was used in a group, two or three participating patients grabbed onto the idea and remained very depressed for the entire group session. Since then, that poem and others like it have not been used for poetry therapy. Entirely pessimistic or defeatist poetry is similarly avoided; however, since many patients are quite depressed, sad poems, particularly those with hopeful or uplifting endings, often provoke strong identification and constructive discussion among group members.

Trite and cliché-ridden poetry is really no good for anyone, so the therapist searches out poems which offer new ways of looking at or dealing with life's predicaments. Unknown authors and unfamiliar lines allow patients an even greater identification with the poetic voice. If they do not know that the poet is a famous person, his words are seen as less didactic, less formidable, and more humanly applicable. This is not to say, of course, that many of the old classics are not useful, but fresh insights coming from fresh voices have a different sort of impact and appeal. Poetry which allows a good amount of space for the interpretation of meaning allows patients to try out new thoughts on others in the group; directly-to-the-point poetry, although forceful, does not stimulate the same kind of experimentation. Philosophical topics which never provide any right or wrong answers always leave a group with a lot of material to be pondered after returning to their rooms or for rehashing in groups of their own.

Certain general ideas which can be found repeatedly throughout the body of poetry available to readers of English have time and again stimulated patients in poetry therapy sessions to introspective work. Some of these which have proven to be most widely applicable in groups which I have led are: ideas about communication, styles of communication, inability to communicate effectively; reaching out to ask for help, admitting one's vulnerability and need for human contact; defense systems, masks and facades people use to protect themselves and keep other people away; relationships with peers, parents and friends; love, styles of loving, giving and receiving love; loneliness, what can be done to overcome loneliness; the difficulties involved in decision-making, making choices among alternatives; taking chances on new modes of behavior, new patterns of thought, risking the security of the old, comfortable ways; self-esteem, self-confidence and the lack of both; reasonable action versus passion-laden behavior; bottling up emotions as opposed to ventilating emotions and success and failure.

HOW A POETRY THERAPY SESSION IS RUN

Probably the greatest task of the therapist is to get patients to attend the groups. It is continually astounding to realize how many people shy away with excuses like, "I don't know anything about poetry," or "I'm not the poetic type," or "I took a poetry class once and hated it." The therapist explains that the poetry group is not a class but a discussion group where there are no right and wrong answers. Patients are assured that no prior knowledge of literature is at all necessary. As it has turned out, a patient usually needs this kind of prodding only once, for, strangely enough, those who fight hardest are almost always those who go away having learned the most.

An air of curiosity generally prevails just prior to beginning a poetry therapy group. Patients are somewhat intrigued by the idea that poetry can be used in a manner that is not boringly academic. Before beginning the session, patients are asked to relax and to clear their minds of all thoughts other than the reading of a poem. Occasionally, some easy relaxing exercises are suggested.

For example, patients might be asked to close their eyes and breathe deeply as the therapist distributes copies of the poem that has been selected for the session. When everybody has a copy in front of him, the poem is read aloud. The therapist is always very familiar with the poem and through his voice can convey whatever emphases he feels are important to the true understanding of the poet's words. Before any discussion begins, patients are encouraged to ask questions they might have about the structure or wording of the poem.

Typical opening questions after the poem has been read are, "How does this poem make you feel?" and "What is your immediate reaction to this poem?" Each member of the group is asked to respond with at least a few words to the opening question, partly to make sure that everyone is paying attention and partly to make verbal and visual connections with each patient. From there, more directive and specific questions are asked and the discussion proceeds.

Following are some examples of poetry which have been particularly effective in my experience. Questions which have been used in the discussion of these poems will be included, as will comments about the poem's effect on the group.

Example

"Directions to the Armorer"*
by Elder Olson

All right, armorer,
Make me a sword —
Not too sharp,
A bit hard to draw,

And of cardboard, preferably.
On second thought, stick
An eraser on the handle.
Somehow I always
Clobber the wrong guy.

Make me a shield with
Easy-to-change
Insignia. I'm often
A little vague
As to which side I'm on,
What battle I'm in.
And listen, make it
A trifle flimsy,
Not too hard to pierce.

* Reprinted by permission; © 1959 The New Yorker Magazine, Inc.

I'm not absolutely sure
I want to win.

Make the armor itself
As tough as possible,
But on a reverse
Principle: don't
Worry about its
Saving my hide;
Just fix it to give me
Some sort of protection —
Any sort of protection —
From a possible enemy
Inside.

1. What kind of person is speaking? What kind of problems does he seem to have?

2. Do you see yourself here?

3. What is the function of armor?

4. What kinds of "armor" do you construct for yourself and how does it protect you? From what?

5. What other kinds of "armor" do you see in this room?

6. Does your "armor" solve or create new problems for you?

"Directions to the Armorer" and the suggested questions lay the groundwork for the discussion of various kinds of defense systems employed by patients and an examination of just how effective or destructive they can be. The terminology introduced by this poem has been particularly useful with patients who tend to balk at such jargonistic phrases as "defense mechanism." Patients have been overheard talking about their coats of "armor" days after the group session in which this poem was discussed. Question 5 has proven to be very provocative in that it gives patients the go-ahead to be aggressively honest with other people in the room. Since it is often much more difficult to recognize the defenses that one employs oneself, the input from other people in the group is frequently very impressive. As good a front as a patient thinks he is putting on, its falseness is usually perceivable to anyone interacting with that patient.

Example

A very intelligent and witty 15-year-old boy was confronted through question 5 by another young student concerning his sarcasm and constant joke-making. After exploring this idea with the group, the boy admitted that his incessant witticisms were his way of keeping people from trying to get close to him, because he really did not know how to be a friend to anyone.

Some of the other defenses which have been pinpointed by patients in response to 'Directions to the Armorer" are outbursts of anger, tough language and "hard guy" fronts, silence, retreat and isolation, tears and indifference. Question 6 seeks to have patients explore the effectiveness of their defenses in a broad perspective. Frequently, they begin to see how many positive experiences their particular brand of "armor" has kept away from them in contrast to the negative ones.

Example

"The Door"*
by Miraslav Holub, translated from the Czech
by Ian Milner

Go and open the door.

Maybe outside there's
a tree, or a wood,
a garden,
or a magic city.

Go and open the door,
Maybe a dog's rummaging.
Maybe you'll see a face,
or an eye,
or the picture
of a picture.

Go
and open the door.
If there's a fog
it will clear.

Go and open the door.
Even if there's only the darkness ticking,
even if there's only the hollow wind,
even if
nothing
is there,
go and open the door.

At least
there'll be
a draft.

1. What is the tone of this poem and how does the repetition of "go and open the door" help create this tone?

* Reprinted by permission of Penguin Books, Ltd.

2. Do you expect a door always to have something behind it? Do you consider a draft "something?"

3. What sort of door is this? What kinds of doors to you see ahead of you?

4. Are you going to open them? How do you feel about opening them?

5. How do you feel about "change for the sake of change?"

Many hospitalized patients have been locked into modes of behavior which have proven time and again to be quite destructive. Often they are unaware of the patterns which their actions have assumed; or if they do see these patterns, they do not know how to break out of them. This poem suggests the possibility of change. A person has a choice about leaving himself open to new opportunities or shutting himself off from them. The insisting tone of "go and open the door" urges the reader to take that first step in a direction which ordinarily might not have even been considered. Responses to this poem can be diametrical as some patients see "doors" as a means of escape, and others see them as a means of protection.

Example

A 30-year-old woman who had been admitted after making several serious suicide gestures, apparently in response to the disintegration of her 10-year-old marriage, was greatly moved by this poem. She identified the door lying in her future as the door to a life of her own, with an identity separate from that of her husband, and fulfilling activities outside the home. During the session her feelings about opening that door changed from one of paralyzing fear to one verging on excitement at the infinite possibilities that awaited her.

Example

"A Poison Tree"*
by William Blake

I was angry with my friend;
I told my wrath, my wrath did end.
I was angry with my foe;
I told it not, my wrath did grow.

And I water'd it in fears,
Night and morning with my tears;
And I sunned it with smiles,
And with soft deceitful wiles.

And it grew both day and night,
Till it bore an apple bright;
And my foe beheld it shine;
And he knew that it was mine,

And into my garden stole
When the night had veil'd the pole;
In the morning glad I see
My foe outstretched beneath the tree.

1. What is anger? What does it feel like? What does it look like?
2. Do you see yourself here?
3. When was the last time you were angry?
4. What did you do with your anger? Do you feel as if you expressed your anger effectively?
5. Is it easy or difficult for you to show anger?
6. Is there anyone in this room for whom you are now feeling, or have recently felt anger?

The discussion of "A Poison Tree" is usually directed at one of two kinds of patients: those who get angry too often or at inappropriate times, and those who do not know how to express anger at all. Many patients, frequently the adolescents among them, have histories of not being able to control aggressive outbursts. For them, anger has often been the primary avenue through which they have dealt with the world, whether or not the anger was justified. Some of these patients in discussing this poem with other group members have come to realize the overkill effect of their outbursts, and have seemed interested in the alternative modes of behavior suggested by their peers.

Example

A 14-year-old girl was in the habit of using a diagnosis of "hyperkinesis" as an excuse for all of her inappropriate actions, including the extreme volatility of her moods. During a discussion of this poem, she was forced by the other group members to admit that she indeed liked and needed to respond with inappropriate fury in many situations because she did not know how to expose her own vulnerability and other, softer emotions. Anger had always been her defense against the more subtle and varied emotions which she was never allowed to express in her family.

Almost the reverse mechanism of the overpowering expression of anger is seen in many patients who are totally unable to express anger even when it would be objectively acceptable. This situation is often revealed in depressed patients or those who admit to carrying around a lot of guilt feelings. Both guilt and depression are said to be the effect of anger which is inappropriately introjected. Many other kinds of patients also, including those with somatic complaints, drug and alcohol problems, or histories of running away from home, have been able to identify buried or misdirected anger as at least part of the cause of their situations.

Example

A potentially very bright 14-year-old girl had dropped out of school during the preceding year, was deeply involved with drugs, heroin in particular, and freely admitted that she fully intended to continue to use drugs after she left the hospital. Her history indicated that her schizophrenic mother and ne'er-do-well father had virtually abandoned her to grow up alone, or at least without parental guidance of any sort. The extreme anger she felt toward both of her parents had never come out; her emotional state remained bland, even when purposely provoked by a therapist. As she began to discuss anger in first an objective way and then as it related to herself, she realized that she feared the omnipotence of her emotions. Her fantasies about the destructive power of her anger in part kept her from expressing it at all.

Example

"The Road Not Taken"*
by Robert Frost

Two roads diverged in a yellow wood
And sorry I could not travel both
And be one traveler, long I stood
And looked down one as far as I could
To where it bent in undergrowth.

Then took the other as just as fair
And having perhaps the better claim,
Because it was grassy and wanted wear;
Though as for that the passing there
Had worn them really about the same.

And both that morning equally lay
In leaves no step had trodden black.
Oh, I kept the first for another day!

* Reprinted by permission of Holt, Rinehart and Winston.

Yet knowing how way leads on to way,
I doubted if I should ever come back.

I shall be telling this with a sigh
Somewhere ages and ages hence:
Two roads diverged in a wood, and I—
I took the one less traveled by,
And that has made all the difference.

1. Do you have a positive or negative feeling after reading this poem?

2. Is there always a "rightness" and "wrongness" in decision-making?

3. Do you identify with the author? How?

4. What important decision-making situations do you see ahead of you?

5. Can you describe your decision-making process? Is choosing difficult for you?

The process of making decisions, not just the major kind, but everyday decisions also, virtually immobilizes some people. Many people find themselves in psychiatric institutions or prisons as a result of making very poor decisions about their lives and never having learned from their mistakes or not being able to choose at all. This Robert Frost poem has been used as an effective tool in discussing the decision-making process, how it was used in the past, and how it might be refined for use in upcoming decision-making situations.

One of the strongest emotions evoked by this poem is regret. It is easy to fantasize about what would have been if another alternative had been chosen; but rather than bemoan past mistakes, the group is asked to focus its attention on present situations about which each of the members has some control. It is important to explore the idea that choice involves loss; in choosing, one must give up something by surrendering an alternative. Once that choice is made, the unchosen alternative does not matter anymore.

Discussing this poem gives patients a chance to explore aloud upcoming decisions that each one foresees for himself and to benefit by the suggestions offered by others. Frequently, a patient realizes that he indeed has a choice about something which he had been resigned to accept before.

Example

A 15-year-old boy was asked to project into the future where he thought he would be if he were to follow each of two possible "roads" that he saw as alternatives before him. Unlike the roads in Frost's poem, the two did not "equally lay," as one asked for more discipline, less frivolity, more attention to school work, homework, and regular hours. The other included gambling, stealing, and sporadic attendance in school—a continuation of the road which had led to his repeated appearances before the courts, and in part, to his hospitalization. The alternatives and their consequences became clearer to the boy who, hopefully, will employ a similar process on his own for looking at decisions a little less near-sightedly in the future.

POETRY WRITTEN BY PATIENTS

Thus far discussion has been limited to patients using and responding to poetry written by other people. Because of the highly charged emotional atmosphere and the vast amount of psychic energy that moves incessantly throughout hospital settings, psychiatric patients frequently try their hands at writing poetry themselves. In my experience with adolescents in particular, poetry seems to be a contagiously popular medium of expression. The creativity which is tapped in the composition of poetry has been compared to the individual's drive toward growth, and indeed, some of the poetry produced and shared by hospitalized adolescents with whom I have worked has corroborated this for me.

Sometimes adolescents will write poetry which lends itself to discussion in the ways the aforementioned poems do. When this happens, with the patient's permission, his poem has been used in the poetry therapy group. The poet's identity is never divulged until after the session is over, and then, only with his approval.

Included here are two poems written by patients who have given permission for using them. Both of these pieces were used in therapy groups with at least as much success as any other poems mentioned here.

Example

"Little House of Loneliness"

Here, waiting in my little house of loneliness
Four walls and a roof enclosing emptiness
I sit on my little footstool in the corner
Waiting
    Waiting for what, I do not know

The not knowing echoes in loneliness
My soul aches with emptiness
Waiting
Only one little door to this little house of mine
One door and a window
I sit on my footstool by the window
Watching
    Many are those who pass by my little house
    Little knowing I am inside
    Looking at them through my window
    Watching
Few are those who notice my little window
For, too busy building their own little houses
They little care how I long for them to see me
Wanting
    Wanting someone to open the door
    Yearning for someone to talk to
    I sit here on my footstool
    Wanting
Fewest are you who walk up to my little house
See me watching through my little window
And knock on my door to be let in,
Waiting, for me
    I sit on my familiar little footstool
    Thinking of my comfortable little house
    While you sit patiently at my door
    Watching me
I walk slowly, with trembling fingers I open the door
You wait patiently and watch it open
Could it be, as you stand before me,
That you, are wanting me?

Example

Untitled

I put on other people
to escape from being me
from seeing me
so I can look happy
look sexy, tough,
look unafraid
look like I've got
peace of mind
everything I don't have
and wish I did
I'm not happy
not sexy, or tough
I'm afraid to look at myself
for what I really am
I have no peace of mind
just confusion and depression
Maybe I should put on me

CONCLUSION

The foregoing discussion is an elaboration of a method of using poetry as therapy which, as it developed, fit itself into the particular context in which it was operating. This method served, in my experience, to stimulate discussion, allow for ventilation, and precipitate identification among group members. The use of nonpsychiatric language helped in establishing the trust and the relaxed atmosphere which are necessary for insight and the ensuing discussion of the conflictual situations underlying emotional disorders. This particular method was used only with nonpsychotic patients, although there undoubtedly are therapists who would feel comfortable using poetry with the entire gamut of illnesses.

As was suggested earlier, poetry may be effectively used in numerous other contexts. A therapist might find that quoting a few lines of a particularly significant verse to an individual during one to one therapy will cut through all of the defensive layers which other techniques had previously been unable to do. Poetry can be used within the therapeutic community concept as a springboard for discussion involving not only patients, but staff and therapists as "human beings" as well. Regular public school classrooms, in addition to specialized therapeutic classes, might benefit greatly from exploring the use of poetry in affective education, a concept which has only recently taken root in certain progressive areas of the country.

It is my firm belief that with an understanding of the dynamics operative within an individual or a group of individuals and a familiarity with a body of poetry, therapists can select poems to be used in a most effective therapeutic manner. In addition, it is possible for patients to realize that even upon leaving the institutional setting, poetry is a tool which can provide them with insight and solace at any moment, not just within the confines of the 50-minute follow-up session.

BIBLIOGRAPHY

Barron, J. Poetry and therapeutic communication: Nature and meaning of poetry. *Psychother. Theory, Res. Pract.* 11: 87, 89, 1974.

Becker, B. Insightful verses. *Am. J. Psychoanal.* 31: 103, 1971.

Blake, W. Poison tree. In Bronowski, J. (Ed.) *William Blake, A Selection of Poems and Letters.* Baltimore: Penguin Books, 1958.

Frost, R. The road not taken. In *Poetry of Robert*

Frost. New York: Holt, Rinehart and Winston, 1969.

Holub, M. The door. In *Man in the Poetic Mode,* Vol. 5. Evanston, Ill.: McDougal, Wittell and Co., 1970.

Lawler, J. C. Poetry therapy. *Psychiatry* 35: 227–237, 1972.

Leedy, J. J. (Ed.) *Poetry Therapy.* Philadelphia: J. B. Lippincott Co., 1969.

Leedy, J. J. The value of poetry therapy. *Am. J. Psychiatry* 126: 167–168, 1970.

Lerner, A. Poetry Therapy. *Am. J. Nursing* 73: 1336, 1973.

Luber, R. F. Poetry therapy helps patients express feelings. *Hosp. Community Psychiatry* 24: 387, 1973.

Merriam, E. How to eat a poem. In *It Doesn't Always Have to Rhyme.* New York: Atheneum, 1964.

Olson, E. Directions to the armorer. In *Man in the Poetic Mode,* Vol. 5, Evanston, Ill.: McDougal, Wittell and Co., 1970.

Rothenberg, A. Poetic process and psychotherapy. *Psychiatry* 35: 238–257, 1972.

Spector, S. I. Poetry therapy. *Voices* 4: 31–40, 1969.

spiritual needs of the psychiatric patient

SR. M. MARTHA KIENING

Much has been written, especially in recent years, about the patient as a person. The emphasis on a nursing approach that not only seeks to identify patients' needs, but also to assist the patient in meeting these needs through effective nursing intervention has gradually evolved into a new pattern. A more systematic, dynamic and sophisticated use of the problem-solving approach has brought forth the Nursing Process with its heavy emphasis on the importance of assessment in reaching a valid nursing judgement and determining the most effective type of nursing intervention. It is evident, then, that an accurate assessment must take into account all of the needs of the patient. In some definitions of nursing these needs are summed up in the term, "bio-psycho-social." Although this term can be understood to include spiritual needs, it is doubtful whether this is always carried out in actual nursing practice. Other definitions of nursing do include attention to the spiritual aspects. An examination of some of the more recent literature on the nursing process gives little evidence of any particular reference to patients' spiritual needs. A number of excellent models for the collection of base line data in nursing periodicals and text books spell out particular needs, but omit assessment of spiritual or religious

needs. At the same time, "The Skilled Nursing Facilities Regulations of the Department of Health of the State of California" not only makes explicit reference to the spiritual needs of the patient, but specifically states that the weekly progress notes shall "be specific to the psychological, emotional, social, *spiritual* (italics ours) recreational needs . . . ." In order, then, to document how such needs are being met, the nurse needs a data base line that includes a clear statement of what is meant by spiritual needs as well as criteria by which she can gauge these needs. Not only must she be able to identify spiritual needs, but she must also be able to incorporate them into the nursing care plan.

The term "spiritual" is often used interchangeably or synonymously with "religious," but the terms are not the same. If they are used synonymously or interchangeably as a basis for assessment of nursing needs, some of the patient's deepest needs may be glossed over or entirely overlooked. Spiritual care implies a much broader grasp of that search for meaning that goes on within every human life and which emerges so much more insistently in the life of the person who is mentally ill.

The White House Conference on Aging refers to spiritual needs as the "deepest requirement of the self which, if met, make it possible for the person to function with a meaningful identity and purpose so that in all stages of life the person may relate to reality with hope." In its simplest concept the word "spirit" is often equated with the "breath of life," the animating principle of the physical organism. The term "spiritual" may at times be rather vaguely understood, but it can be said to encompass those needs which stem from the thinking, feeling, motivating forces which influence us in our search for meaning and our inner strivings toward those goals in life which hold the deepest values for us.

In order for the nurse then, to assess a patient's spiritual needs it is necessary that she use the same skills of listening, observing, exploring, inferring and validating as in any other part of the nursing process. The most significant means that she has at her disposal is the sensitive, purposeful use of the nurse-patient relationship. This relationship should be far more than a sterile problem-solving process if it is to reawaken hope and foster the person's forward movement toward self-actualization and independence. In the words of Sister Corita Dickenson, the nurse-patient relationsip is the ". . . purposeful use of self to help another person grow in ability to face reality and discover practical solutions to problems; it is doing for the person, physically and spiritually what he cannot do for himself, always encouraging his will to take over as soon and as completely as possible. We succeed only when the patient has found sufficient reason to do so, when he has found meaning in life, a life duty to achieve."

Beginning with the patient at the level of his spiritual awareness and of his inner strengths and weaknesses, the nurse enters into a therapeutic alliance with him. The degree to which the patient is willing to enter into this alliance is already a measure of his will to strive toward spiritual and psychological health.

Data base for spiritual assessment is derived from the same sources as the data base for accurate assessment of any aspect of the patient's life. Crucial to this process is, of course, what the patient is experiencing now. Although only the person himself can accurately state what he is experiencing at any given moment (and this may be difficult if not impossible for most patients suffering from the more severe forms of mental illness), his behavior gives clues from which the nurse can begin to make inferences and to explore with him further the meaning of his behavior.

Prescinding from the individual's reaction to his environment at any given time, a series of observations may enable the nurse to begin noticing certain themes and patterns which can form the basis for identifying those spiritual needs to be incorporated into the nursing care plan. Another important source of data is the patient's family or other key figures in his life. They may offer helpful leads as to the person's previous life style and modes of seeking and finding comfort, enjoyment and meaning in his life.

While it is true that the spiritual aspects of the person's life are woven into the psychosocial patterns, some of the more prominent spiritual needs can be singled out here and discussed in relationship to nursing assessment and nursing intervention. The first and most critical indicator of the person's spiritual well-being or lack of such well-being is the degree of hope or hopelessness expressed through his words or behavior. This is so because a spirit of hopefulness is perhaps the greatest single factor which will determine the patient's progress toward regained emotional health. Erikson has described hope as " . . . the basic ingredient of all strength without which we couldn't survive." The nurse will become more aware of the patient's assets and liabilities as the relationship progresses, but the first thing which will usually strike her is the patient's attitude toward achieving his goals in life. The apparent lack of any goals can signal a degree of helplessness that can effectively block any movement toward even the most limited therapeutic objectives. It is hope that keeps alive the desire for and the effort toward survival; hence it is a basic even a life-sustaining force.

Patients may indicate hopelessness in various ways, such as lack of any effort, either physical or intellectual, to move toward a goal or verbalizations of feelings of despair, of having given up. Statements such as, "It's no use," "Just let me die," "It won't work for me; it never does," may indicate a situational inability on the part of the patient to muster sufficient ego strength to meet even basic survival needs. At this time, the nurse will need to meet the patient at this level and to strive in some way to become an alter ego through which he can begin to work his way toward regained hope. A crucial factor here, is the nurse's awareness of her own attitude. If she tries to force the patient into better spirits by overoptimism she may do real harm as the patient will see himself as not being accepted or understood. If the nurse too sees little hope, this will be communicated to the patient and will interfere with even the most carefully planned thereapeutic program.

The nurse's attitude of hopefulness is reflected in the sensitivity and understanding shown by the warm and loving way in which she reaches out to this fellow human being in a spirit of love; the love which stems from a shared humanity and wishes him well. It is based not on the nurse's needs for accomplishment, but on the patient's deep seated need for support and acceptance. Sometimes the nurse's nurturing love can only be expressed by her availability, her willingness to be present and to listen.

The nurturing of hope does not stop, however, with this first step of listening and attempting to convey acceptance and support. Any signs of hope which the patient expresses either verbally or nonverbally are assets; they are strengths which the nurse can affirm and reinforce. By her consistent presence and her quiet refusal to participate in the patient's hopelessness, she begins to lend strength to the person whose own reserves at this time are so depleted. She does, in effect, become an expression of hope until the patient can again begin to reach out toward spiritual restoration and a renewed sense of well-being.

Although, as we have previously seen, the terms "spiritual" and "religious" are not synonymous, they are closely related and somewhat intertwined. Many people express the spiritual dimension of their lives through religious beliefs and practices; indeed it is rare to find a person whose value system is totally devoid of any link, however tenuous, with a Power higher than himself. Since the use or misuse of religious beliefs and practices may have a very important bearing on the spiritual well-being of the psychiatric patient, the nurse needs to be as informed in this area as she is in all other areas of psychiatric nursing.

Clues to spiritual needs can be picked up in various ways by the nurse who has developed an accepting, trusting relationship with the patient.

An elderly lady who sat patiently day after day in the day room of the psychiatric unit was so withdrawn as to be almost mute. She responded only briefly to direct questions and would return immediately to that quiet little world of her own. One day, a nurse heard her humming a tune to herself as she rocked gently back and forth. The nurse recognized the tune as a religious hymn and joined the patient, softly supplying the words. This incident was an opening through which channels of communication were reestablished for this patient. Sharing a familiar area in her life became the means through which she could begin to relate to the strangers and the unfamiliar surroundings in which she found herself. The nurse suddenly became another human being by whom she was accepted and understood.

Although it would seem at first sight that only a "religious" need was being met, it immediately becomes obvious that other spiritual needs were also being signalled. We might conjecture whether a desire for closeness, for understanding, for communicating her loneliness and need for comfort were not also elements of this behavior. The nurse recognized a "reaching out" on the part of the patient and used the presenting behavior as a means of responding to a human being's groping toward another person who might offer warmth and comfort.

Religion in itself has been a somewhat controversial area in psychiatry. Studies have been done and much has been written on both sides by highly respected members of the profession. Most authorities agree, however, that the borderline between healthy and unhealthy use of religion is considerably blurred. For the nurse, the criteria for judging a healthy or unhealthy use of religion must be based on its effects on the patient's level of anxiety and his behavior. Trew offers three characteristics of healthy religion, namely: 1) its " . . . capacity to help us grow in understanding and insight, 2) its ability to develop in us a deeper concern for others, and 3) the provision of some transcendental meaning, some relationship or purpose in life." The difficulty lies in the subjectivity of the religious experience which is, in itself, unique for each individual, including the nurse herself. Some broad guidelines for differentiating the more obviously pathological from the "normal" are a necessary tool in the assessment process. Particularly because of the abstract nature of some of its concepts, religion may become a vehicle for the patient's symbolic acting out of his conflicts.

One patient who made a point of "throwing out" anyone who came into his room with any sort of religious identification is an example of how unconscious conflicts about authority may be transferred and worked through in a religious context. This older man had severed connections with his religious denomination in his early adolescence because of differences with a member of the clergy. When a new chaplain who did not know of the patient's attitude came into his room, the patient told him angrily that he did not want to talk about religion or the Church or any of "that stuff." In fact, the patient told him he might as well leave. The Chaplain asked him pleasantly what he *did* want to talk about. Somewhat taken aback, the patient began to voice his anger at the Church and all religion, but in the course of the monologue, he began to speak quietly of his personal relationship with God and what this relationship meant to him. His was a deep and abiding faith and a highly personalized religion which seemed to meet his needs quite adequately. Disguised under the veil of trouble with religious figures was a lifelong conflict with authority which, needless to say, was not picked up on by the Chaplain. This area of unconscious conflict was one to be dealt with in therapy. Its real basis was not religion, but religion as a vehicle through which it could be expressed and justified for this particular patient.

The highly diversified approaches to be found in the many religions of the world can result in almost as many diverse responses and behaviors. When the behavior a person exhibits raises questions in the minds of the nursing staff, it needs to be explored with him so that false inferences do not lead to ineffective intervention.

A case in point was that of a young woman admitted with a diagnosis of depression. The nursing staff noted that she often withdrew to her room where she sat, looking off into space. Each time this happened, she was reminded that she was supposed to be out in the dayroom with the other patients. Finally, one staff member asked her why she persisted in trying to spend so much time alone in her room. The patient replied that she belonged to a religious group which meditated on the Bible teachings for 1 hour every day. She did not have her Bible with her but was meditating every day, a practice which seemed to give her comfort. The nursing staff recognized how important this was to the patient, but also saw involvement in the ward milieu as a therapeutic goal with high priority. Together, the nurse and patient developed a plan in which the patient could spend 1/2 hour daily in her room as part of the prayer program. A Bible was procured for her. An ongoing observation and assessment of the effect of this plan became a part of the nursing care plan of which evaluation and feedback were important diagnostic factors in judging the patient's progress.

Another set of criteria which may be useful as a basis for nursing assessment can be derived from whether the patient displays maturity or immaturity in his religious orientation and his use of religion. Immature religion shows itself in self-interest, self-justification and magical thinking while the person who has passed from the immature religious attitudes of childhood to the more mature religion of the adult, strives toward transcending childish impulses and desires and redirects them toward the realization of more constructive attitudes and goals.

No matter how understanding and well versed a nurse may be in the area of religion, it will always be difficult to assess her patient's "normal" or abnormal religious behavior with any degree of accuracy. When the patient is a practicing member of a specific religious denomination, consultation with a clergyman of the person's faith can be helpful in assisting the nurse in evaluating the degree to which the patient is distorting or misinterpreting basic tenets or doctrines, often in a way that is detrimental to his own self-realization and growth.

In recent years, many hospitals have instituted departments of pastoral care and of pastoral education through which members of the clergy are helped to recognize and deal with "religiosity" when it presents itself as a psychiatric symptom as well as to work therapeutically with the patient whose spiritual and religious needs can be met by a supportive relationship with a person whose religious orientation is compatible with that of the patient. A clergyman with this kind of background can be of assistance to the psychiatric team and, in many of our larger mental institutions and psychiatric units of general hospitals, is himself a qualified member of the team.

Nurses will often find themselves confronted with situations in which patients are struggling with deep-seated symptoms of mental illness which present themselves as religious ideas, conflicts or behaviors. Since these reflect basic disturbances in personality, they can be significant barometers of the person's mental and spiritual health. Field and Wilkerson refer to this psychiatric phenomenon as "religiosity" and they define it as a "morbid concern for religion which, upon investigation, reveals a basic disturbance in personality."

Important questions to be answered as part of the person's spiritual assessment might be the following: To what degree are hope or hopelessness expressed either verbally or nonverbally? What are his internal strengths and resources and how can they be supported and reaffirmed? What is the person's usual mode of meeting his spiritual needs? Does he spontaneously express any particular attitudes toward or beliefs about spiritual values or about God and His place in his life? Is he a member of any particular Church or religious sect? If so, what is his present relationship and attitude toward his Church? (He may be extremely hostile.) To what degree do his religious beliefs or spiritual values represent a source of strength or comfort? (Do they seem to heighten or reduce anxiety?) If the patient is focusing on religion in an unhealthy or morbid way, or if he seems preoccupied or obsessed with religion what purpose or ends do these behaviors seem to be serving?

Since religion is a highly personalized experience for each individual, there may be a temptation not to deal with this aspect of the patient's life. It is precisely here, however, that the nurse's understanding and judgement may be critical factors in effective intervention.

In summary, we might say that a person's spiritual needs are an important aspect of his personality and should receive as much attention as any other needs. The quality of the nurse-patient relationship is a crucial factor in assisting the patient toward spiritual as well as physical and emotional health.

Observing behavior and listening for clues about the person's beliefs and attitudes toward God and religion are important functions of the nursing process. When a patient expresses a morbid preoccupation with religion that is manifested by bizarre or destructive behavior, therapeutic intervention should be based on an attempt to deal with the underlying conflict itself rather than its surface manifestations.

Whenever feasible, religious practices, visits from key religious persons in the patient's life and expressions of spiritual values should be encouraged and supported to the extent that they appear to be helpful for the patient. Evaluation of their effectiveness must be a part of the overall nursing evaluation process. The nurse should look for signs of reduced anxiety, more appropriate behavior and increased motivation and incentive toward mental and emotional health.

BIBLIOGRAPHY

Dickenson, Sr. C. The search for spiritual meaning. Am. J. Nurs. 75: 1789–1793, 1975.

Evans, R. *Dialogue with Erik Erikson*. New York: E. P. Dutton Co., 1969.

Field, W. E., and Wilkerson, S. Religiosity as a psychiatric syndrome. *Perspect. Psychiatr. Care.* 11: 99–105, 1973.

Roberts, S. Hopelessness. In *Behavioral Concepts and the Critically Ill Patient*. Englewood Cliffs, N. J.: Prentice-Hall, Inc., 1976.

State of California. Department of Health, *Skilled Nursing Facilities Regulations*, Title 22, Division 5, Ch. 3, July 1975.

Trew, A. The religious factor in mental health. *Pastoral Psych* 22 (May) 1971.

White House Conference on Aging. *Spiritual Well-Being*, Washington, D.C., 1971.

Chapter **8**

the role of the patient activities department in psychiatric care

SUSAN PHELPS RHINEBERGER

Early in the course of a nursing student's affiliation with a psychiatric hospital or the psychiatric work of a general hospital, the student will be introduced to a department which will be identified—depending on the hospital's preference in terminology—as Patient Activities, Activities Therapy, Adjunctive Therapy or Occupational Therapy.

Entering the department for the first time, the student might observe patients working at looms or on link belts, competing at a game of chess or checkers, or perhaps participating in body movement exercises. The first impression of one who is unfamiliar with the goals and theories of activities therapy may well be that this is the game room, a place where patients go during "recess." The student may even suspect that the department's purpose is to "keep patients busy and out of the way" between sessions with psychiatrists or administrations of medication.

Such misconceptions about the role of a psychiatric hospital's patient activities department (which for convenience will be the designation used throughout this chapter) unfortunately exist even in the minds of some veteran psychotherapists and other members of the medical professions. The discerning nursing student, however,—through the course of observation and actual participation in the work of the department—soon will discover that the patient activities department is not a place for busy work, but is instead a therapeutic center responsible for important contributions to the treatment and future well-being of the patient.

The size of the patient activities department and its organizational relationship to other departments will vary from one psychiatric treatment center to another. The department may be a unit of a large state hospital, a general hospital, a private psychiatric hospital or a day treatment center. Yet, despite differences in organization and size, the goals of all patient activities departments are the same: to create in the individual patient an increased understanding of himself, and to assist in the development of skills required for functioning effectively in society.

CONCEPT OF COMMUNITY

At any given moment, therapists in the patient activities department of a psychiatric

54

hospital or psychiatric ward will be working with patients from many segments of society: men and women of various ages, adolescents of either sex, individuals who are products of varied ethnic and social backgrounds, people from every conceivable type of home and family situation. The patients will have been admitted to the hospital for treatment of varied disturbances including, among others, depression, anxiety, psychoses, character problems, drug or alcohol addiction, and organically related diseases. Some will have arrived unable to express emotions in a manner acceptable to society; others will have an impaired view of themselves; some are unable to perform the basic activities of daily living; others find themselves unable to participate in family life or a social situation.

Remarkably different though these individuals may be, they are alike in one important respect: each is a member of the community of man. Each arrived at the hospital from a "community" (which may have been as small and restricted as a family unit); each will return to a community (hopefully better able to function) after discharge.

Thus the concept of community is always kept in mind when the patient activities department develops a patient's treatment program.

There are two reasons for this emphasis on community. One is that association in a community or group provides an opportunity for the patient to interact with staff members and practice the everyday social relations which will be required of him after discharge. The second reason is that if a patient can be placed in a community or group situation—one where other patients are making demands of him and can support him in his efforts—then the patient has an opportunity to learn how to feel, think and act in a manner that will be more satisfying to himself and to society as a whole than may have been the case before his hospitalization.

CREATING A LEARNING SITUATION

Immediately after a patient is admitted to a psychiatric care facility, his history and present status are discussed at great length at a meeting which is attended not only by the psychiatrists and psychologists who will be caring for him, but also by representatives of the various departments—including patient activities—which will be concerned with his treatment.

The patient's history will be as important to the patient activities therapist as it will be to other members of the medical team. The history will provide the clues that will help the therapist later understand why the patient may, for example, become depressed or hostile while engaged in a project. Additionally, the history will be a valuable guide to selecting appropriate activities for the patient.

At that initial meeting, a treatment plan is developed. Thereafter all concerned individuals on the medical team—again including the patient activities therapist—will meet daily to discuss the patient's progress and, when necessary, modify the treatment plan.

The first task of the activities therapist is to conduct, in collaboration with the patient, an evaluation which will identify the patient's limitations and assets. This evaluation will provide basic information on such matters as the patient's ability to perform tasks, to be a productive member of a group, and to handle routine activities of daily living. The evaluation also will provide information on his work history and work plans, his recreational interests and his relationships with other human beings.

Once the evaluation has been completed, the activities therapist is in a position to design a learning situation which will meet the patient's needs—needs which may range in complexity from learning how to clean an apartment to learning how to express love.

In creating a learning situation, the therapist will keep in mind the fact that most patients in a psychiatric care facility have some degree of difficulty in facing and handling reality. The activities selected for learning therefore will consistently reinforce contact with reality.

The therapist further will remember that while a patient is in a hospital, the patient will not be functioning in his or her usual role (wage-earner, mother, homemaker). Thus the activities selected will substitute for those functions and approximate those experiences that the patient will encounter after he is discharged and returns to society.

The activities therapist also must make a determination as to whether therapy should take place on an individual one-to-one basis or in a group.

For certain patients—those who have withdrawn from society, for example—one-to-one therapy would be indicated. In general, however, therapy will be more effective if the learning situation takes place within a group or community.

For group therapy to be successful it is not necessary, as might be assumed at first thought, for all members of the group to be at approximately the same level of development as far as task or group-interaction skills are concerned. Such a theory presumes that if a patient is placed in a group where the other members are either far above or far below him in development, then the patient can not or will not function and treatment will be frustrated. Most therapists believe instead that the goals of therapy are better met when the patient participates in a group made up of individuals with varying proficiencies in task and group-interaction skills since this learning situation will more accurately approximate the society to which he will return.

No matter what the patient's level of proficiency in task or group-interaction skills may be, the activities therapist should insist that the patient's participation in a project be at the highest level the therapist believes him capable of. Whenever possible, this participation should include sharing in the process of selecting the group's activity.

There are several reasons why the therapist should insist on maximum participation and sharing in activity selection.

One reason is that in a hospital situation, where all of life's necessities are provided, patients have a tendency to regress from a position of capability to one of helplessness. To fight regression, patient activities therapists therefore firmly encourage participation in structured activities.

A second reason is that if the patient-planned activity comes to a successful conclusion, the patients rightfully can take pride in the accomplishment. And since for some patients this experience may be one of the few times in life when they have enjoyed success, they will have reason to assert themselves even more in the future. If, conversely, the activity fails, the patient will learn to analyze the reasons for the failure, take responsibility for it, and learn to deal with disappointment.

Finally, through active participation, the patient often learns that he is capable of more responsibility than he previously had thought possible.

Many psychiatric hospitals employ what can be called a "step system" to measure the progress of each patient. The heart of the step system is a clearly written statement of graded responsibilities and accompanying privileges through which the patient advances, by order of his doctor, as he successfully meets the responsibilities at each level. The step system is extremely useful in treating adolescents whose problems originated in a broken home or who lived in a situation where discipline was not stressed. For such patients, the step system—with its emphasis on both responsibility and privilege—offers, often for the first time in their lives, an opportunity to understand the consequences of their actions and to learn to realistically put causes and effects in a sequential and reasonable order.

TYPES OF TREATMENT PROGRAMS

Individual needs, abilities and interests always must be considered when a patient's activities therapy program is developed. The following paragraphs describe, in general terms, the types of programs available to the therapist. Because treatment plans and goals often change during the period of a patient's hospitalization, it may become necessary for the activities therapist to substitute or modify programs as required.

Structured Programs

These programs enable the patient to reestablish his obsessive compulsive defenses, reduce the level of his anxiety, and deal with reality. For schizophrenic patients in particular (and to a lesser degree for patients suffering from anxiety reactions) the activities generally will be repetitive with clearly defined rules and methods. An increased amount of responsibility may be given to the patient as he appears able to handle it.

Antidepressive Programs

Depressed patients require firm routines and continued encouragement to remain active. The types of activities selected initially may be limited because of suicidal tendencies. A depressed patient is usually quite angry and one of the goals of activities therapy will be to assist him in externalizing the anger he holds inside. Some antidepressive programs may include housekeeping chores to provide the patient with an opportunity to express feelings of anger or hostility. The depressed patient's program will include strenuous physical activities such as volleyball, exercise and ping-pong.

Resocialization Programs

These programs offer to patients who tend to be withdrawn, seclusive and detached an opportunity to lessen withdrawal behavior and improve their interaction with others. A primary goal will be opening up avenues of communication, and group activities will be stressed.

Projective Materials Programs

Here, the patient is presented with various media available in the patient activities department (watercolors, flowers for arranging, wood for sculpting and so on) and asked to work with them as he chooses and without suggestions or assistance from the therapists. The patient's work is given to the physician who requested the projective work for his interpretation.

Limit-Setting Programs

These programs are designed for patients who exhibit inappropriate and impulsive behavior. The hospital and its staff provide the controls which the patient is unable or unmotivated to set for himself. The staff's attitude and approach—which always must be consistent in programs of this sort—are more important than the modality selected for treatment. The staff should assume a friendly yet firm approach when dealing with patients in limit-setting programs. The patient may be allowed to participate in any activity in which he has an interest, provided he is not allowed to take over the situation. Physical activity, appropriate channeling of the leadership abilities often found in these patients and the opportunity to assume minor responsibilities are essential parts of this treatment program.

Discharge Planning Program

This program is utilized for a patient nearing discharge or for a patient who is in a day care facility. The patient's ability to follow a work routine and accept responsibility is evaluated, and a simulated work situation may be created for him. The program also assists the patient in planning for the use of free time once he is back in the community.

ACTIVITIES THERAPY DISCIPLINES

To meet the goals of treatment, modern patient activities departments employ the expertise not only of occupational and recreational therapists, but also of professionals trained in the therapeutic aspects of dance, art, drama and other fields of creative expression. The forms of therapy most generally employed today are described below.

Occupational Therapy

Occupational therapy is used to assist in the development of more satisfying relationships with others and to assist in the release and sublimation of emotional drives through self-help, manual and creative activities. Occupational therapy activities additionally provide a forum for individual expression and experience in problem solving.

While the list of activities which can be employed in occupational therapy is almost endless, the selection always must be made on the basis of the patient's abilities and needs (a depressed patient, for example, usually exhibits indecisiveness and a fear of failure; he therefore should participate in activities which follow an established pattern and which have easily recognized standards of achievement).

Occupational therapy is useful also as a tool in prevocational training. Through specific activities, it is possible to determine a patient's physical and mental capacities, assess his interests and skills, and evaluate his work habits and his ability to meet others in social situations.

Finally, occupational therapy can provide learning experiences necessary for daily living. Catatonic patients, for example, may require training in such elementary activities as brushing their teeth and otherwise caring for themselves.

Recreational Therapy

Having fun is a basic human need present in everyone. For a psychiatric patient, recreation has special importance. It provides an opportunity to participate in activities he was familiar with when well and assess his capacity for continuing to participate in them. It teaches him to use free time in a meaningful and purposeful manner. It creates a sense of self-assurance, recognition and pride. It helps overcome self-consciousness and develop self-confidence. It gives an opportunity to respond to success and failure. It provides an opportunity to emote naturally. It helps develop socialization skills.

Recreational therapy whenever possible provides an opportunity to participate in social, cultural and physical events both on the hospital grounds and in the outside community.

In selecting appropriate recreational activities for the patient, close consideratior must be given to his age, physical limitations and abilities, and to his past and expressed interests. For patients unable to participate in physically active programs, opportunities must be provided for sedentary activities such as cards, table games and puzzles.

The sk.'led therapist learns much about a patient by observing his actions and reactions during recreational activities. When a patient abruptly decides in the middle of a ping-pong game that he no longer wants to play, the therapist has an opportunity to discuss with him the reasons for his action. Did he, for example, feel threatened by the fear that he might lose? Or when the therapist observes that a patient is slamming a volleyball with unusual force, the opportunity has been created to talk with him about his feelings, to find out why he was nonverbally expressing hostility and anger.

Art Therapy

Art is a nonverbal form of communication through which a patient may project his emotional drives and feelings. Drawing, painting, ceramics and carving are among the activities used to elicit a spontaneous indication of the image the patient has of himself and his life style.

The artwork which the patient creates is often studied by his physician as an aid to diagnosis and is used to determine which therapeutic procedures the patient activities department should provide.

In art therapy, as in other therapeutic procedures utilizing the arts, patients often come together as a group and divide their time between performing the activity and then discussing the feelings prompted by the activity. For example, a patient may first paint a picture and then explain to the group why he painted what he did or what the painting makes him feel. Other members of the group are then encouraged to tell the individual why *they* thought he painted that particular picture and to tell him what his painting means to *them*.

Art therapy additionally provides the patient with an opportunity for relaxation, to develop avocational skills and (as in the situation where a group of patients might work cooperatively on the creation of a large mural) to develop skills in group interaction.

Music Therapy

Music is often used to provide a learning experience in group relationships (as when patients join together to perform in a rhythm band), to develop special interest and appreciation for presented music, and as a means of creative expression. Additionally, music can be employed to stimulate a patient's discussion of his emotions. He may, for example, be asked to explain what he was feeling while he listened to a particular piece of music.

As part of a music therapy program, minor skills on instruments such as the piano and guitar may be taught when this is desirable for the requirements of the overall treatment plan.

Body Movement and Dance Therapy

Body movement and dancing are useful techniques for helping a patient develop skills in individual and group expression and participation. It is, additionally, a method by which the patient may get in touch with his bodily sensations and develop his sense of body awareness.

When appropriate, patients should be encouraged to verbalize the feelings generated by the activity. For example, a patient may attempt to explain what he was trying to express when he moved his body in a certain way, or explain how he felt when he danced with another individual.

Poetry Therapy

Poetry therapy is a still relatively new form of therapy. Basically, the technique is used to help the patient learn to express and interpret his feelings and drives.

Since poetry so frequently expresses universal emotions, a patient engaged in a group discussion of a particular poem often will observe that others in the group responded to the poem exactly as he did and he can thus realize that his problems or feelings are not as unique as he may have thought. There may, however, be times when the poem will produce the exactly opposite effect and leave the patient feeling he is indeed alone in the world. The professional poetry therapist, through training and sensitivity, will quickly be able to note this type of reaction in an individual and use the opportunity to initiate a discussion which will help the patient understand the reasons for his feelings.

Great care must be taken in the selection of poetry to be used in this program. Poetry selected must be on an appropriate intellectual level and relate to the patient's needs and moods. Generally, poetry which dwells on death and suicide should be avoided.

In addition to reading and discussing poetry, patients are often encouraged to express their feelings by writing poetry.

Drama Therapy

Drama workshops can be utilized to act out a patient's emotional problems, or one common to the group. The goal is to help the patients better understand their own feelings and actions and those of others. Because drama therapy should assist the patient in increasing his awareness of reality, the situation being enacted should be a realistic one. Thus, the "drama" might portray a conflict which has developed between a job foreman and an employee because of the employee's refusal to follow orders.

Role playing often is employed in drama therapy. In the hypothetical drama described in the preceding paragraph, for example, the therapist might first play the role of the foreman and then, so the patient may better understand both sides of the conflict, ask the patient to play the part of the foreman. Other members of the group are encouraged to suggest alternate behavior patterns which the patient might have employed in each role.

While many forms of therapy are made available in a patient activities department, the actual selection of appropriate activities for each patient always must be based on his individual needs. For despite the emphasis which has been placed on group activity in this chapter, the truth remains that each patient is an individual and must be treated as such.

BIBLIOGRAPHY

Burgess, A. W., and Lazare, A. *Psychiatric Nursing in the Hospital and the Community*. Englewood Cliffs, N. J.: Prentice-Hall, Inc., 1976.

Corbin, H. D., and Tait, W. J. *Education for Leisure*. Englewood Cliffs, N. J.: Prentice-Hall, Inc., 1973.

Corbin, H. D. *Recreation Leadership*. Englewood Cliffs, N. J.: Prentice-Hall, Inc., 1970.

Kraus, R. G. *Recreation Today: Program Planning and Leadership*. New York: Appleton-Century-Crofts, 1966.

Lowenfeld, V., and Brittain, W. L. *Creative and Mental Growth*. New York: Macmillan, 1970.

Mosey, A. C. *Activities Therapy*. New York: Raven Press, 1973.

Robinson, L. *Psychiatric Nursing as a Human Experience*. Philadelphia: W.B. Saunders Co., 1972.

Chapter 9

the legal rights of the psychiatric patient

D. ALLAN LEVY

More than 100 years ago Dr. Isaac Ray, America's pioneer forensic psychiatrist stated the case for patient's rights very simply, "In the first place the law should put no hindrance in the way of prompt use of those instrumentalities which are regarded as most effectual in promoting the comfort and restoration of the patient. Secondly it should spare all unnecessary exposure of private troubles and all unnecessary conflict with popular prejudices; thirdly it should protect individuals from wrongful imprisonment. It would be objection enough to any legal provision that it failed to secure these objects in the completest possible manner." (Ray quoted by Quen, 1974) But despite the clarity of Dr. Ray's thesis, awareness and concern for the patient's rights had been a long time evolving and have been a long time since in maturing.

The awareness that the mentally ill were people was rather slow in developing in society. After centuries of being seen as possessed or witches, the psychiatric patient began to be an object of human interest during the age of reason. In the western world with the sole exception of Spain where the moors had preserved Roman ideas of treatment, patients from the middle ages had been kept in chains.

Philippe Pinel, generally considered the first westerner to release those chains, was thought mad himself by his contemporaries. Put in charge first of Bicetre in 1793 and of Salpetriere 2 years later, he treated his patients with kindness, opened their windows and fed them a reasonable diet (Alexander and Selesnick, 1966).

In the U.S., humane treatment during the 19th century was associated with Mrs. Dorthea Dix (Curren, 1974). Throughout Alabama she discovered intolerable conditions in the myriad of domiciles for the mentally ill. Consequent to her agitation, Alabama developed a central place of hospitalization, its first state hospital. Subsequently, because of the Wyatt decision which we shall discuss later, this fact becomes one of great irony. Despite all the gains over the past several centuries, the principal progress has been in the past 10 to 15 years. While much has been legislative, most has come about through judicial decisions. This is not entirely capricious for in many instances, it represents deliberate determination to pursue the courtroom route in the effort to bring change by litigation.

THE VOLUNTARY PATIENT

The voluntary psychiatric patient retains the same rights as any other medical patient.

As an adult he is free to come and go as he chooses. His consent to any procedures is essential and he must be fully informed; that is, he must be made aware of all possible consequences of any proposed treatment. Although it is true that in both mental and physical illness dependence and regression, not always unhealthy, often occur. It is the obligation of the professional to allow the patient the right to all decisions about his own person.

Up until the last several years, however, in most states patients could be involuntarily hospitalized if they were seriously mentally ill and in need of treatment. While these decisions were ultimately made by the court, they were usually guided by consulting physicians. Once committed, the patient's stay was indefinite until such time that the physicians in whose charge the patient was, were of the opinion that he no longer needed treatment and was free to go. In California, this situation was changed in 1967; but most states in the union continue to have commitment laws which allow patients to be sent to hospitals involuntarily for mental illness. This trend is changing. Using the Mental Health Act of 1967 of the State of California as an example of laws which are now being adopted, we find that the term commitment has been eliminated, that the court now orders certification, that this certification is for specifically limited periods of time when re-hearings are mandatory and that a patient may be hospitalized against his will only when he is a danger to others or himself or is gravely disabled as a result of mental disorder or impairment by chronic alcoholism (AB 1220, State of California, 1967, pp. 16–22).

In 1975, ruling on the Donaldson case, the Florida Supreme Court said: "The jury found that Donaldson was neither dangerous to himself nor dangerous to others. It also found that if mentally ill, Donaldson had not received treatment . . . a mere finding of mental illness cannot justify a state's locking a person up against his will and keeping him indefinitely in a simple custodial confinement. There is still no constitutional basis for confining such persons involuntarily if they are dangerous to no one and can live safely in freedom . . . nor

may the state fence in the harmlessly mental ill sorely to save its citizens from exposure to those whose ways are different. One might as well ask of the state to avoid public unease to incarcerate all who are physically unattractive or socially eccentric. Mere public intolerance or animosity cannot constitutionally justify the deprivation of a person's physical liberty." (News and Notes: Supreme, 1975) The supreme court has put its stamp of approval on involuntary hospitalization for reasons only of dangerousness to oneself or others. Specifically, the grave disability mentioned in the statutes is not alluded to but we must assume that were this ever tested the concept of grave disability would be included. Generally speaking, the term "gravely disabled" means unable to provide for personal needs of food, clothing and shelter and probably also adequate medical care. However, as must be obvious to some extent, this term is somewhat vague and at times difficult to determine. It has proven to be a knotty problem in certain situations. In an attempt to deal with this and to put the issue on a more specific and sound scientific basis, several physicians at the University of California at Irvine Medical School have attempted to develop objective criteria for the abilities to provide for one's own needs (Wilbert et al., 1976). To a great extent, however, while in most cases this determination is quite obvious, in others it remains somewhat subjective.

RIGHTS OF THE INVOLUNTARY PATIENT

During the commitment proceedings patients have the following rights among others: to have notice of the hearing, to be present at the hearing, to have an attorney represent him, to have evaluation of an independent psychiatrist. In People v. Keith, an Illinois court stated that the civilly committed had no constitutional right to a jury trial. However, once hospitalized, the involuntary patient retains his right to habeas corpus. The procedure allows anyone confined against his will to petition for an immediate hearing on the cause of that confinement (Brooks, 1974, pp. 789–806).

The basic rights of the involuntary patient are spelled out quite clearly in the Mental

Health Act of 1967 of the State of California. They are: the right to wear his own clothes and to keep or to use his own personal possessions and to keep and be allowed to spend a reasonable sum of his own money; to have access to individual storage space; to see visitors; to have access to telephones; to have access to letter writing materials (California Mental Health Act of 1967, chapter 3, article 6).

The American Hospital Association has published a bill of rights which include, "the right to considerate care; the right to have information about diagnosis, treatment and prognosis; the right to information needed to give informed consent to treatment; the right to refuse treatment to the extent permitted by law; the right to confidentiality of communications and records; the right to be advised if the hospital proposes to engage in human experimentation; the right to expect reasonable continuative care and the right to examine and receive an explanation of a bill regardless of the source of payment (*Hospital and Community Psychiatry* 25: 693, 1974).

An important right which must be carefully understood by the psychiatric nurse is the patient's right to refuse treatment. Generally speaking, in the past it had been assumed that if a patient was committed then the hospital authorities could administer whatever treatment they considered appropriate; but exceptions grew to be understood. The first of these included any sort of experimental treatment, the second was psychosurgery and the third was electric shock. It is important to recognize, however, that except as indicated below, patients have a right to refuse all treatments. One basis for this right was established in the case of Winters v. Miller, held in 1971 in New York State. The basis here was that while Mrs. Winters had been legally committed, medication which was forced upon her over her objections violated her right to religious freedom under the constitution. Mrs. Winters was a Christian Scientist (Brooks, 1974, p. 877). However, the doctrine of the patient's right to refuse treatment has spread. In fact, this position was endorsed by the American Psychiatric Association in 1975 when it stated " . . .

except in emergencies if a patient who is competent to participate in treatment decisions declines to accept treatment recommended by staff, we accept the patient's right to refuse. If the physician believes the patient is not competent to participate in treatment decisions, he should ask the court to rule on the patient's competency." (News and Notes: APA, 1975) This position has been followed recently by an opinion from the Attorney General of the State of California who was asked to rule whether a conservator (a conservator may be appointed in California for a certified patient and has the right to arrange for hospitalization, etc. for that patient) appointed under the Lanterman-Petris-Short Act could consent to all medical treatment on behalf of the conservatee. The conclusion reached by the Attorney General, which is an opinion only and not law, but certainly indicates the way that the courts have been going, was "Unless the conservatee is unable to give informed consent by reason of incompetence the conservator under the act may not consent to medical treatment on behalf of the conservatee." (Opinion of the Attorney General, State of California, cv 7Y/327, December 17, 1975) What this means is that even if a court certifies a patient as being dangerous to himself or others or gravely disabled, it does not automatically assume that that patient is incompetent and not being incompetent reserves for the patient the right to decide upon his own treatment. Both the American Psychiatric Association recommendation and the opinion of the Attorney General point to the remedy which to many may seem cumbersome and redundant but nevertheless must be considered. That is, if the hospital administration or the patient's physician feels strongly that this patient must be treated in such and such a way and he refuses them, the administration, doctor, etc., has recourse to going back to the court and initiating incompetency proceedings, which relate to the ability of the patient to make decisions on his own behalf. Without such certification of incompetency, the right to refuse treatment is reserved to the patient. This is a very important right for the psychiatric nurse to know because if she is confronted with the patient who is voluntarily or involuntarily hospitalized but *not* declared legally incompetent and who refuses medication, etc., any attempt to force such treatment is coercive and opens her for suit by the patient.

Another important right was conveyed to mental patients in November 1973. Traditionally, in state hospitals it had been customary for patients, when able, to be put on "work therapy" which means they have been assigned a job of one sort or the other. Generally speaking, they had not been paid for this work since it has been considered to be part of their therapeutic regime. This issue was brought to court, however, and in November 1973, the District Court for the District of Columbia held in the case of Souder v. Brenner that "economic reality is the test of employment and the reality is that many of the patient workers perform work for which they are in no way handicapped and from which the institution derives any consequential economic benefit the economic reality test would indicate an employment relationship rather than mere therapeutic exercise. To hold otherwise would be to make therapy the sole justification for thousands of positions, such as dishwashers, kitchen helpers, messengers and the like." The judge ruled that patients who perform this kind of work must be paid and instructed the Department of Labor to draw up regulations for such work (Safier, 1976). More than 1 year later, the Department of Labor issued regulations governing the employment of patient workers in hospitals and institutions. Basically, the major provisions were that during the initial period of relationship, a year or less, the patient must be considered to be in evaluation and training and must receive instruction for his work and pay that is commensurate with his work; but there would be no requirement for a guaranteed hourly wage. After evaluation and training he would be subject to a group minimum wage of not less than 50% of the statutory minimum wage.

There were other regulations but the thrust of these was not a patient must be paid, although he could be paid less under certain conditions than the Federal Minimum Wage. In addition, the regulation stipulated "that no part of the earnings by a patient worker at an institution can be deducted for the cost of room, board or services. However, the institution may assess or collect a reasonable cost of room, board or other services actually provided to a patient worker to the extent authorized by state law and on the same basis as it assesses and collects from nonworking patients." (News and Notes: Department, 1975) References to the right to be paid decisions refer to the previous state as one of peonage because the advocates considered the mentally ill who were working for no wage to be peons to the state.

CONFIDENTIALITY AND PRIVACY

The need for maintenance of confidentiality of records and discussed material by the nurse almost needs no comment. The principles of medical ethics of the American Psychiatric Association read, "A physician may not reveal the confidences entrusted to him in the course of medical attendance or the deficiencies he may observe in the character of patients unless he is required to do so by law or unless it becomes necessary in order to protect the welfare of the individual or of the community." (Brooks, 1974, p. 1093) This is just as applicable to nurses. The American Nurses Association in its Code for Nurses states, "The nurse safeguards the individual's right to privacy by judiciously protecting information of a confidential nature, sharing only what is relevant to his care." (American Nurses Association Code for Nurses) This right to confidentiality is generally called privilege and basically belongs to the patient who may voluntarily surrender it when he so deems it in his best interest or may lose it under certain specific conditions. These conditions are generally legally accepted in most states. When the waiving of privileges is voluntary it is always wise for the professional to ensure that the person receiving the information is an appropriate one and that the authorization for release of this information is in writing. Obviously, there are times when communication of the patient's record to other mental health professionals, psychiatrists, institutions or insurers is of value to the patient but it is essential to follow the legal requirements to protect not only the patient but the mental health professional himself.

The general exceptions to patient privilege occur either when an examination is directed by the court, when for certain reasons through the death of the patient some material must be known to settle property and other matters, when there are proceedings regarding the sanity or competence of the patient or when the patient presents a danger to himself or others, in which case, the public welfare supercedes the patient's privilege (Brooks, 1974, pp. 1089–1090). Other exceptions are for research, insurance or disability purposes.

A final area in which the patient almost always automatically waives privilege is when his mental status arises as an issue in a law suit which he brings. Generally speaking, the courts have held that the defendant then has the right to examine all pertinent records that he may use to defend himself. An interesting and well known case involving a psychiatrist's refusal to give such information arose in California in 1970 when Dr. Joseph Lifschutz refused to testify to any extent in the case of one of his patient's who had brought suit. One of Dr. Lifschutz's primary causes of concern was that the information might be harmful both to the patient and to the relationship between the patient and his therapist. As a result of the Lifschutz case some procedural changes, at least in California law, have occurred. At the present time it is possible for the psychotherapist to postpone responding fully to a subpoena for his records and to ask the court to decide upon an alternative course. Generally speaking, the courts then may direct either a list of specific questions be prepared, oral deposition, or the records themselves to be reviewed by the court which will then decide whether or not the information is germane to the defendant's case. While this, I'm sure, did not satisfy Dr. Lifschutz nor does it satisfy many psychiatrists who feel that an independent evaluation should be obtained rather than resorting to the therapist's record, it does offer greater protection to the confidentiality of the plaintiff patient than heretofore (Brooks, 1974, p. 1084).

Another interesting case involving the breach of confidentiality of patients occurred around the movie, "Titicut Follies" which was made to expose conditions deemed unsatisfactory in the Massachusetts Correctional Institution in Bridgewater, Massachusetts. The rights of the inmates and patients were to have been protected by their agreeing to be photographed. However, the court subsequently held "that Wiseman had not fulfilled his agreement to protect the privacy of the patients and that some of the 62 inmates identified as shown in the film were incompetent to understand the release. . . . " (News and Notes: Rights, 1975) In addition the court held that "releases were obtained only from 11 or 12 of the numerous inmates depicted." As a result the court granted an injunction against commercial showings of the movie. Recently, another movie, "Hurry Tomorrow" concerning institutionalized patients was filmed in California. Again, as in "Titicut Follies" the apparent motives were beneficent, but again there was a question of consent and it is my understanding that as of this writing, a suit has been filed against this movie also.

The last illustrations more than ever show the dangers in the confidentiality issues. No one would question the lack of ethics in disclosing information for mere gossip or titillation. But in many instances, the person who desires to break the privacy and confidentiality seems extremely well intentioned and on the surface there appears to be no reason for the nurse or doctor to be concerned. These good intentions may vary from collecting data for papers to statistical research for demonstrating deplorable conditions, but in all cases the privilege of privacy confidentiality is the patient's—and only he has the right to waive it.

RIGHT TO TREATMENT

Of all of the patients' rights, probably the newest concept is the right to treatment. In 1960, Dr. Morton Birnbaum published a paper in the Journal of the American Bar Association in which he expounded his thesis of a legal right to treatment for confined patients. In the same issue the editors supported him. Five years later, he repeated the argument in the Archives of General Psychiatry; this time before a psychiatric rather than a legal audience (Birnbaum, 1965, pp. 34–45).

One year later the first case involving the right to treatment, Rouse v. Cameron was heard in the Federal Court of the District of Columbia. Charles Rouse had been committed to St. Elizabeth's Hospital in Washington in 1962 after he had been found carrying a dangerous weapon but was discovered to be not guilty by reason of insanity. The original crime was a misdemeanor carrying 1 year maximum prison sentence. After 3 years of confinement, he petitioned for a release by writ of habeas corpus stating that he had not received psychiatric treatment. In this case, the court of appeal affirmed Rouse's right to treatment but they based that right on statute. Justice Bazelon stated, "the purpose of involuntary hospitalization is treatment, not punishment. After treatment, the hospital is transformed into a penitentiary where one could be held indefinitely for no convicted offense." While Judge Bazelon went on to allude to the question of constitutionality of mandatory commitment without treatment, Rouse was released because the lack of treatment in the District of Columbia violated the law (Fremouw, 1974, pp. 9–10).

However, the issue had been joined and after another case in Massachusetts, the most resounding flash occurred in the state of Alabama. Again, the issue was decided in the courts; however, unlike the Rouse decision, the case was filed as a class action suit on behalf of the residents of Bryce Hospital. The allegations were simply that the level of treatment at Bryce Hospital was totally inadequate (99 employees had been suddenly fired because of a budget reduction) and that in effect, the patients were being held against their will as if they were prisoners. Before the case went to trial, the petition was amended to include residents of another state hospital and the school for the retarded. Before the decision, Judge Johnson asked the United States Justice Department to investigate conditions at the state school (Fremouw, 1974, pp. 12–13). Then basing the right to treatment on

constitutional issues, he stated in his judgement for Wyatt, "to deprive any citizen of his or her liberty upon the altruistic theory that the confinement is for humane and therapeutic reasons and then fail to provide adequate treatment violates the very fundamentals of due process." (Stone, 1974, p. 162) Judge Johnson went farther to state that the right to treatment was constitutional. He put the State of Alabama on notice that it must release its patients or live up to standards which he would set. He then went into great detail to set standards and limits in all areas regarding hospitalization of involuntary patients.

Meanwhile, the case of Donaldson v. O'Connor had been filed in the state of Florida. This was somewhat different from previous cases in that Mr. Donaldson did not file against the state of Florida but rather specifically against the doctor who for a while had been in charge of his ward and later was superintendent of the hospital. He alleged that he had been held against his will with no treatment and specifically with no evidence of dangerousness to himself or others. He alleged that such holding was willful deprivation of his liberty and he not only sought release from the hospital, but he sought more specifically damages from the doctor who had so held him. When this case was tried, once again the court held, "Now the purpose of involuntary hospitalization is treatment and not mere custodial care or punishment if the patient is not a danger to himself or others. Without such treatment there is no justification from a constitutional standpoint for continued confinement unless you should also find that (Donaldson) was dangerous either to himself or others." (Supreme Court, 1975) The jury returned the verdict for Donaldson against O'Connor and a co-defendant and awarded the damages of $28,500.00, including $10,000.00 in punitive damages (Brooks, 1974, p. 1123). The Appellate Court reaffirmed the decision of a constitutionally based right to treatment. It pointed out, "that just because a person can live in better style and more comfortably in a state hospital it does not give the state the right to make that decision for him. It cannot in effect incarcerate him because it desires to raise the living standards of those capable of surviving safely in freedom."

When the Wyatt case went to the Circuit Court of Appeals, the Burnham case was combined with it. In the ruling the Appellate Court avoided the issue of how far courts could go in implementing the right to treatment. As we have seen, Judge Johnson went very far, however, despite the state of Alabama's protests that the district court order had invaded the province of the legislature which was reserved for the state. The Court of Appeals reaffirmed that "It is necessary to provide treatment to those who are involuntarily confined in mental hospitals by the state to make their confinement constitutional. The state may not fail to provide treatment for budgetary reasons alone." (News and Notes: Appeals, 1975)

A newer development in the right to treatment issue pertains not to the right to treatment of the involuntarily confined but rather the right to treatment of voluntary patients. Two cases which to some extent contradict each other relate to this. The first occurred in Massachusetts in 1971 and 1972 when the parents of retarded children at the Belchertown State School filed a class action suit against conditions that were "Shockingly oppressive, unsanitary, unhealthy and degrading. . . . " The court in February 1972, issued a restraining order to prohibit transfer or admission until "Adequate treatment and humane living conditions exist." Subsequently, the state of Massachusetts attempted to have the case dismissed from Federal Court because of a lack of jurisdiction. "The state contended that a constitutional right to treatment cannot be predicated upon a system of voluntary admission." Since all the residents were voluntarily institutionalized at Belchertown, the state said there was no constitutional issue. However, the court did not accept this. It denied the motion and by issuing the restraining order, it suggested the Federal Court's recognition of a right to treatment for voluntary residents of institutions for the retarded (Fremouw, 1974, pp. 16–17).

On the other hand, a few months after this case, Ricci v. Greenblatt had been initiated. This suit in New York State involving the Willowbrook State School was filed alleging something similar (Fremouw, 1974, pp. 17–18). In the Willowbrook case, Judge Judd, "Held there was no constitutional right to treatment although he did order the state to improve some of what he felt to be dangerous and harmful conditions." Previously in the above mentioned Donaldson case, Judge Wisdom similarly had held that the right to treatment was applicable only when the patient was involuntarily confined (Stone, 1974, p. 164). Other cases, however, continued to be brought to test the issue of the noncommitted patient's right to treatment. This becomes especially important in those states where great numbers of patients have been turned out of state hospitals. The proponents of the newer laws on rights to treatment feel that while those patients are no longer involuntarily confined, merely releasing them from the hospital does not relieve the state of its responsibility to mentally ill people. Whatever the arguments may be on either side of this issue one can be certain that the courts have not heard the last case in the right to treatment litigation.

CHILDREN'S RIGHTS

Children have generally been seen by the law as the property of their parents. Thus, they have had few rights of their own. Parents have admitted and extracted their children at their will and the common law rule is usually sufficient for any form of treatment imposed upon the child. Rarely did the court intervene to protect children's interests against those of their parents, a reluctance attributable to the judicial commitment to maintain family unity.

Limitations on guardians, even when state agencies, are greater a U.S. Appellate Court held, "While the parent as legal custodian of his child, may be able to restrict its child's liberty with impunity (subject of course, to child abuse legislation) it does not follow that a state has the same unfettered rights merely because legal custodian of the child. The state . . . is always subject to the limitations of the 14th amendment." (Beyer, 1975) Parents apparently are not.

Recently significant modifications in

these restrictions have been made. In 1967 the Supreme Court in the Gault decision ruled that minors had certain rights at hearings, including right to counsel. Several states have enacted laws enabling persons at age 16 to apply for voluntary admission to mental hospitals without parental consent. A court in Connecticut, a state with such legislation, held that a 17-year-old could be released on his own authority, inferring that capacity to admit implies capacity to discharge. In 1972 a Cook County Court ruled that minors over the age of 13 who had been committed voluntarily by third parties might on their own apply for a hearing for release with all the safeguards of due process.

The most serious alteration in the rights of committed juveniles was determined by a two to one decision of a federal district court in July 1975, declaring the Pennsylvania act authorizing traditional parental power of commitment unconstitutional. Five committed juveniles in the case known as Bartley v. Kremens brought a class action suit. The court not only found the act unconstitutional but "prescribed a panoply of rights that were unprecedented for juveniles admitted to mental health facilities. The court ruled that children of any age are entitled to, and the state is required to provide, a probable-cause hearing within 72 hours of hospitalization, a postcommitment hearing within 2 weeks of commitment, and counsel at all significant stages of commitment. The children also have the right to be present at all hearings, to confront and cross-examine witnesses, and to present Testimony." (Watkins and Roth, 1976) As of this writing the Commonwealth of Pennsylvania had appealed the decision to the Supreme Court and was awaiting its decision.

With emancipated minors, since the family tie is already broken, the child can generally speak for himself regarding treatment in emergencies or serious matters involving public health and welfare.

More progress for children has been made in regard to right to treatment, i.e., Ricci case above. Another circuit court ruled in another case that children were entitled not only to minimum standards of care but also to individualized treatment. In a recent Texas case, the court ordered two state institutions to be closed and instructed the governing body to make radical changes. In an enlightened statement is specified the minimal elements of a treatment program which must aid the youth in achieving the tasks of adolescence including sexual identity, developing intellectual and occupational skills, achieving independence from parental authority, developing a capacity for generally intimate relationships and finally involving a moral code for governing future actions (Kassurer, 1974, pp. 459–461).

In summary, the nurse must remember that the child almost literally belongs to the parents which may at times mean dealing with her own feelings about their decisions.

CONCLUSION

The judicial and legislative advances in patients' rights have not been without their dilemmas. Changes in public policy, fears of the economic consequences of right to treatment decisions plus increasing widening of the requirements to involuntarily hospitalize patients have resulted in a marked lowering of the state hospital populations and the concomitant return to local areas of great numbers of people who cannot totally cope with their illness nor with society's demands. In parts of California, confronted with the stringencies, of the Lanterman-Petris-Short Mental Health Act, local authorities, unable to commit the mentally ill who disturb the peace or are relatively unable to care for themselves within the communities' norms, have had to resort to jail and to the courts. This can hardly be considered an improvement over a hospital setting. Arguments against the right to treatment decisions point out that the consequence frequently is not better treatment. Part of the problem, of course, is the economic consideration, but another part is the result of lack of time to think out and prepare adequate facilities for housing, treatment, medical care, etc., locally.

Similarly the new concepts of patients' rights have produced some bizarre paradoxes in the administration of justice. In some instances, the patient who on Monday was released from the state hospital because there was insufficient justification to decide that he was not competent to care for himself, on Wednesday is found incompetent to stand trial for a felony because of the same mental illness. It seems as if the two halves of society's brain are divided and running off in totally opposite directions. A local California newspaper recently ran a comprehensive and provocative pair of articles on crimes committed by released mental patients. In addition, out of beneficent intent to give greater freedom to all people, the government continues to interfere more and more with the personal freedom of both professionals and patients.

Many of these problems at times seem unsolvable but perhaps for the mental health professional and psychiatric nurse it is important to remember that the patients' rights movement is part of a growing concern for the rights of consumers in general and represents a movement away from the 19th century principle of caveat emptor. Here again contradictorily while insisting that the patient and purchaser be treated like an adult, the government continually treats him more like a child who must be cared for.

Nevertheless it is vital to remember that patients' rights ultimately become our rights, and the legislation and judicial decisions designed to protect patients today protect us tomorrow. But it is also important to keep in mind that ultimately the law can only go so far and that patients' rights must basically be protected by the people who care for the patients. We must decide ultimately how to deal with institutions which dehumanize people and turn conscientious care givers into impersonal wardens. It is incumbent upon all of us to do what we can to rehumanize our medical delivery systems and to continually see our patients as human beings who deserve the best care possible consistent with their rights.

BIBLIOGRAPHY

Alexander, F. G., and Selesnick, S. T. *The History of Psychiatry*. New York: Harper and Row, 1966, pp. 115–117.

American Nurses Association, *Code for Nurses*. New York, 1968.

Beyer, H. The child's right to refuse mental health treatment. *Psychiatr. Annals*. 5: 83–90, 1975.

Birnbaum, M. Some comments on the right to treatment. *Arch. Gen. Psychiatry* 13: 34–45, 1965.

Brooks, A. D. *Law, Psychiatry and the Mental Health System*. Boston: Little, Brown & Co., 1974.

Curran, W. J. Legal psychiatry in the 19th century. *Psychiatr. Annals*. 4: 9, 1974.

Fremouw, W. J. A new right to treatment. *Int. J. Psychiatry Law 2(1) Spring 1974.*

Kassurer, L. B. The right to treatment and the right to refuse treatment—recent case law. Psychiatry Law 2(4), Winter 1974.

News and notes: APA endorses right to care and treatment for all patients. *Hosp. Community Psychiatry* 26: 772, 1975.

News and notes: Appeals court reaffirms right to treatment in Wyatt case ruling. *Hosp. Community Psychiatry* 26: 118, 1975.

News and notes: Department of labor issues rules governing payment of patient workers. *Hosp. Community Psychiatry* 26: 48, 1975.

News and notes: Rights to records law limits student access to psychological records. *Hosp. Community Psychiatry* 26: 321, 1975.

News and notes: Supreme court rules against involuntary custodial confinement of the nondangerous mentally ill. *Hosp. Community Psychiatry* 26: 616, 1975.

Ray, Isaac, quoted by Quen, J. M. Isaac Ray, have we learned his lessons? In Isaac Ray Symposium on Human Rights, The Law and Psychiatric Treatment. Butler Hosp., Symposium Baell Am. Acad. Psy. Law II, 3: 141, 1974.

Safier, D. Patient work under fair labor standards: The issues in perspective. *Hosp. Community Psychiatry* 27: 89–90, 1976.

Stone, A. The right to treatment and the medical establishment. In Isaac Ray Symposium on Human Rights, The Law and Psychiatric Treatment. Butler Hosp., Symposium Baell Am. Acad. Psy. Law II, 3: 162, 164, 1974.

Supreme Court of the United States. J. B. O'Connor v. K. Donaldson. *Int. J. Psychiatry Law* 3: 271, 1975.

Watkins, N. J., and Roth, B. A. Kremens v. Bartley: The case for the state. *Hosp. Community Psychiatry* 27: 707, 1976.

Wilbert, D., Jorstad, V., Loren, J. D., and Wirrer, B. Determination of grave disability. *J. Nerv. Ment. Dis.* 162: 35–39, 1976.

Chapter 10

a practical guide to involving families in inpatient psychiatric treatment programs

DANA L. CONNELL

It takes only one day's observation in a psychiatric hospital to see how many diverse responsibilities for patient care are laid at the door of the psychiatric nursing staff. Individual sessions with patients, groups, medications, nursing care planning meetings, consultations with psychiatrists and other professionals, paperwork, emergencies which disrupt everything; the list could go on and on. How can anyone suggest that nurses should also pay attention to patients' families? "There can't possibly be the time for that; besides, a nurse's job is to care for ailing individuals, not well relatives, too. The relatives can take care of themselves, or if they are really troubled, let the psychiatrist or social worker see them." These are understandable sentiments indeed. And yet, there are a number of sound reasons why family members *must* be included in the

work of nursing staff as well as other professionals on the treatment team of a high quality psychiatric treatment center. Let us break these reasons down into three areas for the sake of discussion: family needs, patient need, and staff needs.

When a patient enters a psychiatric facility his functioning is usually significantly impaired. His family typically experiences a great deal of anxiety and confusion about just what is occurring. Although the individual patient may be the one who is clearly symptomatic, admission to a psychiatric facility is most often a crisis for the entire family. The family has a jumble of anxious questions such as: "What are these changes in our relative? What caused them? Did we? Do we need to change? Will he always be different? Have we 'lost' our relative? How long will treatment take? What *is* the treatment being offered? How does this facility operate? What will be expected of us? What can we expect of the treatment team here? Can they really help us? How can we get the answers to these questions?"

Families need answers to these questions first of all in order to obtain as accurate a perception as possible of their relative's condition. Once they have some tangible information they can begin to sort out their own feelings and consider how to relate to the patient in the current crisis. As treatment progresses new questions arise about aftercare and longer term planning: "Will the patient return to his previous living and working situation, or not? If so, what changes need to be made involving the family? If not, what new plan is appropriate and available? What plan will the family support and what will they reject? Are finances a limiting issue?"

Failure to meet the family's needs for compassionate understanding in their crisis and for answers to their questions results in isolation of the family from the patient (emotionally, if not physically) and from the treatment team. Such isolation makes it difficult, and sometimes impossible, for the most caring family to develop the understanding which will help them relate to their relative in the most constructive way. When the family has a need which is significantly neglected by the treatment team, they may become so angry that they refuse to cooperate with requests later made of them. Such situations are avoidable and have no place in today's psychiatric treatment.

Upon admission to a psychiatric facility a patient may have all the same questions as his family. Generally, these are well recognized and dealt with by the nursing staff and others on the treatment team and will not be further discussed here.

The patient needs to have his family involved in his treatment program because they play such an important part in his life. For many patients, family problems figure heavily in the situation precipitating admission. In these cases, the treatment team must guard against splitting the patient and family into the "good guy" and the "bad guy" or going along with family scapegoating of any member. These are primitive psychological mechanisms. Just because pa-

tients and families use them does not mean that hospital staff members are free to do so! It is particularly tempting to see the patient as a victim of his family. It is crucial, therefore, for all team members to have a clear understanding of the reciprocal nature of family relationships and the part each individual plays in maintaining relationships as they are. This is not simply to say that everyone in a troubled family likes things as they are, but that change may be inhibited by ignorance, fear, anger, or many other factors which must be clarified. In the face of family problems it is important that whatever constructive family ties exist are nurtured during the hospitalization and that problems be carefully and impartially worked with so as to give patient and family the best possible chance to overcome their difficulties.

Sometimes immediate family problems are not central to the issues a patient is struggling with. He may have a physical condition best handled in a psychiatric center or he may be dealing with personal problems which he must resolve himself. Even in these situations, staff recognition of the importance of family support is most helpful to patients and should not be overlooked.

Failure to meet the patient's needs for his family's involvement may leave the patient without a major source of support during a life crisis. If his treatment is established to exclude his family, the patient may also be denied a major dimension of his actual treatment needs.

A treatment team's first admission task is to begin to evaluate the patient's situation in as thorough a way as possible. Many questions will be asked of the patient, and he will be observed very closely. Records from previous treatment will be perused. Appropriate medical testing will be done. It is also important at this time to gather information from family members. Sometimes patients are confused, agitated, stuporous, or otherwise unable to convey much accurate information early in their hospitalization. Family members may then have to be relied upon to provide information about recent events. Sometimes patients are quite able to tell their perception of their troubles but one finds that relatives have a vastly different perception. The first question here may not be so much, "Who is right?" and "How did there come to be such a discrepancy?" The next question then becomes, "How can we integrate the fact of this discrepant information into the patient's treatment program?"

As the evaluation progresses, staff is highly aware of the need to make a working alliance with the patient. In many cases it is as important to develop a working alliance with the family as with the patient, if treatment is to be consistent and successful. Without a strong aliance, there is little reason to hope that a family will follow through on recommendations made to them.

Finally, mental health professionals must remember that while they may be extremely important in a patient's life for a limited period of time, the patient's family will retain far greater power for a much longer time period. There is no percentage in ignoring the family. Denying this to one's self and to the patient does not equip the patient for his future reality.

If then, one accepts the premises that treatment will be more thorough, problems defined more accurately, and treatment recommendations less likely to be sabotaged if families are included in treatment programs, one is still left with the question, "Just *how* shall families be involved?" Let us break this question down into general programs including families and specific treatment modalities including families.

GENERAL PROGRAMS INCLUDING FAMILIES

Orientation

Families need orienting to the treatment center as much as do patients. The larger and more complex a center is, both physically and organizationally, the more this orientation is needed. Orientation should include explaining: the admission procedure, where the patient is housed, the treatment philosophy of the center, the daily routine of the ward, any special procedures or testing necessary for the patient's care, which staff members have particular responsibility to the patient and to the family, and whom within the professional staff the family should contact about various matters.

This orientation may be done individually or in groups, ideally both modalities are used. Individual orienting occurs naturally as families meet with various staff members for evaluation or ongoing informational contacts. Short term orientation groups are extremely useful. These groups are best led by two staff members of different disciplines, each of whom can add a different perspective from his own role in the hospital. One leader should certainly be from the psychiatric nursing staff because this discipline has the most detailed knowledge of patients' daily life in the center. In the group meetings, concrete information may be given by the staff members and corresponding questions raised by the families. This is a good opportunity to clear the air of misinformation sometimes spread through the informal "family grapevine."

Orientation groups should also be expected to be used as a forum for families to air some of their feelings about the recent hospitalization and the events leading up to it. There may be much anxiety, confusion, and anger expressed. It is supportive for many family members to know that others are sharing their own reactions and they are not completely alone with their feelings. They also learn from the adaptations other families are making. A clear example of the usefulness of such a group occurred one evening when a patient's father, who was also involved individually, said to another patient's mother, "I believe what my social workers says to me, but I believe you *more* when you say the same thing because I know you are *living* with the situation." Family members who show a real interest in exploring their relationships in some depth should be referred to other treatment modalities which will be discussed below.

Orientation has been discussed at such length because the time of admission is frequently a crisis in which people are more open to making a working alliance and to making changes in their lives than they will be after the crisis subsides.

Ongoing Family-Staff Communication

During and after orientation, staff should be available to families to discuss the patient's current condition, current treatment plan, and any long range planning which may be necessary. This is usually best done by staff members from different disciplines, each of whom has a different responsibility to the patient and family. Nursing staff may be best able to discuss the patient's daily activities and behavior, the psychiatrist has responsibility for medical information, and the social worker may have responsibility for future planning. Whoever has ultimate authority for the patient's treatment should be clearly designated and available to the family.

When talking with families, it is helpful to share information about which you have knowledge and authority. Frequently, relatives will pour out many questions and press for answers to them all by the same person. It is understandable that they do this when they are under great pressure, but in a multi-disciplinary center, they will usually receive more thorough information by talking with several people. When one's own area of competence is exhausted, the family should be assisted in contacting whomever else they need to speak to. It is unwise to attempt to discuss issues outside of one's area of expertise. This may be tempting for the moment, but will bring many more problems in faulty information than it is worth in the long run. One person should be assigned to help the family integrate the information that they are receiving from various sources. It is, of course, vital that the various disciplines closely coordinate their activities and thinking in interdisciplinary staff meetings.

Patient-Family Visits

In the interst of preventing the patient from becoming isolated from his family, regular visiting should usually be encouraged. This may range from a combination of daily therapy sessions in a high pressure crisis-oriented program to a more liveable once or twice weekly (or less) visit in a longer term setting. Staff support of these visits, on whatever schedule fits a given patient and family, is a message to both patient and family that the staff recognizes the importance of their ties. Whenever possible, visits should include sharing meals, hospital activities (playing pool, ping-pong,

using the coffee shop, etc.), recreational outings, and other activities which maintain or develop aspects of usual and constructive family life. Visits may also provide opportunities to practice certain skills which may need to be learned or sharpened in order to reenter community life, such as: shopping, using public transportation, and transacting personal business. "Working" visits to practice skills or to discuss current family problems are to be encouraged as soon as the patient and family can tolerate them. Such visits are a good way to develop a patient's readiness to leave the hospital.

Because of a patient's condition or extreme family problems, there is sometimes the impulse to bar a family from visiting. This impulse should be considered very carefully before acting upon it. Visits should almost never be denied. Imminent threat of loss of physical control is the clearest reason to prohibit a visit. Any special instructions about what is appropriate for a given visit should be given to the family prior to their seeing the patient. Occasionally, a patient or family member will decide he needs a period of time to sort out his thoughts and feelings before sitting down to talk with his relatives. This decision can certainly be honored as long as a thinking process is more in evidence than an avoidance process. When it seems that a patient is ready to discuss conflictual material, individuals becoming moderately upset or having verbal arguments are *not* reasons to terminate a visit. Upsetting issues must be dealt with, and the hospital setting is a good place to begin the work. Patients and family members may need to talk with staff members about upsetting visits to help them understand what happened and plan for a constructive follow-up visit.

Future Planning

Families should be actively included in aftercare planning for patients. Once patient needs are identified and discussed with a patient and his family, they may be able to make a very workable plan on their own. If that is not the case and professional planning is required, patients and their families should still have ample opportunity to discuss alternatives, reasons for particular plans, financial obligations, and any other questions which they may have. If visits to a new living situation are indicated, they should be planned in sufficient time for both patient and family to integrate the implications of the move.

Special Programs

Consideration should be given to the planning of special recreational activities including families from time to time. This may include holiday programs, dinners, work projects, outings, or any event that is an expression of sharing and good will among patients, families and staff.

Educational programs dealing with current treatment concepts will be appreciated by some families. Others will make good use of carefully selected reading materials which are relevant to the issues with which they or their relative are struggling.

Implementation of various programs and policies such as the ones described above will do much to earn the trust, appreciation, and cooperation of the majority of families seen.

SPECIFIC TREATMENT MODALITIES INCLUDING FAMILIES

When it is apparent that family problems are highly significant in a patient's pathology, one must consider ways to involve family members in active treatment of themselves going beyond the general involvement discussed above. There are numerous ways to do this: individual psychotherapy; couple therapy; family therapy; and a variety of treatment groups—individual, couple, and multi-family groups. Each will be briefly discussed below, but the interested reader is referred to the literature on any particular modality for an in-depth study. A comprehensive treatment program may involve several of these modalities at the same time or different ones at different times in the treatment process.

Individual Psychotherapy

This is the traditional modality of treating family members (as well as patients) and is reflected in the psychiatrist-patient, social worker-family member treatment plan in many settings. It is most useful when the individuals involved are dealing with highly personal issues or are not capable of using a conjoint modality because of such reasons as: extreme personality disorganization, lack of trust, fear, or high probability of physical assault. Particularly early in the hospitalization, the patient may need to do ego-integrative work, while the family member may be able to work on other issues.

In one case, a mother was so excessively intrusive into her daughter's treatment plan that individual sessions were scheduled. In these sessions the mother initially found relief in pouring out her very ambivalent feelings toward her child. She was then able to move on to discusss quite clearly her symbiotic tie to the 12-year-old girl. She described the separation precipitated by the hospitalization, " . . . as if I were left with a gaping wound in my side where my child was ripped from me." As she spoke she could see her need to work on seeing herself and her child as two separate people each with her own life. Her extreme separation reaction could then subside to the level of a mother missing her daughter but tolerating the separation.

Couple Treatment

Couple treatment is frequently indicated within the total treatment plan if the patient has a spouse. Severe difficulty in the functioning of one partner may be precipitated by a significant change in the relationship or may require future changes in the relationship. Couple treatment for parents may also have a place within the treatment plan of an adolescent or child if the youth is reacting to troubles within his parents' marital relationship. A part of family therapy frequently focuses on the marriage itself.

A 15-year-old boy was making no attempt to work toward being released from the hospital. He finally made it clear that he was waiting for his father and stepmother to separate so that he and his brothers could live with their father unrestricted by their stepmother and her children. Couple sessions were then planned in which the couple discussed marital problems which they had been unwilling to acknowledge to each other before. Progress was made and the couple decided to remain together. They conveyed this firmly to the youth who then began to negotiate with them the requirements for his return home.

Family Therapy

Over recent years there has been an increasing emphasis on understanding the family dynamics of a given patient and working out the relevant issues with all family members together. This modality deemphasizes the role of the identified patient as the "sick one" and asserts that the entire family must accept responsibility to change when one of its members becomes dysfunctional. This modality should be considered without regard for the age of the hospitalized patient, but it is probably most commonly used with families of adolescents who will hopefully be returning home. It is frequently used in conjunction with individual treatment for one or more family members.

An 18-year-old girl was hospitalized for a variety of antisocial behaviors. During family therapy sessions she maintained that there was nothing wrong with her and that her parents were "laying trips" on her. It gradually became clear that these "trips" were negative projections from each parent: the mother projected her conflict over safety and goodness versus danger and naughtiness onto daughter, and the father projected his conflict over conventional sociability versus artistic isolation onto the daughter. For the girl, these projections created great pressures which she dutifully acted out. As a result of family discussions about these pressures the parents were able to recognize their projections for what they were and to allow their daughter more space to act as she herself wanted. The girl's comment was, "I'm glad someone finally understands," as she went off to do the "right" things she had been resisting for several years.

Groups

Group therapy is an excellent modality for people who are able to be open enough to work on their problems in the presence of others and who can learn from the situations of others. Group support and group confrontation are two powerful aspects of this modality. Groups may be composed of unrelated individual, couples, or several families.

Family members entering some form of psychotherapy for themselves will sometimes be able to finish the necessary work during the time of the patient's hospitalization. There are other instances, however, in which the patient is discharged before his relatives are ready to terminate their own therapy. In these cases, plans must be made either for hospital-based outpatient therapy or for referrals to community resources which are equipped to provide the appropriate treatment. Such planning should be a part of the overall planning of the patient's treatment program and completes the full range of services to families of inpatients.

BIBLIOGRAPHY

Boszarmenyi-Nagy, I., and Framo, J. L. (Eds.), *Intensive Family Therapy*. New York; Hoeber Medical Division, 1965.

Haley, J. (Ed.), *Changing Families*. New York: Grune and Stratton, 1971.

Luthman, S. G., and Kirschenbaum, M. *The Dyanmic Family*. Palo Alto; Science and Behavior Books, Inc., 1974.

Satir, V. *Conjoint Family Therapy*. Palo Alto; Science and Behavior Books, Inc., 1967.

Sifneos, P. E. *Short-Term Psychotherapy and Emotional Crisis*. Cambridge, Mass.: Harvard University Press, 1972.

Chapter 11

ego-psychologically oriented art therapy

JOHN H. QUINN

Simply stated, art therapy may be defined as the use of a created image for nonverbal communication with the self or others. For example, create an image of how you feel at the moment (on this page with your finger if no materials are readily available). What are you telling yourself? Did you omit anything, add anything, "hear" anything new about yourself? As a matter of fact, did you do it?

As understood here, excepting only speech, gesture and bodily contact, art— graphic art— was man's earliest means of communication. It is an especially sensitive tool for conveying, in symbolic speech, emotions and feelings not to be imparted by words either spoken or written. Modern man, for all his technology, remains basically unchanged in body and psyche, and, for all his paraphernalia of mass media, computer and the rest of it, still finds the old, old tool of graphic art the vessel for communication of the incommunicable.

The art of the past, even back to the earliest known works, remains to this day symbolic speech. This symbolic speech continues to communicate to us part of our past, man's past. Only the artist who drew or incised or painted an ancient picture knows what the picture meant to him: the viewer of his own day or of today "reads" the picture according to his own comprehension and time. Nonetheless, the message remains meaningful, whatever the age.

Early examples of symbolic speech can be found today in Spain and Southwest France in the caves at Altamira and Penne (Tarn). The wall paintings depict—what? A "kill?" Or were they magic formulae for increasing the herd? The realism of the paintings leads one to guess the latter. In any case, after ten or fifteen thousand years, they "speak," their language is clear, universal.

Paleolithic art evolved, in ever-changing forms, each society making its statement, speaking symbolically in its art. Merlin the medieval magician, the shamans of the Mongols and of the American Indians, and other ancient healers used symbolic art to heal the body and the soul.

Nineteenth century psychology formally recognized the role of art as communication. Jung's ranging imagination saw symbolic art as superpersonal, as universal. Having a sensitive, original and positively directed mind, Jung employed a technique called "active imagination." Within the structure of "active imagination," patients are encouraged to write or paint their fantasies, any occupation found to be beneficial in itself and to lead to resolution of inner conflict. As Jung said, many of man's problems are insoluble, yet within the framework of art, reconciliation of our conflicts seems possible, once we perceive symbols for what they are and begin to understand their meaning. Since the work of Freud and Jung, artists and psychologists have gone on to develop new nonverbal therapies through the use of symbols.

Freud made us conscious of our unconscious, of its symbolic "speech," and so pointed the way to art as therapy. As early man communicated with his gods through art, so modern man learned to communicate with his unconscious through art.

It is not our purpose here to envelop "art as communication" in a mystic veil nor to heighten its aesthetic importance nor to judge its quality. Rather, our purpose here is to look at and to treat art as a usual mode of communication, as usual as speech. In other words, art may be useful in the understanding and clarification of human relationships, man to man, man to his world, and most importantly, man to himself.

LOOKING AT ART THERAPY

Painters look at and rank a painting or a drawing or a sculpture as a work of art. That judgment stands whether the creator is known to the painter or unknown, whether the creator be man, woman, child or chimpanzee, normal, bright, disturbed, neurotic or psychotic. Painters "diagnose" works of art in the painterly language of line, form, style, composition and balance.

An art therapist learns a new way of looking at a painting, a drawing, a sculpture: through the eyes and perceptions and with the tools of a therapist. The art therapist is early directed to the work Edith Kramer and Margaret Naumburg. These experienced and highly regarded therapists are both articulate and assured in their statement of the aims, techniques and results of art therapy. In a word, these two women were the 20th century "founders" of art therapy in America.

One need not read far before discovering that Kramer and Naumburg are not in agreement; in their persons and preferences they express the dichotomy within art therapy.

Basically, Kramer stresses the idea of art in itself as therapy in contrast to Naumburg, who stresses the idea of psychotherapy with art used as a tool. Kramer places a high value on the quality of artwork produced, whereas Naumburg feels the quality of the artwork to be of secondary importance, something which usually remains abortive. When Kramer talks of art contributing to the "universal message" (Jung's collective unconscious?), she places herself at a great distance from Naumburg's psychoanalytic (Freudian) point of view and from the ego-psychologically oriented point of view.

PURPOSE OF ART THERAPY

The use of art as a psychological tool may be viewed as nonverbal communication. This form of communication elicits unconscious material and facilitates bypassing of the censor. (In psychoanalytic theory, censorship is the functioning of the ego and superego in preventing dangerous impulses or desires from entering consciousness.) The versatility of art as a tool allows its use with the young or old, with the intelligent and the unintelligent, and throughout the roster of diagnosis. And it is a vehicle to initiate verbal communication from patient to therapist, patient to himself, and therapist to patient. For example:

In a small art therapy group, a 17-year-old female patient (schizophrenic, paranoid) draws a forlorn-looking face. A thick black crayon is used to execute the drawing. The mouth is indicated by a single downward stroke. The nose is tiny. The eyes are omitted.

1. *Patient to therapist* communication: This is a picture of me. I feel very happy today!" The patient communicates (a) the picture is of herself, (b) she is willing to talk about herself, (c) she is indicating that the defense mechanism of denial may be working, (d) that the omission of a body could lead to a discussion of conflictual material of a sexual nature, (e) that she may not really be happy, (f) that by not drawing the eyes there is something she refuses to look at, or that there may be some paranoid ideation, (g) *and* that she may, indeed, be happy today.

2. *Patient to self* communication: "There

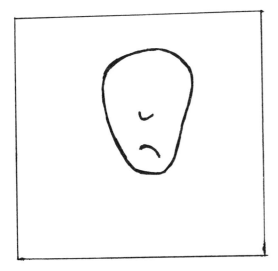

is something about me I don't like," indicated by silently altering the drawing, then by completely destroying the drawing.

3. *Therapist to patient* communication (the communication may take the form of an observation, a statement, or a question): "I notice you destroyed your drawing of yourself" or "The drawing appeared sad to me" or "What didn't you like about your drawing?"

One beginning to an art therapy session is a fast "warm-up" directive such as "Draw a scribble." The scribble makes the putting of pen or pencil to paper easier for the patient. It defuses some anxiety and helps counter resistance to drawing: the therapist may state, "You can scribble, you don't have to know how to draw." The result may be an actual scribble, usually a recognizable drawing. Whatever the result is, it always has some meaning to its creator.

Having made a drawing, the patient will usually be ready to talk about it, thus satisfying a *normal* narcissistic need. One then encourages the patient to free associate to his drawing. Through conversation with the therapist — inspired by and directed to the drawing — the patient may achieve some detachment in his appraisal of himself. With an increased detachment, follows an increase in autonomy and, perhaps, a gain in insight.

At this point, art as a vehicle for verbalization becomes important: 1) questions asked by the therapist about the artwork may reveal symbolic meaning to the patient,

2) patient-to-therapist communication often gives both of them insight, and again 3) patient-to-self "talk" may manifest itself through an additional drawing or mobilization of affect toward the original drawing. (Not infrequently a patient will complete a drawing, pause, then literally burst into tears.)

It is the nonverbal quality of art which makes it a strong therapeutic tool and a nonthreatening one to the patient. The active interpersonal relationship between patient and therapist is not forced. The patient may come early or much later to choosing to share the symbolic meaning of his artwork. Until he is ready for verbal communication, there need be none. Both patient and therapist know the artwork is a communication, thus eliminating much patient anxiety due to a feeling of not "talking." Or, stated another way, a drawing is an immediate symbolic communication.

The length of therapy depends on many factors, among them the readiness and capacity of the patient to confront himself via his artwork. With most patients, the artwork bypasses the censor and breaks through defenses of denial. The art is really there, thus it is very difficult for a patient not to acknowledge it. As patients become aware of the symbolic meanings of what they have made, they gain insight and contribute to their own psychotherapy.

A patient's artwork and accompanying verbalization regarding it should be studied chronologically. They may tell the art therapist in which direction to go in changing treatment/approach: 1) if they indicate progression from pathology to health, 2) if they give warning of regression (example: suicidal ideation).

Artworks are frequently indicative of specific mental illness, e.g., splitting of drawings of human figure indicates schizophrenia; all black and large eyes, paranoia. In general terms, form and content of artworks may differentiate organic and functional disturbances. The form (how an artwork is drawn) indicates neurological disturbances, and the content (subject matter) indicates functional disturbances. (See page 78.) Nonetheless, a series of artworks and the patient's communication about and reactions to them are prerequisites to making a diagnosis. In other words, a person's artwork is his creation and what its significance is to him is real, unknown to anyone else until its meaning is shared. Projection on the therapist's part is a trap to be avoided.

Perhaps one of the most encouraging aspects in using art therapeutically is that it aids in resolution of transference: the patient gradually substitutes a narcissistic cathexis to his art for a previous dependence on the therapist. One can actually "see" the character of the transference in the artworks. The transferences are not only projected

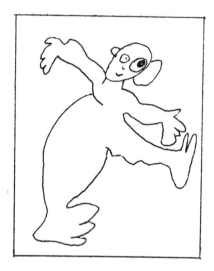

- organic -

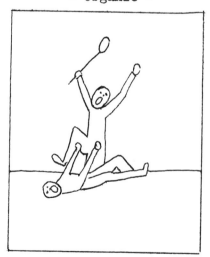

- functional -

visually, but are often expressed verbally. Moreover, the patient can have insight into the original objectification of his conflict when he is able to confront the unconscious imagery in his artworks.

MATERIALS AND SPACE

Structuring of a session and planning the physical space appropriately are both time-savers and useful tools for the art therapist. To be cognizant of the sometimes overpowering internal stimuli in psychotic patients is to appreciate the patients' need for a structured environment. If one works with psychotic patients, space planning is especially essential: boundaries need to be imposed with as little external stimuli as possible, e.g., clear walls, clean paper on tables, evenly spaced chairs, and little noise or interruption.

The materials used by art therapist are flexible and, depending on how they are used, will make for a structured or less structured atmosphere.

Structured materials are especially to be recommended for: 1) early sessions with a new group, 2) when a new member is added to the group, 3) in therapy with a "loose" patient or patients. The structured quality of the material is in itself stable and lends itself to more ready control than does unstructured material. In other words, being itself defined in shape and size and dimension, structured material is less intrinsically stimulating to the unaccustomed patient.

A sound general rule in therapy is to use only structured materials with psychotic patients, with an important exception, noted below.

And a second sound general rule with all patients is to introduce unstructured materials only after *basic trust*, i.e., a good therapeutic relationship with acceptance of firm guidance from the therapist, has been established.

Unstructured materials include oil paints, water color paints, tempera, papier mâché and wet clay, the "loose" materials. By its form, unstructured material demands that the patient control it. Working in one or another of these loose materials is stimulating to any user, and to a patient tends to: 1) "break up" (or "down") inhibitions, 2) encourage the venting of feelings, 3) induce regression and 4) "unrigidify" obsessive-compulsive behavior of the neurotic personality. Successful handling of these "loose" materials requires considerable immediate impulse control, and tends to help the patient "learn" impulse control in other situations and activities.

The important exception to the use of unstructured materials with the psychotic is with those who are paranoid. Patients diagnosed as paranoid do very well indeed with, for example, wet clay. Why? A paranoid patient has, to be sure, a reality testing defect; but he has as well a strong synthetic ego function, which concentrates its great energy on creating delusional systems. This energy, turned to the creative manipulation of wet clay, becomes a powerful tool for sublimation — one might almost say, absorption of the delusional creation — within the reality of three-dimensional and malleable clay.

TECHNIQUES TO INCREASE OR DECREASE STRUCTURE

To give structure to an art therapy session without appearing to be authoritarian or threatening is the platform on which a lasting therapeutic alliance stands, whether with a single patient or with a group. Each art therapist builds his own platform, but there are four "basics."

1. Set a time limit of $1\frac{1}{2}$ hours. Tell the patients at the beginning of the session that it will end in $1\frac{1}{2}$ hours and name the ending time. This eliminates questions and dissatisfaction that the session should be so long or disappointment that it cannot go on longer.

2. Limit or expand the space of the working area to correlate confortably with the number of patients in the group. A large empty expanse (even of white paper or other blank material) can be frightening.

3. Limit the project as to number of colors and/or as to material to be used. There will then not be the distress and confusion of infinite choice. (Even limited choice may be distressing to a disturbed person.)

4. *Be consistent, yet understanding and flexible.*

After a successful therapeutic alliance has

been formed and after the patient has experienced and internalized the "expectations and structure" of the boundaries of an art therapy session, structure may be slackened. In other words, rigid structure is contraindicated when the patient feels safe enough to explore the infinite possibilities of forms, shapes, symbols, etc. that are available within the media used and from his own unconscious.

WHAT IS EGO PSYCHOLOGY

Ego psychology theory represents a shift within the psychoanalytic framework from a drive-oriented to an ego-oriented psychology.

To quote Widroe, "After 1923, when Freud introduced his structural hypothesis dividing the psyche into the id (the mechanism for generation and storage of drive energy), the ego (the apparatus responsible for modification and control of drive energy), and the superego, certain psychoanalytic theorists began to direct their attention away from the problems of drive discharge and more toward the problems of drive modification. Intrapsychic conflict was discussed less in terms of undischarged drive energy and more in terms of a poorly adjusted or inadequately developed control mechanism. The functions of the ego were viewed less as 'resistances' to drive energy discharge and more as potentially successful harmonizing agents, seeking maximal gratification for the entire organism within the limits imposed by the environment."

And, "the major difference" (between a drive-oriented and an ego-oriented psychology) "is that the proponent of ego psychology, by concentrating on the ego as the main structure of possible therapeutic change, will tend to differentiate ego functions more explicitly and hence considerably broaden his therapeutic approach."

WHY EGO PSYCHOLOGY AND ART THERAPY "FIT"

The ego is supported in art therapy by encouraging secondary process over primary process thinking, i.e., by supplying external controls. The nine ego functions are described here individually for clarity in discussion, although in fact each ego function blends into and affects every other. For example, a gross defect in any one of the nine ego functions interferes with the others and may block encouragement of autonomy in the patient.

The ego functions are herein listed with a description of how each receives support through a patient's participation in the experience of using art self-exploratorily.

REALITY TESTING

Art therapy is used to help a patient with defective reality testing to change visually his point of view: *to help him to see what is really there.* For example, three blocks of wood—one square, one round, and one triangular—are placed on a table (otherwise empty and bare). The directive is, "Draw what is on the table." Once the drawing is made, the patient may talk about the objects drawn and the drawing itself, which allows for reality testing. If this is successful—if he draws the objects actually on the table—he may be given further directives, such as to draw other single objects in the room: single, but unset-off as are the blocks. Thus, the patient may begin correction of faulty visual reality.

SELF-OBSERVING EGO FUNCTION

Self-observation is an inevitable aspect of making a work of art insofar as the patient watches his artwork take shape and form under his own hands. To this extent, he looks at himself, and makes observations based on the drawn images of his own action, thoughts and feelings.

If in the therapist's judgment it will not be too threatening an act, the patient will be asked to draw a self-portrait. When this is done, self-observation is carried to a point well beyond the earlier drawing.

The directive in a group may be, "Connect a line from your drawing to another's on the table." Having done this, most patients then go on to compare their drawn line to one or more other patient's drawn lines, thus releasing further self-observation.

AUTONOMY

A work of art is an original expression. A patient, like any other artist, feels a narcis-sistic urge to talk about his accomplishment—a healthy autonomous act. Patients are regularly asked to sign each completed work: thus it becomes more autonomously "mine." And the fact of completion itself is autonomy-building. A cycle (start-change-stop) has this autonomy-building factor even if the cycle consists only in drawing a single line (pen or paper-create line-pen off paper).

OBJECT-RELATIONSHIP

Creating a drawing or a painting allows the patient to expand beyond himself: he "owns" his own work. This is further reinforced when he signs his work.

If the therapist judges the patient's anxiety level to permit it, he directs the patients to "Draw the group." When the patient can do this, he is in fact acknowledging other group members as "real," as objects within his ken of reality. And the therapist himself picks up important clues.

IMPULSE CONTROL

Impulse control is nurtured through starting the drawing or painting or sculpture, working on it, not destroying it, and completing it. Impulse control is especially encouraged when an unstructured material such as wet clay is used. With sublimation art leads to "healthier" defenses, thus greater impulse control.

THOUGHT PROCESS

Understanding and following the directive, then talking about the finished piece, allow opportunity for the patient both to listen to logical speech sequence and to respond. Also, repetition of symbols—unless it be of a perseverating nature—offers "visual sequences."

SYNTHETIC EGO FUNCTION

This ego function is aided by regularity of the scheduled art therapy sessions; the patient knows the day of the week, the hour, and the place. Often, the material is re-used with patients who have a defective synthetic ego function, adding to the continuity they associate with the art therapy sessions.

In drawing or painting or sculpting, emphasis is placed on breaking down the subject matter into shapes and putting it back together. For example, the directive, "Draw something remembered by connecting one line to another line until you have your image," may elicit a bizarre drawing of a house. The house is redrawn in individual shapes, e.g., the foundation, the walls, the roof, etc. Next, the house is properly "rebuilt," in a sense; a whole and realistic image of the patient's remembered house is created both on paper and in his mind—all in an ordered and organized fashion.

DEFENSE MECHANISMS

With creating a work of art, defense mechanisms may be broken through without trauma to the psyche; the art provides the "searcher" and uses external controls. The media covers the id material.

CONSCIOUSNESS

Creating art allows for this ego function to protect the ego by focusing attention on acceptable objects—in this case, the objects being nonthreatening, self-created images. One may often observe a patient with a "groggy" affect literally "brighten up" while concentrating on his work.

MODIFICATION OF DRIVE ENERGY

Drive energy may be modified using art as the vehicle; it takes the form of sublimation. Basically, sublimation through art comprises four stages: 1) a displacement process, 2) delayed gratification, 3) catharsis and 4) a socially accepted manner of expression. Ernst Kris, discussing the value of spontaneous art, states, " . . . the regressive behavior can be meaningfully channelized, the onslaught of the id loses some of its boundless potential since control tends to be recaptured by the ego, a recapture which takes place in the shaping of the material." In other words, with the "channelizing" (displacement and delayed gratification), the id loses some of its potential (catharsis) and the ego recaptures the control (sublimation) which takes place during creation and completion of a work of art.

An *example of sublimation* would be a young female patient putting into aesthetic form—a beautiful bowl of flowers—what had begun as a crude release of aggression—a "shit head"—against her mother. The girl displaced her aggression against her mother onto the clay, received delayed gratification in so doing, and experienced exhilaration both expressed and shown nonverbally while working on the sculpture, indicating catharsis. And a beautiful bowl of clay flowers is socially acceptable as a form of expression.

To illustrate the use of ego-psychologically oriented art therapy the "art work" of Donna, an anorexic, is presented.

BODY IMAGE, IDENTITY AND AUTONOMY

Given the thesis that for lasting therapeutic gains anorexics need first to alter misperceptions and misconceptions of body image, the following two art therapy sessions with anorexic patient Donna are discussed: 1) a body image-oriented session and 2) an identity-oriented session. In both sessions, the faulty ego functions of reality testing, self-observing ego, autonomy, and object relations are investigated through Donna's drawings.

The question, *"What is body image?"* has been defined and re-defined, yet its meaning remains elusive. The Oxford English Dictionary (1964) describes *body* as "the physical or material frame of man or of any animal; the whole material organism;" for *image*, "an artificial imitation or representation of the external form of any object, especially of a person." (Like a mirror image.) Body image is a feeling or a visual form we create "in our mind's eye" of bodies: 1) how our body appears to us, 2) how we perceive others as viewing our body, and 3) how we perceive others' bodies. This three-fold concept helps to uncover the patient's attitude to his own body, how he experiences and perceives it. It also suggests clues to his ego, e.g., deformed or intact reality testing, self-observing ego functions, autonomy, etc.

How do anorexics perceive their body image? Using massive denial, an anorexic may feel his body as magical, capable of many feats, even as indestructible and in need of no nourishment to survive. The body appears "normal" even when in an extremely emaciated state. Often, ownership of the body is denied.

How and why is art therapy useful in treating anorexics? The person who draws a person, an object, cannot use denial of the drawn image (it does not disappear); it is difficult not to accept ownership of a drawn image. Drawing an image is a way for an anorexic to differentiate himself from his environment and to affect it rather than to be affected by it. The drawing helps the patient see more clearly a changing concept of what is really drawn, of what is really there. The drawn body image also promotes a synthesis of body image and promotes secondary process from primary process by giving external controls (uses art to cover id material and to build tolerance to frustration).

A drawing is immediate symbolic communication without need for speech. But, once drawn, the patient then feels the need to verbalize the significance of his drawing, this need catering helpfully to the anorexic's narcissism.

The drawn body image becomes a "healthier" defense through allowing sublimation: displacement (onto art), delayed gratification, catharsis, and a socially accepted means of expression, in this case a work of art.

In looking at the drawings elicited by the two-part body image/identity directive, it is well to remember Bruch's comments on the study of body image: "The deviant body size itself is related to or even the result of disturbances in hunger awareness, or of *other bodily sensations.*" (Italics mine.) Bruch includes in the study of the body image: 1) correctness or error in cognitive awareness of the bodily self, 2) accuracy in recognizing stimuli coming from without or within, 3) sense of control over one's own bodily functions, 4) affective reaction to the reality of the body configuration and 5) one's·rating of the desirability of one's body by others. For the anorexic, all of these points are defective.

BODY IMAGE-ORIENTED ART THERAPY DIRECTIVE

The patient, Donna, was handed nine sheets of paper (eight, 8½ x 11, and one, 16 x 16). The directive was two-part in order: 1) "Draw a body part on each of the eight smaller sheets of paper. Plant it so that every part of the body has been drawn before you run out of paper." 2) "On the large sheet of paper, draw a complete person." After each drawing was done, there followed a discussion of it.

Drawing #1: *A head:* "A head is for thinking; it looks empty; my head feels empty."

Drawing #2: *Eyes:* "Eyes are for seeing; sneaky eyes to watch for what people do behind my back; for getting irritated."

Drawing #3: *A nose:* "A nose is for smelling, for bumping into things with."

Drawing #4: *A mouth:* "A mouth is for smiling, for talking, for kissing."

Drawing #5: *An arm:* "It is my right arm; for doing things with."

Drawing #6: *A torso:* "A torso is for feeling."

Drawing #7: *Legs:* "Legs are for walking."

Drawing #8: left blank: "I've done all the parts."

The obvious omissions are Donna's left arm, her ears, breasts, and the genital area. (Note that 'eating' for the mouth and 'standing' for the legs were not mentioned.)

Of the omitted breasts, Donna stated, "Why does it have to be a girl, or be me?" When the omitted ears were discussed, Donna said, "I guess I don't want to hear something." *For the omitted left arm, Donna's response was "I really didn't draw my left arm, did I?" and "I wonder why I'm detached from it."* When questioned whether her arm was detached from her or she was detached from the arm, Donna silently began tapping her left arm with the pen she had been using for the drawing. As the intensity and frequency of her hitting her left arm increased, she was asked, "Why are you hitting your left arm?" Donna stated, "I don't know . . . maybe I used it to block blows when my mother hit me . . . or maybe I hit her with my left arm."

For the second part of Directive 1, Donna drew a figure from the head to the feet. (See page 00, Drawing A.) In this figure drawing (which Donna said was of herself) there are the following differences from drawings of the first part of the directive. The ears are included and the sneaky eyes are omitted; "If I listen then I guess I stop looking," said Donna. The mouth is closed; hair, breasts, clothes, and the left arm are added. Of special note in the figure-drawing are the line quality, the inclusion of all parts, and *the grotesquely attached left arm.* After Donna had drawn the head and neck with solid single lines, she drew in the left arm, and from there down in the drawing the line quality fragments, indicating anxiety and lack of consequent control. The deterioration of the lower three-fourths of the drawing was commented on by Donna and she was asked where the lines started getting "shaky" (her word). At this point Donna said, "I wonder if I'll ever know what's wrong with my left arm," and was ready to end the session, as she was visibly shaken.

In addition, in Donna's "composite" drawing of the directive, "Draw a body part on each of the eight smaller sheets of paper. Plan it so that every part of the body has been drawn before you run out of paper," we see some interesting results in comparison to her "total" drawing.

The "composite" drawing indicated psychotic ideation of a paranoid flavor. The censor—due to the nature of the art therapy directive—was bypassed, as were the defense mechanisms. In one sense, unconscious material was dramatically increased due to a diminishing of a strong synthetic ego function (each body part not allowed to be drawn one after another on one page).

IDENTITY-ORIENTED ART THERAPY DIRECTIVE

In the following session, identity-oriented directives were given. Upon arriving for the session, Donna immediately began telling of a verbal fight she had had with her husband, which, upon his leaving, had ended with her saying, "You are telling me how *I* should feel . . . . If I want to feel sad, I'll feel sad!"

The directive was, "Drawn a similar incident in your life" (Similar to the argument with her husband). In her drawing, Donna portrayed herself striking her mother on the head. Donna immediately said of the drawing, "Now my mother has the large left arm." After the next drawing, of "How

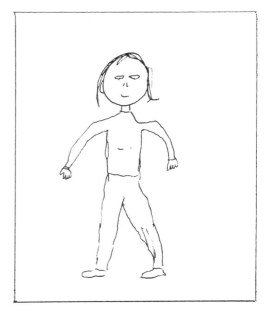

Drawing A: "a complete person—me."

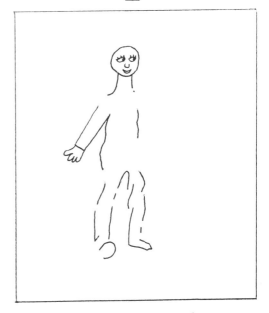

Drawing B: composite of 8-part drawing of a person

close you feel to your husband, your father, your mother, to any other specific person, and to yourself," Donna completed the directive three times, each time stating, "I don't know where to put my mother, or me," yet she put herself and her mother on the same place on the line and said, "We're in the same space."

Donna became anxious at this point. She drew herself as a small girl and said, "I drew myself as a little girl." The next directive, "On a sheet of paper, draw yourself as large and your mother as a little girl," Donna was utterly unable to draw, even to attempt this. She said, "I can't do that. I can't bear drawing both of us in the same space."

The next drawing was at the frustration level Donna could confront. It was, "Draw yourself as a large line and draw your mother as a small line." She drew the two lines, saying, "That's me (the small line) underneath my mother," i.e., she had graphically communicated to herself her confusion as to whether she is herself or her mother. Of this, Donna said, "That was a slip."

The next drawing was a repeat of the previous directive, "Draw yourself and your mother." Donna smiled after completing this drawing and said, "I really need the barrier between us!" (It had a large line between the figures.)

Her last drawing of the session represented "the two paths I have." When asked if she could label each path, Donna said, "No, I never though of that . . . traveling, I suppose." Looking over the series of drawings, Donna said, "Maybe each path is an identity and I have a choice."

DISCUSSION OF BODY IMAGE AND IDENTITY-ORIENTED DIRECTIVES AND DRAWINGS

Bruch states that the sense of fullness the anorexic feels after eating a small amount is a "phantom phenomenon, a projection of memories of formerly experienced sensations."

To go further, it would appear that persons diagnosed as having anorexia nervosa, primary, have psychologically regressed — over a lifetime — back into the womb, as if unborn. This leads to their lack of body image and the feeling that they do not need to eat to survive since — unconsciously — they are being nourished by their mothers. And further, that the defense mechanism

of identification with the aggressor results in an almost total symbiosis with the mother, leading to — unconsciously — their feeding themselves by way of the umbilical cord. In other words, they are their mothers and they are also inside of themselves, connected with the nourishing cord. (Forced feeding, with a tube, is frequently observed to be pleasurable for anorexics and is, possibly, a secondary oral [feeding] gratification.)

The body awareness technique (of the preceding directive) was used to reality test, piece by piece, Donna's body and to aid her in acquiring ownership of it. When Donna asked, "Why am I detached from my left arm?" rather than asking, "Why is it detached from me?", and when Donna projected her bizarre left arm onto her mother, one could exchange the word *arm* for *mother*, and have her ask, "Why am I detached from my mother?"

Donna's anxiety increased as she confronted the reality of owning a body. Her drawings indicate her growth through their imagery, i.e., amorphous images, little girl figure, and teenage or young woman figures. She is realizing she has a body and it is not her mother's.

Donna' decision not to eat in order to feel better about herself tells us of (indeed, shows us) her deep inner dissatisfaction. Perhaps the inner dissatisfaction may have come from Donna's life situation, her lack of proper body concept, and little self-identity other than through identification.

Donna ended a particular session by saying, "I don't know who I am, but at least I know I'm not my mother!"

Three drawings of Donna were completed in an art therapy group consisting of Donna and two other female patients.

The first warm-up directive, "Draw the first thing that occurs to you," elicited a drawing that Donna called "traveling." It was of a car "stuck" on a "bumped" road. Although Donna called this drawing "traveling," one saw the car in the drawing as being "stuck," a fact pointed out by the other group members. Donna agreed and said she herself felt "stuck" in life, returning to her belief that she reacted to the entire world and wasn't capable of acting upon it.

The directive for the next drawing was, "Draw yourself as you see yourself now and draw yourself as you *want to be*."

In discussing these drawings, Donna both realized and expressed that the figure on the left looked like "a little baby in bed with a large ball on the bed." The figure on the right was "free," she said, and looked older, "about the teenage years." This graphic presentation of Donna's self-image and her wish for a future teenage self-image again dramatizes her faulty reality testing. It displays, also, her wish to be "free," to gain autonomy, to grow, albeit only to the teen years.

The similar stance of the two figures indicates a growing sense of self-esteem in that the "wish figure"—on a solid base line—is an enlarged version of the baby figure: the wish to grow, yet remain intrinsically the same individual.

The next drawing of Donna's was called, "As young as I can be." It had an umbilical cord-like line directed toward the baby's mouth.

The other group members commented on the "umbilical cord" and, at first, Donna denied it, saying it could be a blanket. Moments later, Donna said embarrassedly, "It might be an umbilical cord." This led

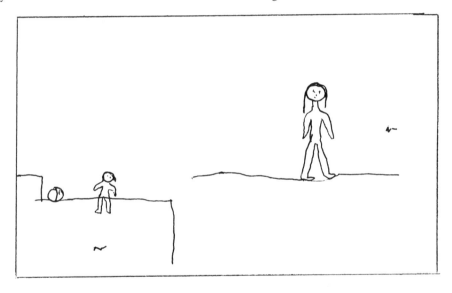

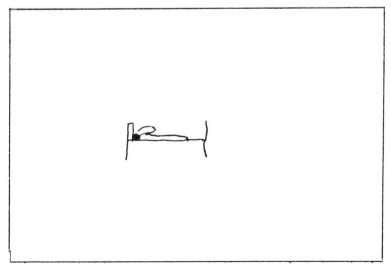

the group into a discussion about independence, responsibility, self-esteem, body awareness, growing and depending, a discussion to which Donna contributed—for her—enthusiastically, if cautiously.

The three abovementioned drawings—with Donna's explanation of their meaning—indicate a deep desire for autonomy, the main drive in all primary anorexia nervosa. The drawings also indicate failure to learn the normal areas of human life so essential for 1) communication, 2) functioning in the world and 3) autonomy and self-esteem sufficient to confront the world rather than constantly responding to it without any self-actualization and with inevitable resentment of it and oneself. If one sees oneself as a baby in a crib, what control over the environment is available, and what opportunity for "practicing" at living a life—indeed, for learning the tools with which to live?

The struggle for the anorexic is mighty, defense mechanisms strong. Massive denial is used to prevent confronting the bizarre bodily needs (or lack of needs) in a world in which he feels helpless, in which he "acts to" rather than "upon." The helplessness of this schizophrenic reaction—if it may be so called—makes even the struggle itself appear ambiguous to the anorexic.

In Donna's case, she said, "I have anorexia nervosa." If she gave up that illness, what would be left? In a sense, Donna has to be born and grow through childhood a second time. She has to attain an identity and her own autonomy. As Donna struggles to give up what she "has"—anorexia nervosa—the resulting void is large.

In summary, it has been suggested that art as a form of therapy can be advantageous. It has also become manifest that if art therapy is to be recognized as a useful profession, art therapists (present and future) *must* have some sort of theoretical and psychological base which will enable them to jump from the art-elicited unconscious material to verbal therapy. Otherwise, the individual art therapist will find himself floating amongst an overwhelming visual presentation of unconscious material, without the means to use it therapeutically. The aim of this chapter is to demonstrate the amenability of art as therapy to function from an ego-psychological base, something which may well appear both logical and useful to other art therapists in the field.

In the case of Donna, art has been used as a therapeutic tool to evoke unconscious imagery, to increase awareness of the human need for "feeling."

May it not be so for any person who has a "problem"? And may not the void of loss *seem* greater (as in Donna's case) than the relief from psychic pain? Perhaps one role of art therapists is to aid those in pain to help themselves, through filling that presumed void with creative expression—in a word, art!

BIBLIOGRAPHY

Bruch, H. *Eating Disorders: Obesity, Anorexia Nervosa, and the Person Within.* New York: Basic Books, Inc., 1973.

Kramer, E. *Art Therapy in a Children's Community: A Study of the Function of Art Therapy in the Treatment Program of Wiltwyck School for Boys.* Springfield, Ill.: Charles C Thomas, 1973.

Kris, E. Schizophrenic art: Its meaning in psychotherapy (Book review). *Psychoanal. Q.* 22(1), 1952.

Naumburg, M. *Dynamically Oriented Art Therapy: Its Principles and Practice.* New York: Grune and Stratton, 1966.

Widroe, H. *Ego Psychology and Psychiatric Treatment Planning.* New York: Appleton-Century-Crofts, Div. of Meredith Corp., 1968.

PART 2

Community Mental Health

the nurse in community mental health

JERI E. RYAN

In 1963 Congress passed the Community Mental Health Centers Act. It was a victory for sanity's sake. Courageous men and women had fought long, hard battles against ignorance, terror and ennui. Nineteenth century psychiatry had progressed slowly, often suffering set backs, the victim of internal struggles and debates, the whipping boy of outraged citizens and political parties. The intransigent beliefs about the cause of mental disorders or insanity died hard as scientific research gained importance. Indeed, the myths of that time remain with us today in the form of prejudice, guilt, and moralistic and judgmental overtones.

World Wars I and II heightened awareness of psychic trauma and propelled the country into a new era in this field, demanding investigations, treatments and results. The Community Mental Health Centers' Act began the process of decentralization by dismantling the old system. The legislators turned to the people and in effect declared "the mentally ill patient is your family member, your neighbor, your employee, your citizen. We have housed him too long in our large cumbersome, outmoded state hospitals or asylums. Our limited knowledge, our protective concern, our downright fear banished him to remote areas where he was confined and stripped of those very things which integrate his personality. Isolation, regimentation and questionable treatments have not cured him. Or even helped him very much. He has become a burden to the taxpayer, to the institution, and most tragically, to himself. But that is past history. A new day has dawned."

Modalities of treatment such as individual and group psychotherapy, crisis intervention and the breakthrough in psychotropic drugs indicated strongly that prolonged hospitalization was no longer necessary and in many cases could be eliminated entirely. Pandora's box had been opened and the evils had escaped. With the lid closed, hope remained inside the gift given those patients who left the herding system and returned home. The former patient had come from his family, his job, his community. The scientific body had convinced the law makers that some relationship or link exists between these elements and the patient's confused state of mind, his disorganization or madness if you will. Somehow his mental or emotional reorganization must take place in his natural surroundings.

The Mental Health Act presupposed that mental health centers would use knowledge and skill as well as creativity in fulfilling the mandate to care for this segment of its population during the reentry phase following hospitalization. Working cooperatively with local communities, it would assume responsibility for improving those elements of life which foster health through various avenues of prevention.

Subsequently, through federal funding and grant-in-aid to states, counties, and cities the revolutionary concept began to take shape and form and to clothe itself with fashions appropriate to the dignity of man. Buildings with adaptation in design began to appear. Professional and paraprofessional staffs were mobilized. Often a multidisciplinary team resulted which could readily utilize specific skills of its members. The university was considered by many to be a necessary component to the plan if top-notch recruitment of future professionals was to be realized. Also, such an alliance with the university would provide clinical teaching for its faculty and experience for its students. Research and evaluation could be associated with this group and the benefits which would accrue would be invaluable. General, local hospitals were approached to accept contractural agreements for short term, inpatient hospitalization for the acutely ill thus including existing facilities into the schema. Progressive groups began to work with well established public health departments and joined forces to promote health education especially through consultation, evaluation and research.

More than a decade later we can look with some pride at the accomplishments of many community mental health centers and satellite units dotted across the country. "Some pride" because in certain locales the decentralization process envisioned at its inception appears to be working quite well. Continuity of care is a priority, community involvement is high and a modicum of health seems to pervade suggesting that primary prevention as perceived by Caplan (Caplan, 1966, pp. 1–31) has been a mutual goal of the health team, the educators, the guardians of public safety and the individuals who make up the given community.

Without a full scale study, however, it is impossible to take accurate readings of the total system in action. Relying on current investigative reports, published usually at the behest of local governing boards responsible to the tax-payers, reveal, in some instances, serious deficiencies within the system. For instance, the continuing philosophical debate as to health care constituting a "right" for every person and therefore supported by public funds serves as a deterrent to seriously accounting for numbers of clients whose cost of care is reimbursable. Proponents of this stance are often professionals who champion the cause of the poor and disadvantaged. The adversary then becomes the administrative arm of the system which has been given the authority and responsibility to carry out the regulations and guidelines of the funding agencies and must therefore be accountable for its actions.

Historically, superintendents or administrators of health care facilities have been professionals, usually physicians. With the proliferation of Schools of Administration, the picture is changing somewhat. Nevertheless, in mental health centers, the chief administrative officer is frequently a clinical psychiatrist. Etzioni describes the dilemma:

When people with a strong professional orientation take over managerial roles, a conflict between the organizational goals and the professional orientation usually occurs (Etzioni, 1964, p. 179).

This dilemma takes on new dimensions in an age of the consumer, of informed consent and patients' rights. The professional, especially desiring to use foremost clinical skills, can no longer ignore or turn a deaf ear to these concerns. At least not in a public service agency such as community mental health. It has become increasingly clear that clinical assessment, diagnosing and treatment are but one part of the larger plan. The local community mobilizing against the rising crime rate, the high cost of living and the ever diminishing natural resources look to professionals to work with them in providing consultation, emotional support and direct intervention of social problems. Whether individual clinicians respond to such demands remains a question. Some feel the scope of community interaction is far too broad and they are not prepared to enter into such an alliance; attempting to do so only dilutes their effectiveness as clinicians. Others may feel it is precisely what the members should be doing as a team in program planning and are disheartened by colleagues who cannot seem to move beyond first base, who continue to treat solitary illness and bother not at all about primary intervention through community involvement.

And so the question arises, what is community mental health? What does it really mean? The answer depends in large part on the person or persons questioned. A clinical nurse specialist, requesting time on an agenda of a local citizens' community meeting asked these questions of the assembled group. Puzzled looks prompted additional questions such as, "If someone in your family became mentally ill or a neighbor's behavior was such that you realized some type of psychiatric help was needed, where would you go for assistance? For the most part, people stared back in startled silence. Nonverbal messages of anxiety were loud and clear but only a few were able to suggest that calling the police would be one way to get help while others felt that taking a person to an emergency room in a nearby hospital would be best. This particular community group represented a newly developed area in a large cosmopolitan city. Interested, intelligent people from different socioeconomic, ethnic and cultural backgrounds had formed the ideal locus for assessing problems dealing with their schools, after-school programs, neighborhood crime, consumer rights concerning open space, transportation and other city services which would contribute to the comfort and efficiency of living. These interested citizens had been meeting twice a month for more than 2 years in the elementary school cafeteria. Duly elected officers and committees worked diligently, giving freely of their time, energy and skills to upgrade their circumscribed locality. They were justly proud of their accomplishments. For example, they had developed a working "co-op" to assist one another in purchasing food and other commodities at lower costs, a real boost to the senior members on fixed incomes. Yet, in their overall planning, the problems of health care in general and mental health care in particular had not been addressed in any way by this group.

A quick show of hands at the meeting described, indicated that the majority did not know that they were a part of the city's catchment area, that they had legal protection of their rights regarding mental illness or that a host of services were available for a variety of problems, especially services which could prevent illness of many forms through educational programs, consultation services and community involvement on advisory boards from their district.

On the other hand, item #5 on the agenda, "Your Local Community Mental Health Program," represented years of attempts on the part of the Community Mental Health Center for entrance into the group's tightly knit council. Many requests to address the board, the open meetings or special interests groups had been put off, discouraged and even denied because of "more pressing problems." Visits had been made by members of the mental health team to local merchants, clergymen, school principals, physicians, den mothers, attorneys and others. Some appeared personally interested and concerned but felt unsure about the climate of the citizens' group. Others displayed a sense of suspicion or disbelief, citing personal experiences with city or county facilities involving health problems. The age-old symptoms of fear and prejudice were evident.

Progress was slow and a certain sense of hopelessness had invaded the mental health team. Primary prevention, consultation, research, education and evaluation were simply big words written by the prime movers of the concept of community health; it was much easier to become engrossed in the small population of the acutely ill or the wider, garden variety of recycled chronic patients. Nevertheless, the team effort continued, faint-hearted at times. The outpatient unit itself was a new addition to the community and perhaps what appeared to be unconcern or a stand-off position on both sides was in reality a normal pattern of behavior.

Neither group had been informed of the other's position, goals, objectives or projects. The community mental health center had been established with marginal input from the local group which became evident the evening the center was allowed time to present its case. The shortcomings of this community "case history" are glaring.

Congressional acts can establish systems for the public's good or safety or health. It can legislate guidelines for matching funds and set priorities. But it cannot enforce the human ingredients of communication, of trust, of sharing, of participation. Such bridges must be built by the people themselves and by those working within the facilities providing specific services to the citizenry.

The reader might legitimately ask what has all this to do with community mental health nursing? "A great deal!" is the writer's spontaneous response. Filling out forms is recognized today as a part of life which one cannot escape. Occupation: "Community Mental Health Nurse." "Clinical Nurse Specialist." To the nursing community these titles may have significance but to the general public, the word "nurse" is probably the one recognized as having some identifiable meaning. This was surely the case at the meeting mentioned earlier since a clinical nurse specialist representing the community mental health center was the introduced speaker. The word "nurse" seemed to be the title acknowledged by most nonverbal nods.

The psychiatric nurse working in one or several areas of the community mental health system can be isolated, examined and tested in order to determine traits, specifics, or commonalities with other nurses. However, this approach becomes constricting and limiting since it removes the components essential to the definition of nursing practice for this particular group. This is not to say that the nurse cannot practice apart from other members of the mental health team which include psychiatrists, psychologists, social workers and paraprofessional or community workers. On the contrary, individuality is essential if multiple skills are to be utilized. Nevertheless, it is the concept of the collective, or the team's approach which is the hallmark of community mental health services in this country. Where this is lacking, programs are not viable and proscribed services are waning if existing at all.

Therefore, it would follow that any consideration of the nurse's role must be viewed against the backdrop of mental health pro-grams planned within the local community. Because this has not always been the case, some consider community mental health nursing as the same old thing with a new label. Others who have attempted to learn more about the system itself or who have participated in specific programs may see it as a freeing and exciting step into the future. A degree of autonomy and independence is offered to the individual and simultaneously to the team in a way seldom experienced in large, bureaucratic institutions. Because of the different disciplines represented, a colleague relationship often results and the nurse, perhaps for the first time, is aware of the freedom from the often oppressive and constricting hierarchical structure characteristic of nursing in hospital inpatient settings.

Looking at the multidisciplinary team members whose professional education contributes in no small way to their management of patient care, the nurse alone stands apart from the group. A license to practice nursing is the accepted credential to participate as a team member. Generally, it is hoped that the selection process will propose a nurse with a baccalaureate degree in the case of a staff position and a master's prepared nurse for the role of clinical nurse specialist. While it may be true that many nurses are highly skilled and have considerable on-the-job training and clinical experience, the prerequisites remain a strong nudge, not a mandate. To be sure, the Division of Psychiatric and Mental Health Nursing of the American Nurses' Association is attempting, in a commendable manner, to challenge nurses to assume more responsibility in their scope of practice by advocating higher degrees and certification as mental health nurses and clinical specialists. Nevertheless, in many parts of the country a "nurse is a nurse is a nurse."

And nurses practice nursing. A criticism of nursing? Yes. But also a challenge because within the team concept of mental health care, nursing has unlimited possibilities. This relatively new form of nursing care or practice emerged only in the 1950's. Until that time, nurses were engaged marginally with patients in large state hospitals acting as assistants, caretakers, and monitoring treatments and medication. They were not involved to any great extent in direct therapy. With the advent of community mental health facilities nurses began to be recognized as vital members of the psychiatric community. This has proved to be a refreshing and liberating experience for many nurses who have had or sought additional education in this fascinating field.

In most community mental health programs, nursing requires an advanced degree, as was initially stated. But not with the consistency of public health nursing which years ago delineated its standards. It is a common belief today that almost anyone can "do" therapy. Of course this is hazardous and can be deleterious to the client or patient as well as the would-be therapist. However, lacking substantial scientific evidence regarding the cause and treatment of mental illness after so long a time, we are witnessing a heyday of charlatans, of the occult, of unbelievable fads aimed at quick, easy cures. The stakes are high both in psychic trauma and pocketed wealth.

Viewing this phenomena, nurses may once again see themselves as rescue workers. Licensure justifies many things under the law. It can never justify lack of preparation at a high level, supervised practice, evaluation and clinical competence. In practice, it is not uncommon for community workers, for instance, to relate extremely well to individuals, to families, and especially to community groups. Frequently their innate experience, their ethnic or cultural identification cannot be contested. It is invaluable. Does it substantially move people toward wellness? Probably yes, in many instances. Nevertheless, these particular insights or skills are utilized within the team structure to identify problems, to work in conjunction with others who can differentiate symptoms, who can interpret behavior and who can judiciously initiate treatment plans, follow through and evaluate their efficacy. These parameters demand of the clinical team member a basic education at the master's level with additional preparation in intrapsychic phenomena, crisis intervention, family therapy, health teaching, consultation, research and evaluation. Not every practitioner can be proficient in all

these areas, but such work points out that nurses who have come from staff positions in hospitals treating patients with acute mental illness need additional preparation to work effectively in the complex areas of community mental health. Some continuing education courses are addressing these issues surrounding power and politics, community involvement and consumer participation.

It is hoped that nurses will avail themselves of additional knowledge through courses dealing with leadership, organizational theory, cultural, ethnic, and religious studies. Heightened awareness in these areas would prove beneficial to all professionals in the field of mental health.

If the community mental health nurse is to enjoy a colleague relationship in the true meaning of the word (as opposed to a sense of camraderie) a high degree of independence and autonomy must be established. It is difficult, in spite of ANA's current position, to understand how this can be realized fully without the commensurate educational preparation of team co-workers.

Because the current picture of community mental health nursing does not admit of large numbers of nurses entering the field the question of placement becomes a serious one. Funding remains tentative and frequently in jeopardy which necessitates shifting or eliminating positions. Mental health units which are a part of the Civil Service Commission allocate positions through a ratio system concerned with several disciplines working in concert to form the team. Private hospitals do employ nurses, but their roles are somewhat limited or timeworn and do not seem to express significant creativity. Clinical nurse specialists, on the other hand, are considered to be a luxury in many institutions and therefore utilization of these qualified nurses remains low. This is certainly not true in every hospital or clinic, but institutions feeling the pinch, now the crunch of high cost medical care, cannot consistently afford this level or nursing, or they have not been convinced by the nursing community of their substantive value. Criticism of this statement may follow, but the truth remains that for the most part, nursing has not united to establish its unique role or contribution to the degree that it cannot be replaced by others and for less money. In university-related hospitals, nursing is faring better and clinical competence is recognized more and more. The clinical ladder is becoming a reality. In general hospitals, in smaller community hospitals and in clinics the traditional model remains for the most part. Breakthroughs are noted in the journals and are heartening. Some progressive institutions are encouraging nurses to continue their education and allow time for this purpose. Many, however, cannot deal with a system which presents them with nurses with more and less education, more and less clinical experience, yet demanding the same salary for all. Again, this disturbing element is a thorn in the side of care-giving centers which do not deal with other professionals in such a manner.

Where then does the psychiatric or mental health nurse practitioner gain experience, pursue graduate studies, engage in research or retain a clinical position? Students enrolled in educational settings might answer that it has become increasingly difficult to find a niche in which to study, to observe, to complete research. Others attempting to find jobs are turning more and more to private practice and are attempting to work through legal restrictions inhibiting their services. Third party payments are being considered and may evolve if proponents are able to establish nursing knowledge, care and practice as a value apart from medicine. Such practitioners utilize consultation on a mutual, collaborative basis with physicians.

In the meantime, qualified nursing practitioners are working in acute care hospitals, rehabilitation units or nursing homes. Many await the opportunity to participate in psychiatric outpatient units, crisis centers, specialty units such as drug abuse programs or extended care facilities. Some have managed to find positions in public health nursing but the waiting list remains long. Does it seem likely that there will be a shift in the mental health community to allow for increased numbers of nurses within its ranks? Much will depend on the status of the mental health field itself and the funding processes which will be forthcoming as a

new political climate pervades Congress which may be more aware of the voice of the consumer than in previous years.

At the present time, the newly elected President is attempting to unite a fragmented country which displays wounds of war, scandals, and deprivations of many kinds. High unemployment, rising cost of living and the alarming crime rate would indicate a need for more services to people struggling with these problems. On the other hand, mental health and mental health professionals are cited as culprits for many of the ills of our modern society. It will take enlightened, charismatic leaders to turn the tide at this juncture. Recent high court decisions on human rights may place stringent demands on many public servants including mental health professionals. The present system is already being replaced by a more perfunctory, detailed, bureaucratic one which demands accountability in the extreme. Neglect of some areas of the original concept of decentralization such as administrative and fiscal responsibility as well as consultation, education and research are significant factors in newly imposed restraints.

Since nursing represents the largest single group providing health care in its myriad forms, it would seem appropriate to encourage a certain creativity wherever it occurs. If it is unlikely that psychiatric nursing will provide positions for large numbers of practitioners, we must examine the concepts of that care and see if they can be applied elsewhere and to greater advantage. Acute care settings would be an example in point. Nurses working in acute settings find themselves under incredible pressure, unending stress. The coronary patient often represents a mirror in which the nurse sees a reflection of her own inner tensions, pressures and fatigue. Recently a student submitted a paper about the deathbed in the coronary care unit. Every day a deathbed for someone. It is a disturbing account and raises questions about endurance, survial and mental health practices of nurses functioning at a rate equal to athletes, athletes without the physical and psychological training for their participation. Would it not be helpful, is it not imperative, that such nurses be equipped with more than basic tools of psychology? Dealing with the self is at the heart of understanding human behavior. Knowledge and practice can be translated into meaningful and useful supports for the nurse, for co-workers, for patients, families and significant others. It is challenging to propose that a psychiatric clinical nurse specialist, available to a group of acute care units, providing assistance, consultation, emotional support and a solid inservice program could reduce fatigue, stress, absenteeism, turnover rates as well as foster individual and collective growth through mental health principles.

This proposal could be utilized in any setting. How often nurses complain that their job is not as exciting as working in acute care, that their patients provide little challenge because of their routine care, their neurotic behavior or their chronicity.

The whole point of human interaction, that vast wealth of vibrant life which can exist between persons lies dormant in many patient units today. The myth that therapy of whatever type holds rewards for the few needs to be dispelled. To be sure, certain psychological states require skilled intervention and that is the role or at least one role, of the psychiatric clinical nurse specialist. Nurses, in general, can learn and use mental health principles, psychosocial skills of communication and interpersonal relationships to a high degree. Such skills open doors for many patients which would otherwise remain closed forever. Crisis intervention is not a sacrosanct formula to be used only at identified centers. The death of a loved one presents a crisis daily in hospitals everywhere. How nurses deal with such a crisis *is* the issue. Are they simply following the procedure manual and dealing with the human elements as best they can? Could they learn how to deal with grieving family members in more appropriate ways if such methods became a part of their nursing practice? Recognition of such states as depression, anxiety and acting-out behavior is often lacking among those who care for the medically ill, those undergoing surgery or those whose life style must radically change when they leave the hospital.

Nurses returning to the university to complete their education could share and bring valuable input to bear on the learning process which could include pathological states and methods of treatment. Recognition does not necessarily mean intervention, but it is essential if consultation or referrals are to be made appropriately. Knowledge of the public health system and the mental health services offered to the community could become viable and continuity of care could become a reality.

DeYoung and Tower note in their interesting study that the "it" or "X factor" is the humanistic element in what we call nursing (DeYoung and Tower, 1971, p. 95). Increased research, nursing research, may unearth more of the "it" as it attempts to build its unique body of knowledge. Perhaps it is in the humanistic approach that nursing will have a unique contribution and that the "total person" will become just that and not a concept divided into minute parts, rarely studied much less encountered as a "whole" person.

In this sense, then, community mental health nursing joins the body of nursing to foster the "X factor" or educated caring as a concept worth pondering. It seems to have its roots deep in its past history but its branches demand more if it is to continue growing.

BIBLIOGRAPHY

Caplan, G. *An Approach to Community Mental Health.* New York: Grune & Stratton, Inc. 1966, pp. 1–31.

Caplan, R. B. *Psychiatry and the Community in Nineteenth Century America.* New York: Basic Books, Inc., 1969.

Carter, F. M. *Psychosocial Nursing.* New York: Macmillan Publishing Co., Inc., 1976.

DeYoung, C. D., and Tower, M. *The Nurse's Role in Community Mental Health Centers: Out of Uniform and Into Trouble.* St. Louis: C. V. Mosby Co., 1971.

Etzioni, A. *Modern Organizations.* Englewood Cliffs, N.J.: Prentice-Hall, Inc., 1964, p.79.

Etzioni, A. *The Semi-Professions and Their Organizations.* New York: The Free Press, 1969.

Fagin, C., McClure, M., and Schlotfeldt, R. Can we bring order out of the chaos of nursing education? Am. J. Nurs. 76: 98–107, 1976.

Kalkman, M. E. *Introduction to Psychiatric Nursing.* New York: McGraw Hill Book Co., Inc., 1950.

Lewis, E. P., and Browning, M. H. *The Nurse in Community Mental Health.* New York: The American Journal of Nursing Co., 1972.

Morgan, A. J., and Moreno, J. W. *The Practice of Mental Health Nursing: A Community Approach.* Philadelphia: J.B. Lippincott Co., 1973.

Peplau, H. E. *Interpersonal Relations in Nursing.* New York: G.P. Putman's Sons. 1952.

Chapter 13

the psychiatric nurse specialist in private practice

BEVERLY J. HENDLER

Role expansion for registered nurses as practitioners is a relatively new concept in nursing. The expansion of the registered nurse's role has evolved because of a number of influencing factors. Some of these factors include: the shortage of primary care physicians (although this is a controversial issue from time to time), the involvement of the federal government, the women's liberation movement, the increasing complexity of acute hospital care, the reforms in the education of health professionals, the demands and expectations of the consumer for better and more comprehensive health care and the growing support for physician's assistant programs.

There is no doubt that a great deal of time, effort, and energy has gone into the planning, development and implementation of the nurse practitioner programs. The establishment of the nurse practitioner role has, as might be expected, been a slow and exhausting process. There are several factors that have contributed to this slow progress. First, an important area that was overlooked in the early stages of developing this expanded role for nurses was the proper introduction of this new category of health care provider to the public. A crucial part of this introduction should have included the adequate education of the health care consumer, and health professionals in all

disciplines, to this new type of practitioner. Failure to adequately inform the public about the purposes and advantages of utilizing nurses as primary care providers resulted in the creation of some unnecessary confusion, opposition and, unfortunately, resentment.

The confusion occurred because of a lack of clarity regarding the nurse practitioner's level of functioning—e.g., her capabilities and limitations, the lines of authority and responsibility in the clinical or professional setting and the degree of theoretical and clinical preparation for this new role.

Experience has demonstrated that some patients who have been referred to a nurse practitioner for care and treatment have been unwilling or reluctant to see a nurse for the purpose of therapy. Some patients have vehemently stated that they "want to see a doctor because the doctor can take care of me better." The clients are oftentimes unaware of the nurse practitioner's level of expertise and capabilities.

Opposition to the nurse practitioner program has come from a number of sources. Surprisingly, some of the strongest opposition has come from people in the nursing profession. Their opposition has been primarily related to a lack of understanding about this new role.

Other groups that have opposed the establishment of the nurse practitioner role include administrators in the health services, physicians and the majority of the third-party payers who deny payment to nurses for nursing care.

Obviously, the confusion and opposition that have been focused on the nurse practitioner movement have eventually created resentment in large segments of the health care delivery system.

It is important to point out, however, that some of the negative attitudes and opinions that were formerly expressed by many individuals concerning the nurse practitioner approach to patient care are changing. Current evidence reveals that the nurse practitioner movement has had a positive impact on specific areas of the health care system in this country. Consequently, the nurse practitioner has begun to gain respect, acceptance, and status from health professionals in other disciplines. Equally important is the increasing positive recognition the practitioner is beginning to receive from clients.

The term "nurse practitioner" is the general designation for the individual practicing as a nurse practitioner, nurse clinician, and clinical nurse specialist. The nurse practitioner in psychiatric nursing is referred to as an "advanced practitioner" or "nurse specialist." For the purpose of this chapter the term nurse specialist or advanced practitioner will be used when referring to the nurse practitioner in psychiatric nursing.

PREPARATION FOR THE NURSE SPECIALIST ROLE

The nurse specialist is prepared to deliver primary care to patients. In order to do this, she must possess advanced knowledge and skill that will enable her to make sound clinical judgements regarding patient care. A nurse in this role must be able to conceptualize client care and apply the nursing process in the care and treatment of patients.

The advanced practitioner usually holds a master's degree in psychiatric nursing. There are some exceptions to this, however, in that there are practitioners who hold diplomas and have completed a nonacademic practitioner course. A few nurse specialists have earned doctorates.

THE NURSE SPECIALIST IN THE CLINICAL SETTING

Maukasch (1975, p. 1834) defined three settings in which the nurse specialist might practice. These include:

1. In institutions concerned with inpatient or ambulatory care. The majority of practitioners are found in these settings. It must be kept in mind that the practitioner is given a great deal of professional autonomy in these kinds of settings. The function of the nurse specialist in the institutional setting is to work collaboratively and interdependently with other health professionals to develop patient care objectives, to plan and implement care and to mutually evaluate outcomes. Nurse specialists in the inpatient or ambulatory care agencies have been more readily accepted than nurse specialists in the settings described below.

2. In solo practice, either self-employed, or as a member of a group of nurse practitioners. Nurses involved in this type of practice have received the strongest opposition from health professionals. Again, many physicians and certain segments of the nursing profession have expressed most of the opposition to the nurse specialist in solo practice.

This author strongly opposes this type of practice for the nurse specialist. The practitioner in this setting has achieved a level of autonomy that will probably not be observed in any other setting. Most nurse specialists in all settings welcome the autonomy that they have achieved in their practice. However, empirical evidence has demonstrated that some nurses in solo practice have occasionally become confused about the limits or boundaries of their autonomy. The outcome of this confusion could conceivably direct the solo practitioner toward a philosophy of visualizing her "autonomy" as a license to practice medicine rather than staying within the scope of nursing. It is this type of autonomy that could potentially jeopardize the future of the nurse specialist concept.

Autonomy in nursing, if utilized properly, can present many advantages to the nurse specialist. It offers the individual an opportunity to be flexible, creative, and to grow personally and professionally. However, this obviously cannot be at the expense of another person, particularly the client and the system of delivering health care.

The nurse specialist functions by performing nursing and complementing, when necessary, the physician's doctoring. The nurse specialist who confuses the two roles can potentially create serious problems for herself, the patient and her colleagues.

One of the primary arguments voiced by many nurses who oppose the solo practitioner is the fear that individuals who are not adequately prepared clinically and theoretically will "set up shop" and do more harm than good in caring for clients. Obviously, the nursing profession, especially the nurse specialist program, does not want or need to be represented by incompetent, unqualified nurses who could possibly damage the continued growth and expansion of the nurse specialist concept of administering care. One or two serious mistakes on the part of the solo practitioner in caring for patients could cause a profound regression in the nurse practitioner movement.

To allay these fears, to protect the nurse specialist and to provide for continued professional growth, the nurse specialist should include professional supervision in any plans for private practice.

Supervision of the health professional is a crucial element of any practice. An individual who fails to include supervision as an active part of that practice takes the risk of retarding her professional growth by failing to improve or enhance her skill and knowledge as a practitioner. This would ultimately affect the caliber of care she gives her clients.

This author is concerned that the nurse specialist in solo practice might let the ego balloon of private practice blind her to the need for establishing and maintaining adequate and ongoing resources for the supervision of her work with patients.

The nurse specialist in solo practice usually has limitations placed on her in terms of having sufficient referral resources. The primary effect of insufficient referral sources is that the nurse specialist in solo practice is hindered in establishing, maintaining or expanding her practice.

In addition to the problem of having insufficient resources of referrals, the nurse specialist in solo practice usually has difficulty receiving payment from third-party payers for her services to patients. The reluctance or unwillingness to pay the nurse specialist in solo practice possibly stems from the fact that the nurse is prepared to do nursing and, unlike the physician, she does not practice medicine.

3. In self-employed, interdisciplinary groups. The nurse practitioner in this setting may be a partner or an employee in an incorporated practice. She practices collaboratively and interdependently with other health professionals in the group.

Nurse specialists who practice in an institution or as an employee or partner in an interdisciplinary group will have a more positive effect on the continued expansion of the nurse specialist's role than the nurse specialist in solo practice. Members of society, particularly the majority of the health care providers, are less willing and eager at the present time to accept the latter type of practitioner. The type of practice in which this author is involved is as an employee in an incorporated medical group. The practice is limited to psychiatry. There is only one nurse specialist currently employed in the group.

The services offered by the medical group include inpatient and outpatient psychiatric treatment and care. Specific types of care available to the client include individual counselling for inpatients and outpatients, discharge planning for hospitalized patients, posthospital follow-up treatment, outpatient group psychotherapy, marriage and family therapy and home visits. Outpatient group psychotherapy and home visits are done exclusively by the nurse specialist.

The nurse specialist in private practice has her own client case load. She functions as the primary therapist for the majority of the patients referred to her.

The advanced practitioner is responsible for the careful, thorough assesment of patients as well as the formulation, implementation, evaluation and revision of the plans and goals for a patient's treatment.

In addition to functioning as a primary therapist for clients, there are occasions when the advanced practitioner practices as a co-therapist with a psychiatrist.

Whether she practices as a primary therapist or as a co-therapist, she does so under the direct supervision of a physician. The point must be stressed that the nurse specialist has the professional autonomy that is needed to function as a primary care provider. The members of the medical group emphasize the importance of working collaboratively and interdependently with each other. The advantage of this approach is that it offers the nurse specialist easy access to supervision, it eliminates the potential for the practitioner to practice medicine rather than to practice nursing, and it enhances patient care.

Most of the clients that are seen by the advanced practitioner are referred to her by the physicians in the medical group. Occasionally patients are referred for therapy by health professionals or agencies outside the medical group. The diagnostic classifications, problems, and symptoms that are presented by the clients are quite diverse.

The advanced practitioner's level of educational preparation is more specific for that role. The distinct theoretical and clinical preparation enables the nurse specialist to be quite versatile in her ability to problem solve and to function effectively as a resourceful primary care provider. The resourcefulness or versatility of the nurse specialist permits her to serve a more useful function with a medical group. In specific kinds of clinical situations the advanced practitioner has an important edge over the psychiatrist or psychologist. The following clinical example will illustrate this point:

Example

Mrs. Thomas, a 68-year-old woman was referred to the nurse specialist for posthospitalization follow-up care. She has been widowed for 1 year. Her nuclear family includes a married son, who resides in the bay area and with whom she has had little contact over the past several years, and a sister who lives on the east coast. The patient was born and lived most of her life in the Midwest.

After the death of her husband the patient became almost immobilized because of depression. She stayed in bed almost constantly and went through periods when she would not eat or take care of herself physically. She refused to see any of her friends and would not answer her telephone most of the time.

Mrs. Thomas' son went to his mother's home and demanded that she return to California with him. After much persuasion she agreed to do so.

On arrival at the bay area she was placed under the care of an internist and was referred to a psychiatrist for admission to the inpatient service of a psychiatric hospital. She was hospitalized for approximately 4 weeks. Her progress while in the hospital was good. It was decided during her hospitalization that she would move to California permanently since the support systems in her hometown were relatively nonexistent.

The nurse specialist's involvement in Mrs. Thomas' care was quite extensive. First, after the psychiatrist had set a discharge date for the patient, the nurse specialist was involved in formulating the plans for follow-up care. 1) The patient needed to find appropriate housing accomodations in the area. The nurse specialist assisted the patient and her family in accomplishing this task. 2) The son requested some guidance as to how to deal with his mother after her permanent move to the bay area. Therefore, the nurse specialist met with the patient, her son and daughter-in-law, on a weekly basis for family therapy. 3) The patient needed to have available resources for becoming more actively involved socially. As a result of her involvement with similar patients, the nurse specialist was able to gear the patient to senior citizens groups, bridge groups and other social organizations. 4) The nurse specialist saw the client at home weekly to determine her progress and level of functioning in the home. This also offered the patient another support system. 5) As a part of her follow-up care, Mrs. Thomas attended an outpatient psychotherapy group in which the nurse specialist was the group leader. 6) The patient was seen weekly by the psychiatrist for the specific purpose of monitoring her medication regimen as well as serving as an important source of support for the client. The psychiatrist and the nurse specialist had a great deal of open exchange of information with each other about the patient. Needless to say, this was an important component of Mrs. Thomas' treatment and care.

The versatility of the psychiatric nurse specialist is further demonstrated in her ability to do physical assessments and to administer physical nursing care to patients in addition to carrying out her responsibilities related to the care of clients with psychosocial problems. This type of nursing approach is particularly pertinent to the care of the geriatric patient.

Example

A 70-year-old married, retired restaurant owner was referred for psychiatric hospitalization and treatment following an acute depression which culminated in a serious suicide attempt. The reason he gave for the suicide attempt was related to his concern and fears about his physical problems. The patient has been under the care of an internist for 1 year because of severe hypertension, frequent urinary tract infection, angina and "poor circulation" in his lower extremities. Prior to his discharge from the hospital the patient was referred to the psychiatric nurse specialist for posthospitalization follow-up care. The patient was initially seen at home on a weekly basis.

Each time the patient was visited at home a careful assessment and evaluation of his physical and psychological condition was done. The evaluations were reported to his internist and his psychiatrist. The client was seen at intervals by his internist and psychiatrist.

Involving the patient in his care was mandatory so that he would follow through with the necessary measures that would help control his physical problems. This was facilitated more effectively because the nurse specialist gave the patient careful instructions regarding the treatment plan pertinent to the client's physical and psychological problems.

When caring for a patient with these kinds of problems the nurse specialist is in a better position to spend more time with the client in comparison to the amount of time the physician can give him.

The nurse specialist can sometimes offer a valuable service to patients that a physician cannot serve because of the specialist's accessibility to clients. An example of this is the nurse's availability to do home visits, a function that is very rarely done by physicians. An important benefit of this service is that many patients receive the care that they need and that they might not otherwise receive if a nurse specialist was not available.

Example

A 15-year-old female who had recovered from a psychotic episode was sent to the County Children's Shelter to await disposition to a foster home. Because the services at the Children's Shelter were limited, the patient could not have transportation to see her doctor on a weekly basis. Therefore, the nurse specialist was involved in the patient's care by making visits to the Shelter on a weekly basis to assess the patient's condition, to function as the patient's primary therapist, and, consequently to serve as a source of support for her.

Again, the patient's progress might have been endangered or halted if this important service had not been available.

The nurse specialist can be effective in the treatment of clients who seem to have difficulty relating to physicians.

Example

A 50-year-old woman, the wife of a prominent physician, was admitted to the hospital because of depression and chronic alcoholism. In therapy sessions with her psychiatrist she seemed to be determined to avoid exploring conflictual issues in her life. She was generally quite pleasant to her physician but would not engage in a discussion about her intrapsychic conflicts.

Because of her lack of progress in therapy, the psychiatrist asked the nurse specialist to see the patient to try to establish a therapeutic alliance and to determine whether the client might relate better to a nonphysician professional.

During the initial interview with the nurse specialist it appeared that the patient was rather guarded with regard to the information she divulged. However, in subsequent sessions with the nurse, the client shared more information that was necessary and useful to the development of a meaningful treatment plan.

The most significant information related by the patient focused on her relationship with her husband. For years they had not been close and had merely shared a house together. She described him as an intimidating person around whom she felt insecure most of the time. Part of her feelings of intimidation had to do with the fact that he was a physician and she believed herself to be intellectually inferior to him. She had transferred these thoughts and feelings to her psychiatrist.

Because the patient found it easier to talk with the nurse specialist and deal with some of the conflictual issues surrounding her life, she was able to make some progress in her treatment.

The nurse specialist functioned as the primary psychotherapist for the client. The psychiatrist's primary involvement was the monitoring of the patient's medication regimen.

A question that is often raised is how the involvement of two therapists affects the therapeutic outcome of a client's care. Empirical evidence related to therapeutic outcome has demonstrated that the involvement of two primary therapists has had tremendous therapeutic results. It is important to stress that involving two therapists in a patient's treatment should be decided upon only after careful evaluation of the patient. The rationale(s) for this should be clearly defined when the patient's treatment plan is formulated.

The nurse specialist's involvement in the treatment of hospitalized patients is generally as a co-therapist. The psychiatrist and the nurse specialist work very closely with the hospital staff to formulate, implement, evaluate, and, when indicated, revise the patient's treatment plan and goals for treatment. The co-therapists place tremendous importance on the daily feedback received from the hospital staff regarding the patient's progress or lack of it. It is apparent that all persons on the treatment team must work collaboratively and interdependently regarding the patients' care. This was clearly demonstrated in Mrs. Thomas' treatment. Without this exchange of information, a workable and effective treatment plan cannot be established and maintained.

SUPERVISION

Earlier in this chapter, reference was made to the importance of supervision of the nurse specialist's work with clients. Again, it must be emphasized that supervision is an integral part of the nurse specialist's practice.

The nurse specialist will sometimes encounter a client problem or situation in which she has had no experience. It is important that competent, experienced resource persons be available to her for instruction and guidance in managing these difficulties with which she is confronted. This is particularly true for the beginning advanced practitioner.

Supervision will offer the advanced practitioner a source of support and is beneficial in terms of helping the nurse to become more confident and, subsequently, to become a more effective nurse specialist.

Supervision is generally more useful when the individual is willing to look at all aspects of the work that is done with a given patient. Naturally, this means that an individual will be vulnerable to criticism. Nonetheless, intensive exploration and examination of the way in which one participates in a patients treatment is imperative for avoiding unnecessary errors in a patient's treatment and for determining ways in which a client's care might be enhanced.

To reiterate, the philosophy of the incorporated medical group in which this nurse specialist is employed is to practice collaboratively and interdependently with each other. Therefore, supervision is quite accessible to this nurse. The nurse has been given a clear, direct message that she can contact another member of the group any time there is a question about her practice or a patient's condition.

An important element that makes for effective and meaningful supervision is the attitude of the supervisor. Supervisors who instruct and guide without humiliating, intimidating, or unnecessarily embarrassing the supervisee are far more effective than the supervisor who teaches by employing scare tactics in the supervision sessions.

Creating the proper atmosphere for supervision increases the liklihood that the supervisee will benefit from the experience. Included in this proper atmosphere is the relationship between the supervisor and the supervisee. The relationship must be one in which the two individuals can openly discuss and share opinions and information relative to the treatment of patients. Implied in this statement is the need for mutual trust and respect for one another as health professionals.

It is usually important to have a scheduled appointment for supervision so that both parties have sufficient time to deal with issues that are pertinent or about which there is concern. In addition to this, the supervisee should be prepared for the supervision session by outlining topics, questions, or areas of concern regarding her work with patients so that maximum benefit can be gained from the supervision period.

SUMMARY

Regardless of the opposition that the nurse specialist movement has received to date, this author believes that the addition of the nurse specialist to the health care system is a viable component of future nursing. The advanced practitioner can make a valuable and significant contribution to the delivery of health care in this country. Her best contribution can be demonstrated in her versatility, flexibility as a practitioner and her accessibility to clients. She can contribute by being a change agent for the health care system by promoting the idea of more comprehensive patient care. In order to make these contributions, the advanced practitioner must have adequate theoretical preparation, have sufficient and well-rounded experience as a clinician, demonstrate leadership and teaching ability, be willing to take risks, be assertive and develop the confidence to make sound decisions that affect patient care. Furthermore, to function more autonomously in the treatment and care of patients, the nurse specialist must demonstrate that she is qualified, competent and capable of practicing in this manner. Otherwise, she will be a "specialist" in name only.

BIBLIOGRAPHY

American Nurses' Association, Congress of Nursing Practice. *Nurse-Practitioner, Nurse-Clinician, and Clinical Nurse-Specialist.* Kansas City, Mo., The Association, May 1974.

Bullough, B. The Influences on Role Expansion. *Am. J. Nurs.* 76:1476, 1976.

Cleland, V. Nurse clinicians and nurse specialists: An overview. In *Three Challenges to the Nursing Profession.* Selected Papers from the 1972 ANA Convention. Kansas City, Mo.: The American Nurses Assoc., 1972, pp. 13–26.

Lewis, E. P. The new breed. (Ed) *Nurs. Outlook* 22:685, 1974.

Mauksch, I., and Rogers, M. Nursing is coming of age—Through the practitioner movement. *Am. J. Nurs.* 75:1834, 1975.

The nurse practitioner question. (Interview) *Am. J. Nurs.* 74:2188, 1974.

Chapter **14**

the personal touch in crisis intervention

LARS F. WILLIAMSON

Open Door Ministries is a Christian organization which operates a rap center/coffeehouse on the waterfront in Sausalito, California. In addition to this coffeehouse program, Open Door Ministries is actively involved in the operation of the only mobile crisis intervention team in Marin County. (Marin County is located in the San Francisco Bay area, just north of the Golden Gate Bridge, and has a population of about 255,000 people. The San Francisco Bay Area claims to have the highest suicide rate in the nation.) By mobile, we mean the crisis team will go out to see the person wherever he might be—at home, on a streetcorner, in a bar, or in a hotel. The foundation of the crisis work done by the team from the Open Door is based upon the concept of the value of the individual and the reality of human physical, phychological and spiritual needs.

Open Door operates out of a small unpretentious building on the waterfront, away from the main stream of traffic. It is staffed entirely by volunteer counselors, both professional and lay, and is financed solely by private and anonymous donations. The simple food and beverages available to clients also are donated. Activities take place there by the light of candles, most of which are made by the volunteers. Those who come to Open Door are met by a warm and inviting environment. Most sit comfortably on large pillows scattered about the carpeted floor.

The following description of the rap center facilities and operation is given to show how the crisis follow-up is handled by the program there. It must be remembered, however, that the center is neither a crisis "drop-in" center nor a psychiatric halfway house. It caters to "normal" people, as well as those who are seeking help. This provides an opportunity for normal and not-so-normal, people to socialize, with no lines drawn between them. Everyone, and anyone, is welcome. Open Door Ministries does not offer group therapy.

Although technically the approach is through an agency, it is not a typical agency approach. It is a one-to-one personal relationship in counseling and an informal "be yourself" atmosphere at the rap center. Everyone is respected as a person and ·is given the right to do almost anything, even if it means doing nothing. In other words, at Open Door there is no expectation imposed upon the person to participate in any particular way. Each person is free to associate—or not associate—with whomever he pleases. There is no pre-planned program, no formal entertainment, no group sessions, no radios or television sets. There is a piano, a guitar, bongos, chess set, free coffee and tea, soup, and whatever other food benefactors may donate. Outsiders often wonder how it is possible to operate a successful program without some type of entertainment or planned activities. At Open Door, emphasis is upon people relating to people. Most of the clientele soon find themselves talking to others, and even the most shy and withdrawn soon "come-out" and begin relating to others. While differences of opinion may often arise, as with any interpersonal relationships, people usually do find themselves accepted for themselves, and this seems to instill in them a feeling of importance and of being a person of real worth. Perhaps this is the key to the therapy that "just happens."

In summary, Open Door is a place where people can go to relax, meet people and enjoy themselves. Most of all, it is a place where counseling may be found, if it is wanted, but it is not necessary that one be defined as "sick," in order to come. This is unique and unlike the Suicide Prevention Centers, Mental Health Crisis Units, Halfway Houses, Hot Lines and most drop in centers where the main criteria for using the facilities is to "have a problem." However, the atmosphere has been found to be so therapeutic that the crisis team operated by Open Door Ministries usually refers its clients to the rap center as a place of follow-up. Even some of the staff from the county mental health unit have commented on the positive changes which they have seen in some of their clients after they have started coming to the Open Door.

CRISIS AND CRISIS INTERVENTION

What is a crisis? In broad terms, a crisis in a person's life, or in a family, may be considered to be the result of any event or series of events which seriously disrupt the life sequence of that person or family. Thus, and this is an important concept, there is no universal situation which constitutes a crisis for all individuals.

Crisis intervention is the coming into the lives of people, or a family, at the time of a crisis, with the goal of getting the person, or family through the crisis, and into a reconstructed, redefined, and/or rediscov-ered life style.

In the type of crisis intervention work which is being done through the Open Door, there are three basic phases: 1) initial contact and evaluation of the situation, 2) planning with the person for the immediate future and obtaining a definite commitment and 3) follow-up and long range planning, based upon a more detailed evaluation of the individual's needs and capabilities.

There is no absolute, clear-cut separation between these phases. However, phases 1 and 2, by necessity, nearly always occur during the first meeting with the person, with phase 3 beginning a day or so later. Later these phases will be demonstrated by example.

A wide variety of knowledge is invaluable, especially in phases 1 and 2, in looking for "handles" to hang onto in helping one through a serious crisis. Many times the only way in which rapport can be established between counselor and counselee seems to be through some seemingly insignificant similarity between the individual persons, or through some interest they share. On several occasions, this interest has been cats, motorcycles, photography, place of birth, schools attended, flying airplanes, works of art or antique collections. In these "life and death" situations, any, and all, topics are considered fair game.

The knowledge acquired to move effectively into phase 3, surprisingly, is a general knowledge. It is the knowledge of all sorts of community resources, volunteer programs, job opportunities, AA and drug abuse programs, singles groups, medical and mental health facilities, etc. It is sometimes beneficial to be familiar with some of the philosophies of various local psychiatrists or counselors, so that an appropriate referral might be made. An example of this would be a hesitancy to refer an immediately, seriously suicidal person to a psychiatrist who believes in prescribing lethal doses of pills "just to show that he trusts the patient." Believe it or not, this has happened more times than anyone likes to remember.

With any type of counseling, one main job for the counselor is to redefine the situation. This is especially true in crisis counseling. When a person finds himself in a crisis, he usually has developed a point of view which has two major characteristics: it is distorted and it is generalized. Both of these aspects of the crisis attitude will be explored in more detail. First, the individual tends to make things seem worse than they really are. Common occurrences, or events which happen to many people, are viewed as personal affronts, or as something which has been directed against the particular person involved. Troubles, which are in fact, at least somewhat under control of the person are considered inevitable. Many of these situations, which constitute everyday occurrences, would warrant only passing consideration for people who are "together" emotionally. Examples of these are: the rent is due, people are coming to dinner, a son is graduating from college, a daughter is being married, it is necessary to go shopping. Even these everyday events are beyond the person's ability to handle. The results are circular: e.g., one has a traumatic experience and becomes somewhat depressed. It must be noted that the "trauma" may not be immediate, but something currently occurring may trigger memories or thoughts of past conditioning or events which begin the chain or cycle of events leading to the present crisis. Because he is depressed, he doesn't eat properly and doesn't sleep well. This makes him less able to cope with the situation, and he becomes more depressed and loses more sleep, and on ad infinitum. It has been well substantiated that physical conditions have a psychological effect and vice versa. (Walker, 1975, p. 68; Meyer, 1975, p. 75; Horn, 1976, p. 44).

The second aspect is related to and is an outgrowth of the first. The person generalizes in a negative manner—*no one* cares about him, *everything* is wrong, *nothing* works out, and he has *never* been happy. In fact, the only person who may *seem* not to care may be the person who is most important to him. Most things really may be O.K., except for a few very important areas (marriage, job, or family). In fact, he may have had *years* of a very happy, satisfactory marriage or life.

These characteristics have been pointed out here because at least a general understanding of these concepts is vital to the approach which has been found to be exceptionally effective in this ministry.

Other important factors in crisis intervention are specific characteristics of the *counselor* inherent in him—warmth, empathy and genuiness. (Truax et al., 1966, pp. 395–401; Truax et al., 1966, pp. 10–11). Other characteristics can, and must, be learned, such as the ability to listen. Even more important are the capacity to hear (this might be equivalent to "reading between the lines"), knowledge (technical, as well as general) sufficient to be able to evaluate the person in the light of his overall situation and make recommendations that will enable the counselor to move in a positive, productive direction, the ability to ask the appropriate questions to allow an appropriate evaluation and a general "skepticism" as to the reality of the client's evaluation of himself. The ability to listen can be learned, and in a formal sense, the basics involved can be taught. However, one only becomes a really adept listener through practice. Listening and hearing involve not only awareness of words, but also, to a great extent, body language. The use, here of the term "body language" refers, not so much to large body movements—such as crossing the legs, folding the arms or leaning toward or away from the counselor—but more to reactions, such as balling of the fists, squinting eyes, slight nervousness, etc. Facial expressions, especially momentary, fleeting ones, tell much about the person's feelings about the questions and/or the subjects mentioned.

Through Open Door Ministries, crisis intervention is handled on a strictly personal level, although in each case the three distinct phases are still evident. The immediate goal is to make certain that the person in a crisis is capable of surviving the next 24 hours. Although this goal is achieved in as many ways as there are crises, several common important factors are still involved.

1. The concept of the worth of the individual is of primary importance. It is this spiritual concept which really forms the basis for the operation of the Crisis Intervention Ministry, as well as the coffeehouse/rap center program, itself.

2. Each person is a separate individual who interprets his life and situation in a

specifically personal way. His interpretations are never projected in total onto another person, neither is he evaluated according to a stereotyped model person.

3. Fortunately, in spite of the above concept, all people within any culture have enough general similarities to enable the crisis intervention counselors to learn from experiences with one person, and apply their lessons to another.

While the 24-hour period has been mentioned as the criterion for success in crisis intervention, there is a follow-up program which begins about this time. It is felt that if a person is extremely lethal at a specific time, and he can be brought to a state where he will survive another day, the immediate crisis has been averted! This does not preclude a recurrence if something is not done to change the person's situation: hence—follow-up!

Usually the follow-up begins with getting a commitment from the person for a visit or call to the rap center on the following night. In the meantime, the situation has been analyzed by the staff as much as possible, and some type of referral decided upon, if it is deemed necessary. When the client calls, he will know that someone has been concerned enough to help him work out his problems. He also will discover more support from the rest of the rap center staff who have been made aware of the situation. Also, as discussed earlier, the person will meet other nonstaff people who will be accepting and supporting to him.

As with any counseling program, in crisis intervention work, one must be aware of the needs or problems. In the case of Open Door Ministries, the request to go to see someone usually comes from the local Suicide Prevention Center. However, calls also come from other agencies and private individuals in the area. Normally these requests are made after an agency counselor has devoted extensive time and effort in trying to talk the caller into a "better place," and it has become evident that only a personal encounter with a helping person will "turn the tide."

After initial contact and a turning point has been reached, sometimes the person will initiate a call at another time. These problems often can be dealt with by phone. This becomes even easier the second or third time, because the caller knows that, if necessary, someone will come in person to be with him. Because this has happened already, it strengthens the "handle" that someone really does care about him. The uniqueness of the "mobile" nature of Open Door Ministries *is* going whenever needed.

Examples of the application of this personal approach may be seen in the following illustration:

Joe X.: Referral from a suicide prevention center. His 10-year-old son has died in Europe the day before. His wife is in a mental hospital in Texas. Joe was in a bar, and a friend had called the suicide prevention center. Joe intended to go to his hotel room, get his gun and shoot himself. He had to die in order to go help his son who was "calling him."

Phase 1. The Crisis Intervention Team went to the bar and met Joe and his friend. It was quickly determined that Joe did not have a gun with him, and he really did not want to hurt anyone, except himself.

Phase 2. During a long conversation it was discovered that Joe really didn't want to kill himself, except that was the only means by which he could "help his son." The counselors' only resource at that time was to insist that his son was actually all right, and there was nothing Joe could do for him. After many hours, Joe began to feel that the counselors really meant what they were saying. He decided that he wouldn't kill himself that day if he were allowed to go home. However, he would not relinquish the gun! He felt a real obligation to the people who had given so much time to him, and he promised to phone the rap center the following night.

Phase 3. Joe didn't call back! He was a foreign correspondent for a major news service, and it was discovered that he had been re-assigned that day. Thus Phase 3 was not really carried to completion, and it was a long time before the results were known. About a year later, a message was left on Open Door's answer-phone saying, "This is Joe X. I'm in town for a few hours, and just wanted to say thanks. Everything is fine now."

In Phase 2, especially, it was necessary to zero in on the specific problem. Rather than regard his symptoms (aural hallucinations—hearing his son calling) as insanity, and taking him to the local mental health unit—where he would not go willingly—the problem was discussed openly, and logical reasons for this distressing occurrence were given to him, i.e., concern and grief over the loss of his son. But it was not feasible to allow him to define the solution in the way he was doing it! By personally dealing with his feelings and problems specifically, he was made to believe that possibly: 1) his son was all right and 2) he couldn't really help his son, anyway. Joe was allowed to have his feelings, express his thoughts, and still be treated as a person, with dignity and respect. He was made to feel that the counselors actually did understand and sympathize. He knew they wanted him to live, and he was helped to feel that his son would be taken care of without him. A short, but intensive, personal relationship developed which kept the man alive for the time, and which he acknowledged through his phone call a year later.

MANIPULATION: A COMMON FEAR OR A VITAL GAME

In crisis intervention, as in most of the "helping professions," one of the major "fears" expressed by counselors is that of being manipulated. Rather than dreading the occurrence, or avoiding it at all costs, manipulation should be considered in the following context.

Manipulation is a natural part of the crisis counseling process, and when kept under control, it is a game which must be played. This enables it to be turned to the counselor's advantage, rather than fighting it, while dealing with the person in a crisis.

The game of manipulation is comparable to a chess tournament where each player attempts to force his opponent into a series of moves from which he cannot extricate himself. Each player attempts to control the game, and thus cause his opponent to submit to defeat, or concede the game. However, there are several subtle, though significant, differences between chess and manipulation.

First, in manipulation, there may be more than one winner. In fact, if the game is well played, both players will win. The counselor wins by maneuvering the person into the

place where he can no longer play the game, or realizes that he can no longer benefit from playing. A serious danger here is that this may often lead to a potential secondary crisis where the person feels that his last defense is gone or that his last attempt to get help has failed. At this point, the counselor must be prepared to offer the counselee alternatives to giving up. Also, benefit will be realized if the counselor can make it clear that he still cares about the person and is trying to help. In fact, this is a good time to emphasize that it is easier and more enjoyable to work with the person when he is past the game stage and can be more "up front," or open in the relationship. This emphasis will reinforce the positive "non-gamey" position and provide definite incentive to stop the manipulative practices. It is vital that the major communication at this point be through action, in addition to the verbal. In other words, saying "I care," is not as effective as actually being available to help!

The counselee wins by finally getting past the place where he feels that the only way he can get help is by doing drastic things to force people into "helping" him—in short, manipulation. He then is in a place where he can be directed into a more productive life or referred to the most appropriate resource available.

On the losing side, while there is one way for the counselor to win, there are two ways to lose. If the person gets worse, leaves therapy without making progress, or commits suicide, the counselor looses. He also looses if the counselee keeps him in the manipulation process so that he (the counselee) make no progress, thus does not have to get better.

Thus, rather than being a really negative trait or process in crisis intervention, manipulation should be considered a normal part of crisis work. The ideal situation is one in which the counselor manipulates the person into the place where he is willing to try the suggested means to get his problems resolved and his life straightened out. It should be stressed, here, that manipulation by the counselee is generally not a totally conscious process. Its processes, based on some fact, are often subconscious in nature.

The goal in this "game" is for both the person in crisis and the counselor to win.

The following atypical example, although an extreme case, was chosen because it shows graphically the extremes to which people can, and will, go in playing this "game." It must be remembered, however, that most people are much more subtle and covert in their playing.

Ronald Q.: Referred to the Open Door Crisis Team by a Bay Area Suicide Prevention Center.
"Hello, Suicide Prevention."
"Help! I'm dying!" Sound of telephone dropping — receiver bumping against wall — then silence.

"Hello, Open Door."
"I'm really sick. I need someone to come get me. I'm in the City (San Francisco).
"Where in the City?"
"I'm at Fort Miley." (U.S.P.H.S. Hospital in San Francisco)

"Operator."
"Operator, help me! I'm going to kill myself!" Operator plugs him into a crisis line.

Ronald had spent much time and expended considerable energy in manipulating nearly every agency in the San Francisco Bay Area. In fact, in less than 2 years' time it became impossible to make a referral with which he was not intimately familiar. Not only had he heard of the agency, but he could quote names, addresses, telephone numbers, hours of service, and give a description of the programs that were available.

Ronald came to Open Door on a referral from a Suicide Prevention Center, and almost immediately he began his quest for attention. He said he liked the place, but we should have a security alarm system — "I can design one." He discovered that one of the staff members was a "Ham" operator, and Ron's father "was a 'ham' and operated a radio broadcast station in Ohio" — this could not be verified. Ron "had worked for several years for the phone company in San Francisco" — their personnel office had no record of his name. He had also "designed and operated numerous 'blue boxes' on the phone company system," but he insisted that he was not a 'phone freak' — this likewise could not be verified. Although he promised to supply Open Door with a 'blue box,' no such device ever appeared.

Ronald was an incessant talker, and his lines of "achievements" and criticisms (little of it being constructive) of people and agencies were interminable!

Among the escapades which were attributed to him was the one which became known as "messing up the bathroom." (It must be mentioned here that the rest room at Open Door was maintained primarily by the clientele, and having an outside entrance was made available for their use on a 24-hour basis. The clientele mentioned were mainly waterfront people in Sausalito, and they were not predisposed of putting up with a lot of foolishness from adults.) "Messing up the bathroom" consisted of a series of antics beginning with stopping up the toilet, through plugging the sink and leaving the water running, to defecating on the floor and unscrewing the light bulb. While it could not be proven, it was known that Ronald was the culprit. The response to his actions was extremely negative; there were threats of dire consequences, including bodily harm, to the unfortunate soul who had done the damage. These remarks and threats, while never directed at Ronald, were always said in his presence. This action was followed by a lengthy discussion with him, by one of the more imaginative clients, about a plan to catch the vandal. The details were every bit as wild as anything Ronald had proposed in his numerous contacts with the various agencies. It involved portable T.V. cameras hidden across the yard and infrared film cameras to photograph the unwary villain in the dark. His ideas were even solicited. The "messing up the bathroom" game stopped!

Another of his games was to come to Open Door, stay 10 to 15 minutes and leave. He would go next door to a pay telephone and call the Suicide Prevention Center and demand that they contact Open Door and tell them to talk to him! The response to this by Open Door's staff was to "come on very heavy with him" — making it quite plain that he would not be dealt with politely and courteously unless he responded similarly. If he wanted to talk at Open Door, he could approach the staff directly. On the other hand, the staff began to initiate conversations with him only when he acted civilly. Note: this did not preclude trying to help him with specific problems when he needed help.

During the times when he was not "doing his trips," he received attention and conversation, including being told that it was much nicer to talk with him when he wasn't doing "crazy" things. He began to respond more suitably, rather rapidly. While he was not denied his right to be weird, he was only given what he wanted when he gave up his strange behaviors.

Ronald's response, while not immediate, did begin shortly, and progressed rather rapidly. He began to attend Open Door less, and his calls there and to the other agencies declined rapidly over the next few months. He still calls Open Door occasionally, and seems quite "together." The nature of his calls is now more social—"just calling to say hi," "I'm doing O.K.," "I got a job," etc.

In short, it was through involvement with Ronald's game, making it unprofitable for him to try to manipulate people, that he was maneuvered into a position from which he could only win by changing in ways the counselors desired. Finally, through filling his needs only when he was "up front," Ronald was brought around to a socially acceptable means of communication and healthier interpersonal relationships. Everyone won the game of manipulation!

These concepts of manipulation are rather unique and have not been found in any reference source dealing with this phenomenon in the counseling process. They have, however, emerged through repeated experiences during the past 5 years of crisis intervention counseling at Open Door Ministries. Although unconventional, they have repeatedly worked successfully in practice for us.

SUMMARY

Crises are a normal part of life. When they become severe enough—that is, when a person becomes seriously incapacitated in all, or a major portion of his life—it is necessary to apply professional intervention techniques. It must always be remembered that crises are very personal events and that a specific thing which precipitates a crisis in one life may be inconsequential in another. While there is no usual thing which constitutes a crisis, there are similarities between the symptoms, or reactions, exhibited by persons in crises. The ability to "sense" stress or underlying reactions coupled with rapid recognition of the symptoms and the determination of the severity are essential for efficient crisis intervention. A general knowledge of a wide number of subjects is extremely useful in establishing the necessary repport with the person—any subject, no matter how seemingly insignificant or irrelevant, can be useful in making this connection. Above all, warmth, genuiness, empathy and a sense of calmness and confidence are essential for the crisis counselor. This is especially true when he is a member of a "mobile" team which cannot depend upon the resources of a crisis center to provide the assistance of personnel, drugs and restraining gear in the event of an emergency.

BIBLIOGRAPHY

Adams, J. E. *Competent to Counsel.* Nutley, N. J.: Presbyterian and Reformed Publishing Co., 1970.

Aguilers, D. C., and Messick, J. W. *Crisis Intervention: Theory & Methodity,* 2nd ed., St. Louis: C.V. Mosby Co., 1974.

Collins, A. H. *The Lonely and Afraid,* New York: Odyessey Press, distr. by Bobbs-Merrill Co., 1969.

Horn, P. (Ed.) Physical problems can masquerade as mental problems (News Line). *Psychol. Today* 10: 44, 1976.

Keith-Lucas, A. *Giving and Taking Help,* Chapel Hill. N.C.: University of North Carolina Press, 1972.

Lun, D. *Responding to Suicidal Crises.* Grand Rapids. Mich.: Wm. B. Eerdmans Publishing Co., 1974.

Moyer, K. E. Allergy and aggression: The physiology of violence. *Psychol. Today* 9: 76, 1975.

Oats, W. E. *Where to Go for Help,* Philadelphia: Westminister Press, 1972.

Parad, H. J. (Ed.) *Crisis Intervention.* New York: Family Service Association of America, 1965.

Truax, C. B., Frank, J. D., and Imber, S. D. Therapist empathy genuiness and warmth and patient therapeutic outcome. *J. Consult. Psychol.* 30: 395–401, 1966.

Truax, C. B., Fisher, G. H., and Leske, G. R. Empathy, warmth, genuiness. *Rehabil. Rec.* 7: 10–11, 1966.

Walker, S., III. Sugar doctors push hypoglycemia. *Psychol. Today* 68, 1975.

Chapter **15**

understanding suicide

RICHARD REUBIN

SCOPE OF THE PROBLEM

Not only does suicide represent a paradoxical contradiction to the axiom that self-preservation is the first law of life, it is also a form of death that is taboo. Suicide attempts are still illegal in nine states, and in 18 states abetting a successful suicide is considered a felony.

Despite adverse attitudes toward suicide, it represents a major public health problem. Indeed, suicide ranks high among the 10 leading causes of death in the United States today; in California it ranks seventh; among young people under age 35, it ranks second or third. Moreover, it would appear that as more medical advances are achieved, the current mortality rate will decrease. Accidents, homicide, and especially suicide will continue to advance in their rank of leading causes of death.

It is estimated that in the United States this year, 50,000 people will commit suicide, and more than 500,000 will make unsuccessful attempts. While these statistics are impressive, there is strong evidence that official statistics on suicide are substantially underestimated. For example, where suicide is socially or legally disapproved, the victim or his relatives may attempt to conceal evidence that the death was a suicide. Also, even if no one attempts to conceal the cause of death, suicide is often difficult to distinguish from an accident or homicide. In some instances, especially in areas where coroners do not employ psychological autopsies to ascertain the cause or probable cause of death, many of these equivocal deaths may be classified as "undetermined" on the death certificate. Similarly, another statistical bias is encouraged as physicians and coroners do not operate from a universal definition of suicide. For example, one coroner may not classify a death as suicide unless witnesses were present, another, only if a suicide note was found, and another only if the deceased were older than 13 years of age.

While it would seem appropriate to view suicide statistics as under-reported and with some degree of skepticism, it does not follow that suicide rates are completely unreliable. Rather, it is suggested that comparisons made in variations of rates will be more meaningful when interpreted in terms of relativity rather than absolutes.

THEORIES

Regardless of statistical accuracy, suicide is a major public and mental health problem. It is interesting to note that no other creatures on earth are known to bring about their own demise with such deliberation and purpose as man. While some other species (lemmings, certain whales and porpoises) may be seen to engage in self-destructive behaviors, their premeditation of the act cannot be measured.

Suicide is a universal phenomenon among

men. It occurs in nearly all cultures and crosses all racial, religious, socioeconomic and sexual lines. Indeed, it represents an archetype recorded since man's earliest history.

The study of the nature of man and the search for meaning in human existence cannot overlook the phenomenon of suicide. Each scholar who has endeavored to theorize about human behavior and personality has, by necessity, developed a theory explaining the nature of suicidal behavior.

While there is no complete or universally accepted theory of suicide, significant concepts from four major theoretical orientations will be briefly discussed. These will include sociological, psychoanalytical, behavioristic, and humanistic views on self-destructive behavior.

Sociological Theory

In 1897, Emile Durkheim conducted the first scientific investigation of suicide. Collecting and analyzing demographic data, Durkheim delineated three distinct categories of suicide: egoistic, altruistic and anomic.

According to Durkheim an egoistic suicide involves an individual who suffers from feelings of alienation and interpersonal strife. Such an individual typically finds no meaning in life and his ties with society are either negative or nonexistent. Examples of egoistic suicides might include: the self-inflicted death of a recluse or hermit who lives in isolation from his social milieu; the existential philosopher who finds no integration with his physical or social existence and whose beliefs uncover no reason or meaning for continued existence; or the political or religious activist who willfully sacrifices his life in a symbolic and potentially violent protest.

Altruistic suicides are described by Durkheim as occurring under circumstances where group needs are paramount and override the need for individual survival. In these instances, the suicidal individual demonstrates especially strong ties with his social milieu and his life is willingly forfeited for the benefit or survival of others, i.e., country, group, family, or significant others. With a great sense of national patriotism

and social integration, Japanese kamikaze pilots volunteered to fly explosive-laden planes on missions whose sole purpose was to execute a suicidal crash dive upon a strategic target. On a tribal level, altruistic suicides can be seen in the Eskimo and some other American Indian cultures. Not wanting to be a burden to the clan, aging and no longer productive individuals separate themselves from the nurturance and support of the clan and wander off alone in anticipation of their certain demise. Similarly, examples of altruistic suicides in contemporary society may be found in the self-sacrificing parent who heroically and intentionally intercepts death so the children are not physically harmed.

Perhaps most common to our contemporary society is what Durkheim classifies as an anomic suicide. Anomic suicides are triggered by a loss of social cohesiveness and/or a disturbance in social status. Self-destruction is sought when previously achieved social integration and individual norms dissipate in the wake of a significant loss or great disaster. Self-destructive acting out in response to such losses as death, divorce, or separation from a loved one, chronic debilitating illness, environmental upheaval, ensuing unemployment, downward mobility or a sudden drop in socioeconomic status accompanied by feelings of low self-esteem, despondency, guilt, shame or disorientation represent typical examples of anomic suicides.

Psychoanalytic Theory

In his pioneering work in psychiatry, Sigmund Freud devoted considerable attention to the phenomenon of suicide. Most significant in his writings on the subject is his hypothesis of two instinctual drives which constantly vie for control within each person's psyche. Freud names these drives "eros"—the life instinct, and "thanatos"—the death instinct. Self-destructive ideations are viewed as the result of the intimate and constant interaction between eros and thanatos. Ambivalent feelings of wanting to live and wanting to die are alternatively experienced as each force waxes and wanes in subconscious control and strength.

Freud postulates that eros and thanatos

are shaped and influenced during early developmental phases or critical periods. For example, Freud provides that the conflict is first expressed during infancy in an internal struggle with feelings of helplessness, frustration, anxiety and fear of abandonment. Freud contends that a predisposition to suicide is usually associated with the failure of important ego functioning acquired during this early stage of development.

Another important Freudian conceptualization regarding suicide is the relationship between depression and unexpressed rage. In his work with suicidal and depressed people, Freud found that depression typically involved unvented or mischanneled anger intended for someone else that is turned back on the individual. From this, Freud concluded that suicide was intrinsically involved with the desire to kill someone.

Another psychoanalyst, Karl Menninger, divided Freud's death instinct into three subdivisions. According to Menninger, every suicidal person possesses some degree of three wishes, one of which is most predominant: the wish to kill; to be killed; to die.

As attested by Freud, when the wish to kill is predominant, the suicidal crisis involves misdirected or unvented anger and the self-destructive act is seen as releasing the pent-up rage or the seeking of revenge. Predominant feelings may be, "I'm so angry, you shouldn't treat me like that . . . I'll show you, you'll be sorry when I'm gone. I'll kill myself."

When the wish to be killed is predominant, the suicidal episode involves intense feelings of guilt or worthlessness. Typical feelings manifested in conjunction with this wish might be, "I'm such a bad person, I've done such a horrendous thing, I don't deserve to live."

Representing the most potentially lethal of the three wishes, the wish to die involves seeking escape and giving up. Statements such as, "I can't go on; I can't fight or try anymore; Life is not worth the struggle or pain," may be seen as common verbalizations of this wish.

The stronger the wish to die, the greater the likelihood of a successful suicide. Young people are seen to exhibit more often either the wish to kill or the wish to be killed—and, while they may actively engage in suicide attempts, they usually survive. Older people, on the other hand, more often exhibit the wish to die. Attempts by the elderly appear more serious and are more often lethal. Indeed, the elderly represent the population with the highest incidence of suicide.

Behavioristic Theory

While suicidal behavior may be seen to run along family lines, it is neither a genetic trait nor inherited from one generation to another. Behaviorists, however, view suicide as a learned behavior which can generate familial predispositions to self-destruction. Just as other behaviors may be reinforced or extinguished from external input, symptoms of depression and suicidal ideations can be similarly influenced by the responses of others. Suicidal behavior may be learned and encouraged by reinforcement or modeling to affect gratification in three areas: 1) to gain attention and support while lessening demands and expectations; 2) to control or manipulate a significant other; and 3) to cope with severe stress.

Just as some children may learn to benefit from the "sick role" where inordinately more attention and sympathy are offered and parental expectations and demands are markedly reduced, similar reinforcements may be derived from depressive symptoms. As the depression becomes more chronic in nature, however, the desired and expected reinforcement may ultimately diminish from fatigued significant others. To rejuvenate the lost attention, suicidal threats may be manifested which usually generate greater support, at least for a time, from loved ones. The threats too, after a time, may lose impact and the attention seeking individual becomes forced to demonstrate the sincerity of his suicidal communications. A minor suicide attempt may follow. Again, reinforcements may be received, pressures relieved and attention gained. However, the pattern of desperate suicidal gestures becomes established. With each successive suicide attempt, the likelihood of rescue and survival diminishes. While the intention was to gain attention and support, many such situations end tragically in actual suicidal death.

Another method of providing reinforcement for suicidal behavior is that of modeling. An individual can learn that suicide threats can be powerful tools in manipulating another's behavior. The suicide threat is used to control another by evoking their sense of guilt, responsibility, or concern. Controlling the behavior of another through threats like, "If you leave me, I'll kill myself and it will be *your* fault," can be quite disconcerting. Successful manipulations may provide inherent reinforcement for the behavior, but when the seriousness of the threat is challenged and action is forced, lethal acts often result.

Suicide may not only be taught as a way to gain control or attention, it may also be viewed and learned as an acceptable and efficient way to deal with severe stress. In this sense, suicide is viewed as a reasonable alternative in problem solving endeavors. Just as when a parent is absent from the family home after a divorce, separation, or death, a child may assume responsibility for the loss. Exhibiting such feelings as, "If only I had behaved better, or kept my room cleaner, then daddy would still be here," a child may make similar associations regarding the suicide of a parent or significant other. Such incidents have lasting effects, and while the child may eventually resolve feelings of responsibility for the death, suicide is maintained as an alternative for coping with stress. Later in adult life, especially at a time when major losses or stresses are incurred, come memories of how the deceased parent handled things when they were going through pain and hardship. Indeed, the frequency of suicides within certain families gives great credence to the powerful impact such incidents have on significant others, and especially those who experienced the loss at a young and impressionable age.

Humanistic Theory

Within the humanistic theory, suicide is accepted as an inalienable right and an option available to every individual. It is contended that suicidal ideations and thoughts of death, as well as postulating the reactions of one's survivors, are universal contemplations among men. Moreover, suicide is viewed as an innate alternative to alleviating extreme levels of stress.

Each individual is seen to possess a unique tolerance to differing levels of pain and stress. When this threshold is approached, suicidal thoughts become manifest as an obvious alternative to continued existence in the seemingly intolerable life situation. As the stress continues beyond an individual's natural tolerance, feelings of helplessness and hopelessness for alleviating the pain become paramount. Still ambivalent about living and dying, suicide may be viewed at this time as the only viable alternative for changing intolerable life circumstances, reducing inordinate stress and relieving seemingly unending psychic pain. Unable to discern any other alternatives while in a state of "tunnel vision," the distraught individual seeks not death, but relief from psychic pain through a suicidal demise. Thus, humanists would view verbalizations of suicidal intent as serious messages which must be met with active support and direct interventions from concerned others. Indeed, early intervention which provides hope, alleviates pressure and seeks viable alternatives to seemingly intolerable life situations can effectively diminish suicidal risk and forestall ominous tunnel vision.

CLUES TO SUICIDE

Suicide Can Be Preventable

In what may seem to be a cry for help, nearly all seriously suicidal people attempt to communicate their intentions prior to the accomplishment of the act. If these clues to suicide are observed and acted upon by the significant people in the suicidal person's environment, changes in his life can be initiated which result in a lower, less lethal suicide potential. Less lethal alternatives may become viable to the suicidal person through the supportive and directive efforts of either a therapeutic relationship or a relationship with an empathetic and concerned significant other.

Relatively small changes, or even the possibility of future change in a seemingly hopeless life situation, can diminish the individual's suicidal potential considerably. Since suicide represents a self-directed aggression with a large component of ambivalence toward successful acting out, it appears to be more easily preventable than other modes of death. In fact, nearly every successful suicide could have been prevented through an awareness of the prodromal clues and the appropriate involvement of others during the crisis period.

Suicidal Communications

One of the most widespread and dangerous myths about suicide is: "People who talk about suicide won't commit suicide." Almost all suicidal people give clues to their suicide; often, however, the clues are not perceived until after death has occurred. In particular, suicidal communications are directed toward others in at least 80% of all self-intentioned deaths. These communications may serve to gain attention; place blame and engender guilt; ventilate pain or anger; manipulate another; test allegiance, love or concern; or prepare others for the imminent death. These communications are often directed toward significant others who are perceived as supportive and caring.

Clues to suicide may be observed in four areas: 1) verbal (direct and covert); 2) behavioral; 3) somatic; and 4) psychodynamic.

Verbal Clues

Direct verbal clues include statements like: "I am going to kill myself." "I want to die." "I won't live through this." "I am going to jump from the bridge." More covert statements might include: "It won't matter much longer." "After Saturday everything will be OK." "What's the use." "I'm worth more dead than alive." "I won't be a problem much longer." "I give up."

Behavioral Clues

At times suicidal danger may be interpreted on a behavioral rather than verbal level. Behavioral clues may include: any recent change in behavior, especially when depression lifts "for no apparent reason;" putting affairs in order, drawing up a will, writing farewell notes, giving away personal possessions; sudden changes in personality; difficulty in concentration; inability or unwillingness to communicate; neglect of appearance; withdrawn, rebellious or irrational acts.

Somatic Clues

Somatic clues to suicide are often symptomatic of the self-destructive person's depressed affect and may include any of a great variety of physiological complaints, i.e., eating or sleeping disturbances, psychosomatic complaints, headaches, muscle aches, irregular bowel movements, inordinate medical fears, etc.

Psychodynamic Clues

Suicidal intent may be demonstrated through the expression of emotional clues. Repressed anger, sexual anxieties, deflated self-image, irritability, hostility, hallucinations, delusions, despondency, unexplained mood changes, feelings of helplessness and hopelessness, agitation, apathy, guilt, shame, confusion, embarrassment or tension may, indeed, be significant precursors to self-destructive behavior.

When clues are perceived, it is vital that as a concerned other or as a helping professional, suicide is openly discussed. Whenever it is suspected that a person may be contemplating suicide, it is imperative that the concerned other approach the subject directly and openly so that the distraught person is given complete permission to discuss feelings, plans and motives. While suicidal feelings are frightening to the person having them, opportunities to bring out details of these feelings, especially when treated with seriousness and concern, can often diminish the likelihood of self-destructive acting out. Unfortunately, many helping professionals and lay people fear bringing up the topic of suicide (regardless of the clues they have perceived) for fear of implanting the idea in another's head. Suicide is much too permanent and decisive a decision for the power of suggestion to initiate. Indeed, the mere mention of suicide, or the question, "Are you thinking of killing yourself?" is not sufficient to take hold in a person who is not already thinking about ending his life. Moreover, if the person is contemplating suicide, the willingness shown on the part of the concerned other to talk about this tabooed form of death can be a great relief to the individual who has been immobilized with feelings of self-destruction.

LETHALITY ASSESSMENT

Suicidal communications may at times be manipulative tactics aimed at controlling the behavior or actions of a loved one or friend. All people who give clues to suicide or threaten the act do not actually commit suicide.

Many assessment scales have been developed to predict the seriousness of suicide potential. One such scale found to be effective by the Marin Suicide Prevention Center is based on actuarial (statistical) prediction. The scale includes 10 factors which statistically predict those people who are most likely to commit suicide within a 2-year period. Each of the factors on the scale is given equal weight, and when summed provide the following rankings: 1 to 3, low risk; 4 to 6, moderate risk; 7 or above, high risk. The factors included on this scale are:

1. Age and sex
2. Recent stress
3. Symptoms
4. Suicide plan—method available
5. Prior suicide attempts
6. Medical status
7. Communication
8. Life style
9. Alcohol
10. Resources

Age and Sex

While there has been much publicity regarding the rise in youthful suicide rates, older people are still vastly more likely to commit suicide than younger or middle-aged persons. In general, suicide rates increase proportionally with advancing age.

While women make two to three times more suicide attempts than do their male counterparts, men successfully commit suicide at a rate nearly twice that of women.

A suicidal communication from an older male tends to be most dangerous, from a young female, least dangerous. A suicidal communication from an older woman, however, is more dangerous than that of a young boy. Young people do kill themselves, however, even if the original purpose may have been to manipulate and control other people and not to die.

Recent Stress

Stress may arise from either interpersonal or intrapersonal factors such as the loss of a loved one by death, divorce or separation; loss of a job, money, prestige or status; physical illness or impending surgery; accidents; threats of legal or criminal prosecution, etc. At times, increased anxiety and tension appear to result from apparent successes, such as a promotion on the job and increased responsibilities or upon reaching a long term goal.

Stress must be evaluated from the suicidal person's point of view. What might be considered minimal stress by a concerned other might be felt as severe stress by the individual experiencing it. It is necessary to evaluate the degree to which the suicidal person is reacting to the stress. In general, acute stress constitutes greater suicidal potential than chronic stress. That is, a recent loss is more stressful than a loss which occurred some time in the past. However, while an acute stress constitutes greater immediate danger, there is also a greater probability for successful resolution than with a more chronic situation.

While a given stress is usually not the underlying cause of a suicide, it often acts as a trigger. Usually the triggering stress to a suicide attempt represents the culmination of a build up of many minor conflicts

Symptoms

Significant symptoms related to suicide potential are often displayed in response to the stress involved. These symptoms may include depression accompanied by sleep disturbances, appetite disturbances, weight gain or loss, social withdrawal, loss of interest, apathy, severe feelings of hopelessness and helplessness, feelings of physical and psychological exhaustion or psychosomatic complaints; psychotic states characterized by delusions, hallucinations, loss of contact or disorientation, or paranormal experiences; agitated states where feelings of tension, anxiety, guilt, shame, rage, anger, hostility, restlessness and pressure are common. Of most significance is an agitated depression in which the suicidal person feels a great need to act out and alleviate the pressure of a seemingly intolerable life situation.

Suicide Plan — Method Available

Suicide is not generally an impulsive act. Much thought is given to specific details of method, location and timing. It is important to assess how much thought has been given — what, if any, method has been chosen, and whether that method is readily available. The more thought out the plan, and especially one which involves multiple or lethal available methods, the higher the suicide risk.

Prior Suicide Attempts

A history of one prior suicide attempt increases the suicide risk. A first attempt is often given more contemplation than subsequent ones. It would seem that after making a prior attempt the suicidal person has transgressed the barrier of harming himself and has relinquished the taboo against suicide. Indeed, statistics show that almost all successful suicides have a history of at least one prior attempt.

Medical Status

Suffering from a severe depressive affect, most suicidal people develop some physiological complaints. Indeed, nearly three-quarters of successful suicides have visited a medical doctor within 4 months prior to their death. Moreover, the debilitating and painful experience of a long term, chronic ailment; the anticipation or prospect of imminent surgery; or the fear of (and often self-diagnosed) terminal illness contributes greatly to increased feelings of helplessness and hopelessness. The suicide risk rises proportionately with an individual's negative prognosis for relief of symptoms and pain. Moreover, the risk of suicide may increase further with the deterioration of relationships with medical professionals, hospitals and significant others.

Communication

The ability and willingness of a depressed and suicidal person to communicate openly and deal effectively with others reduces the risk of acting out and provides an opportunity for active intervention by others to alleviate the suicidal crisis. Indeed, the greater the number of people who have established and maintained an open and communicating supportive relationship with a suicidal person, the more favorable the prognosis. Over time, however, as the situation becomes more chronic in nature and symptoms of depression and pain are not alleviated, communication and relationships with significant others tend to deteriorate.

While withdrawn communication and apathy may be merely a symptom of depression, or even at times a manipulative cry for attention, it signals an increased suicide potential. Feeling alone and abandoned, the suicidal person may reach a point where communication with his significant others in particular, and the world in general, seems futile and is withheld. Blocked communication may also result when previously involved and concerned others, feeling exhausted, helpless, or blackmailed, ultimately "burn out" from the constant and draining emotional demands on their time and energy. In either instance, the results are similar; less communication occurs between the depressed person and his world, and the likelihood of suicidal acting out becomes greater.

Even if the channels of communication remain open between the suicidal person and his significant others, the manner of communication can also be an important indicator of suicide potential. An individual who is able to continue functioning and communicating on a reality-based level is less likely to commit suicide than a person who has lost his hold on reality and has episodes of seeing visions, having delusions or hearing voices calling him to his death.

Life Style

While a stable life history may indicate that a person has coped successfully with life's stresses in the past, an abrupt change in life style can increase short term suicide potential. Job changes; moving; loss of a loved one through death, divorce, or separation; the prospect of financial problems; downward mobility; ill health; criminal involvement; or social humiliation can disrupt an otherwise stable existence and engender desperate feelings of despondency, loss, or shame and may contribute to suicidal acting out. However, in time, as the individual adjusts to the change and the situation becomes resolved, the suicidal risk may diminish considerably.

People who live a chronically unstable life style involving multiple short term marriages or relationships, jobs, environments, causes, friends, etc. represent higher long term risks. Moreover, people who live alone, abuse drugs or alcohol, are homosexual, transvestite, or transsexual, are members of sub-groups which show higher suicide rates than do their more traditional counterparts.

Alcohol

While alcohol is often used as a medicine to ease pain and provide escape from stress, it follows depression as the second most common adjunct to suicide. Regardless of whether alcohol use represents a chronic problem or a seemingly temporary combatant to increased stress, it is noted in approximately 65% of all successful suicides.

Alcohol consumption may be seen to increase suicide lethality in three ways: 1) as a depressant, it can reinforce and heighten feelings of helplessness and hopelessness; 2) decreasing inhibitions and fostering disorientation, alcohol may provide temporary courage for impulsive acting out; and 3) the synergistic effect resulting from the combination of alcohol and barbiturates provides a lethal and all too available method of self-destruction. Indeed, whenever alcohol is involved, the potential for suicide is increased.

Resources

The availability of an individual's personal resources is often critical in determining his suicide potential. Resources which may be helpful in alleviating a suicidal crisis may include a job, adequate finances, religious beliefs, animals, hobbies, or anything which has previously added meaning and

quality to the person's life. Most important resources, however, are people: family, friends, co-workers, helping professionals, and concerned others can often be the determining factor in a suicidal crisis. Suicide potential diminishes proportionally with the number and quality of concerned others actively involved in the suicidal person's life.

CLINICAL MANAGEMENT

Therapeutic involvement with an acutely suicidal person can often provide the helping professional, family or friends with more rigid demands and responsibilities than those typically imposed by people with other sorts of problems. Indeed, dealing with an acutely suicidal person may be a slow and at times unrewarding process, and a suicidal crisis can often be as traumatic for those trying to help as for the individual going through it. Feelings of anxiety, fear, frustration, depression, concern and anger are not unusual when attempting to deal therapeutically with severely suicidal people.

In the context of a therapeutic relationship, and especially one dealing with the prospect of suicide, the helping professional's attitude toward death and self-destructive behavior is of great importance. Moreover, the ability of the helping professional to deal with the possibility of a client's imminent death depends, in large measure, on the professional's own reconciliation with death in terms of his personal philosophy. Indeed, helping professionals' orientations toward suicidal behavior reflect not only their theoretical bias, but too, their personality and experience.

Helping professionals must carefully evaluate and understand their own attitude toward death and suicide before they can sit quietly and without anxiety next to a client who is contemplating suicide. If their own ability to face death is a major problem in their life, and further, if they view death as a frightening, horrible event, they may be unable to face a suicidal crisis calmly and helpfully with their client.

Helping professionals, who are filled with anxiety created by the anticipation of a possible self-destructive act by their clients, may be prevented from adequately inquiring into their suicidal ideations (feelings or plans). Sound and personally acceptable theoretical, philosophical, and scientific attitudes toward death and suicide, on the other hand, may help overcome the fear and pain of loss inherent in dealing with suicidal people and may further serve as defensive and reparative agents for the professional intervening in suicidal crises.

Practical Knowledge Required

While theories of suicidal behavior may provide a conceptual approach to the phenomenon, they are neither sufficient nor always necessary for the practical handling and management of self-destructive people. Sensitivity, warmth, interest, concern, and consistency can provide meaningful help to a suicidal person within the framework of any theoretical system. Regardless of theoretical bias, it is important to be cognizant of the various therapeutic techniques and agents which have been developed to reduce the suicide potential and enhance the process of recovery. Indeed, the reason some helping professionals are reluctant to intervene in suicidal crises may lie in their lack of practical knowledge and their unfamiliarity with the problem.

Although there is no systematic formulation of therapeutic techniques which can guarantee a successful intervention in a suicidal crisis, some guidelines may be set for the helping professional to deal most effectively in managing these cases.

Be Active and Directive

Overwhelmed by feelings of helplessness and hopelessness, suicidal people may envision that nothing can change their situation and that they are alienated from those around them. Perhaps the central theme in intervening in a suicidal crisis is to maintain an active, directive and especially involved role throughout the crisis period. When clues to suicide are perceived, they need to be confronted and openly discussed. Details of suicide plan, method, and timing must be determined, and steps must be taken to separate available methods from the self-destructive individual. At times the overwhelmed person will benefit from a reduction of responsibilities. In such instances, it is essential to initiate temporary interventions which will remove the need for decision making and reduce outside obligations.

Involve as Many Resources as Possible

Involve family, friend, co-workers, physicians, clergy, therapists, etc. The more people who can demonstrate their concern, the better the prognosis, and also the greater the relief from singular responsibility for the helping people involved. It is very easy to get burned out by the inordinate demands for attention when the professional is the only one dealing with a suicidal person.

Make Contracts—Let the Suicidal Person Know You Are Concerned and Available

Stay in close contact with the suicidal person. If possible do not let him remain alone during the acute crisis. Remove available methods for suicide. Gain a promise that the person will not make an attempt (today, in the next week, or until he has tried some agreed upon alternative first). Most importantly, gain a contract that he will call you before he acts on his suicide plan. Share with the person how terrible you would feel if he killed himself.

Acknowledge Suicide as an Alternative

Treat all suicidal communications seriously. Suicide *is,* and needs to be acknowledged as, an alternative, but one to be used only when all else fails. If the suicidal person has focused on his death as the *only* solution to his seemingly hopeless life situation, it becomes important to help broaden this person's perspective by presenting or developing more viable alternatives. Relatively small changes, or even the hope of eventual change may, at least temporarily, alleviate the acute crisis. Remind the suicidal person that although suicide may be an alternative, it is a most final one. Reinforce that suicide be reserved until all other alternatives have been tried first.

Discuss Ambivalence

Acknowledge that a person has the power and ability to commit suicide, but that it is the final choice. Confront the suicidal person with evidence of his ambivalence about living and dying. In most instances it is not death that is truly sought, but rather relief from pain. Reinforce that there is a part of the suicidal person that wants to live. Underscore the person's importance to his significant others and affirm the remaining positive aspects of his life. Commit yourself to working with the part of the person that wants to live.

Provide Hope

Support the fact that the suicidal person has not always felt this badly. Encourage discussion of times when he felt more hopeful. Remind the distraught person of his resources and provide hope that things will not remain this intolerable forever. Create as much action in positive directions as possible in order to demonstrate how things are likely to change. Direct discussions to times in the past when the person felt badly, and focus on what happened then to help alleviate the situation. While it may be tempting, avoid offering false hope or platitudes such as: "You're still young and you have your whole life ahead of you," or "You're such a strong person, I know you can get through this." Such statements do not provide support, rather they diminish the depressed person's confidence and trust in the concerned other.

Determine What Has Provided Meaning in the Past

Often the suicidal person has been living in an unhappy life situation for some time prior to the onset of an acute suicidal crisis. Reinforce and focus on whatever has provided meaning in the person's life to allow him to have lived this long. Especially important aspects are those which have provided feelings of self-esteem, self-worth and pleasure. Such experiences may be derived from children, grandchildren, lovers, friends, relatives, hobbies or even social causes. In some instances, only the concern for the welfare of a loyal pet may be found to provide sufficient reason to continue living. If such is the case, reinforce the concern by asking the suicidal person, "What would happen to 'Fido' if you killed yourself?"

Explore Death Fantasies

At times suicidal people have unrealistic fantasies about their death. They may envision that they will be able to attend their own funeral, or be able to experience the reactions of their survivors. Let the suicidal person know that as far as we can tell, this is not so. Avoid philosophical debates about death issues, but work to negate or deromanticize their notions about death. Point out that death will come to all of us eventually, and further that no one knows what death is like, we know only that it is not like being alive. Moreover, discuss the possible consequences of an aborted suicide attempt where the individual may become maimed or helpless as the result of an unsuccessful suicide attempt.

Discuss Reactions of Survivors, Especially Children

Discuss the possible reaction the suicide will have on the person's family, friends and especially children. Share the fact that suicide was once considered to be a genetic trait as it seems to run in families. While we now know that this phenomenon is not genetic in origin, it does seem to be a learned way of coping with stress. Ask the suicidal person if he is aware of the possible consequences his suicide would have on his loved ones; most certainly he does not want to inflict this trauma on them.

Discuss Responsibility

Discuss the fact that the ultimate decision is his. No one can stop a person from taking his own life. Suicide may often be used as a manipulation to control the behavior of another. When this occurs, it is important to tell the suicidal person that you do not want him to kill himself, but that you will not accept the responsibility for his death, that it is ultimately his choice, and although you care greatly and see hope for his situation getting better, you cannot prevent him from acting out. Be sure to then discuss the person's ambivalence and other concerns delineated in this section.

Reinforce Professional Help

Bring in new resources. Consult local suicide prevention centers which can provide consultations, intervention, treatment and referrals. Reinforce the fact that with professional help the suicidal person may be able to find relief from his pain and be able to institute changes more quickly and efficiently. However, be sure not to provide false hope. Therapy is no magic answer, and the individual will need to be motivated to work with the mental health professional and to give the endeavor sufficient time to produce symptom relief.

BIBLIOGRAPHY

Allen, N. H. *Suicide in California: 1960–1970.* State of California: Department of Public Health, 1973.

Durkheim, E. *Suicide: A Study in Sociology,* (2nd ed., 1930), translated by Spaulding, J. A. and Simpson, G. Glencoe, Ill.: Free Press, 1951.

Farberow, N. L., and Shneidman, E. S. (Eds.), *The Cry for Help.* New York: McGraw-Hill Book Co., 1961.

Freud, S. Mourning and Melancholia. In *Collected Papers,* Vol. 4. London: Hogarth Press, Ltd., 1949.

Menninger, K. *Man Against Himself.* New York: Harcourt, Brace and World, Inc., 1938.

Mitchell, M. E. *The Child's Attitude to Death.* New York: Schocken Books, 1967.

Resnik, H. L. P. (Ed.). *Suicidal Behaviors: Diagnosis and Management.* Boston: Little Brown and Co., 1968.

Shneidman, E. S., and Farberow, N. L. (Eds.). *Clues to Suicide.* New York: McGraw-Hill Book Co., 1957.

Chapter **16**

alcohol abuse
and
the family

CAROL EDGERTON MITCHELL

The American family, our traditional support system, reflects our culture's stress and strain. Both analytic investigations and sensitized experience point to its indices of cumulative stress: mounting reports of child abuse, accelerating divorce rate and, even, cumbersome numbers of our "worried well," those family members whose somatic ills stem from troubled psyches. Both a cause and an effect of interpersonal tension, alcohol abuse needs to be considered in any assessment of family stress.

An estimated nine million Americans, or 7% of our adult population, abuse alcohol (Alcoholism in the United States, 1974, pp. 3-5). Conservative estimates suggest that, with each of these individuals, the lives of five "significant others," — child, friend, spouse, employee, sibling, parent — are intricately interwoven. Significance of the problem involves every family. The interrelationships of community, personal and family disorganization attendant upon alcohol misuse are inescapable. The financial toll, over 25 billion dollars a year (Alcoholism in the United States, 1974, pp. 3-5), includes the cost of burned buildings, automobile injuries and deaths, drownings and industrial accidents (Baker et al., 1974, pp. 318-324; Dietz and Baker, 1974, pp. 303-

311; Hollis, 1974, pp. 8-10). Since alcohol damages every body system, costs for such treatment and convalescence must be included. Physical implications and treatments are expanding. Only recently, severe congenital anomalies associated with use of alcohol during pregnancy have been identified. The brain damage and musculoskeletal defects are irreversible (N.I.A.A.A., July 29, 1976). Alcohol abuse within the family distorts communication and alters essential behavior patterns. It has been identified as causative in almost 40% of divorces (N.I.A.A.A., March 30, 1976). Parental alcoholism is also associated with child neglect (especially when alcohol incapacitates the mother) and child abuse (N.I.A.A.A., October 6, 1974). Whether from learned behavior or genetic predisposition, children of alcohol abusing parents often repeat the cycle. Young people's drinking seems to have increased, as does that of the elderly. Their and others' personal distress compounds the cost analysis but eludes total summation.

Alcohol is our favorite drug. We use it to ease social relationships, to dull pain and to deflect anxiety. Its contribution to our economy is evident in its advertising portion of all levels of media. Less evident, but more generous, is its 10 billion dollar contribution to federal and state taxes (Becker, 1977). One has only to politely decline alcoholic beverages for a single month to estimate alcohol's position in our patterns of living. Yet, the line between use and misuse, social drinker and alcoholic, is often obscure. Debating the intricacies of a diagnosis can obscure the need for intervention and serve as sanction for acceleration of "the problem" until it merits an unequivocal diagnosis. Cutting through these categorical ambiguities, the National Council of Alcoholism has devised an exhaustive physiological and behavioral criteria system for diagnosis and also has defined the condition quite simply, as a state of "pathological dependency on ethanol." The disease is chronic and progressive; both physiological and emotional signs and symptoms mark its three main stages as: early (drink and live), middle (live to drink), and late (drink to live) (Mitchell, 1976, p. 513). Neither age, sex, nor economic status clearly differentiate the victims. While a genetic predisposition to alcoholism has been identified, environmental variables seem to trigger the condition. Certainly, family and other support system stability is a mitigating or, conversely, an instigating factor. When comfortable traditions establish a regulatory framework for drinking behaviors, alcohol abuse lessens. Conversely, culturally mobile groups whose traditional frames of reference are disrupted, show higher incidence of abuse.

This disruption may be the significant factor in the alcohol abuse evident in mobile, nuclear families. Both geographic and economic mobility have fractured their stabilizing framework. Ours is a restless — almost nomadic — society. Migration tends to strip away familiar support systems and to introduce additional demands for adaptation even while it obscures the new group norms that are necessary for cultural integration. The social restraints inherent in familiar networks, the perceived self-responsibility associated with "being known," rather than anonymous are lost; presentation of self in an unmeasured setting is the new necessity. Each family member must negotiate an "operating space" in the new environment. Economic mobility does much

the same. Even in a society where upward progression is the expectation, if not the fact, the "rules" for managing its demands may be unknown. Stresses normally accompany change. Yet, changelessness in a changing world can be equally stressful. Geographic stability when the significant others leave; economic stability while others progress; these are the reverse side of the coin and are equally demanding. Alcohol is a popular over-the-counter drug for stress: its short term "tranquility" is evident, its long term disruptions are obscure.

Mobile or static, challenges abound as a family negotiates the ordinary and extraordinary events of living; when these adaptation efforts are distorted by alcohol abuse, the normal challenges become threatening obstacles. While alcohol use is socially sanctioned by many families, its misuse is feared and stigmatized. Through stigmatization, the guilt, anger or apprehension experienced by the observer is redirected and focused upon the victim, or alcohol abuser. While this lends a certain comfort, a sense of "You, not I," safety to the observer, it also encourages acceptance of negative role by the stigmatized. As a family system mirrors the collective image of its members, the stigma of one member is generally shared by the others. The label, alcoholic, threatens both individual and family status and encourages denial and mutual evasion by its members. A family that is able to seek appropriate assistance for most threats to its well-being may close ranks in secrecy when the threat is alcohol abuse. Individuals within that family may repeat the process, shielding their own awareness from a fellow member's stigma-threatening problem. The energy that might go into adaptive change is, instead, channeled into a system of mutual deception. Group and individual withdrawal from community contacts may be an important part of this reaction. When each contact is seen as a threat of discovery and stigmatization rather than an opportunity for help or improvement, it will be avoided. Children learn to meet their friends away from home or, perhaps, give up having friends. Parents and spouses do the same. Avoidance, resentment, guilt, hostility, depression: the tightly circumscribed emotions grow from each other and spiral into increasingly maladaptive behavior.

Myths prosper in such an atmosphere of ambiguity. For man is a fairly rational creature and derives a sense of power from his perceived control of his environment. The unknown threatens. Even as does the wider culture, each family develops a system of myths designed to explain the unexplicable. "If it's any problem at all, it's Dad's, and no concern for me or anyone else." "Alcoholics are skid-row bums, my wife's no alcoholic." "Junior high drinking; no way, those kids are too young for alcohol." These myths mask the unknown; they bridge ambiguity and represent their pseudo-reality as a manageable, controllable Truth. This comfort factor encourages their self-perpetuation even while their substitution of half-known for unknown discourages the eventual discovery of more-known.

Attitudes intertwine with myths, providing rational/emotional templates for personalized behavior. If the myth advises that alcohol is "joy juice," and that drinkers are merry, then the family's attitudes covering happiness, pleasure principle, good times and responsibility weave into their perception of both the myth and the reality of their own — and others' — alcohol usage. The myth-attitude alliance offers short-cut, well patterned interaction responses. Like habits, these customary responses are almost automatic, rising by cue and comfortably avoiding any arduous exploration for reality. As with the myths, there is a generalized cultural sharing of the attitudes which, in turn, tends to encourage their wider acceptance as indisputable.

Myth-attitudes form a powerful duo. They clutter relationships with their distorted reality and interfere with problem detection and solution. Particular interventions are needed to stem their negative impact. For family or individual, a strategy design includes: 1) detection of alcohol's myth-attitudes, 2) examination for factual versus mythological content, 3) analysis of significance, 4) communication of findings and 5) evaluation of the response.

1. Pat answers, blanket statements and global generalizations are all hallmarks of myths. Their attitudinal component is evidenced by a consistent mental state. The diagnostic emotional twinge may be fleeting, censored by cultural "oughts and shoulds," but its honesty and consistency advise of its reality. Attitudes are durable and tend to persist even after the pseudo-facts that supported them have been discounted. They can yield to thoughtful analysis.

2. Examine the statements for factual or mythological content. Detective work is indicated here, for actuality may seem elusive. Yet, alcohol abuse is of such increasing concern that information sources are now sprinkled throughout the community. Since facts and figures in an individual's data base are fairly amenable to change, knowledge offers a potential leverage necessary for modification of deeply entrenched attitudes.

3. Through analysis, the significance of the myth-attitudes partnership can be determined. Their endurance is meaningful when seen in context of the effect they create, the sanctions they imply for family, individual or community behavior. The sanctions emerge as a major cause for the myths' self-perpetuation; their analysis can suggest areas for intervention.

4. Myth-attitudes are symbiotic. The removal of one party's contribution cuts off the process of interdependency. But the short-circuits need to be publicized. For while solitary knowledge is particularly vulnerable to self-doubt, openly shared knowledge is more contagious than the murmured secrecy of mythology. Sharing promotes physical and emotional energy.

5. An honest objectivity is the best safeguard of myth eradication lest new myths substitute for old. The dynamic cycles of insight are responsive to new understanding even as the brittle stereotypes of myths are staunchly defended from fearful change. Response of the individual or family unit should illustrate a freeing of energy, once bound in emotional defense, for problem solving and mutual growth.

STRATEGIES IN ACTION

An analysis of some representative alcohol myth-attitude combinations reveals their interactional patterns. These "Fact and Fancy," "Tried and Only Truism," conditioned responses have directed family and community efforts to cope with ambiguity of alcohol abuse. These myths are common; not universal; enduring; not eternal. Accessible to our five-step intervention strategy, they yield fresh insight into the dynamics — and challenge — of alcohol abuse while they also suggest alternatives for action.

Myth I: There's No Cure for Alcoholism; It Is a Hopeless Situation.

Attitude. Includes inadequacy, resignation, boredom.

Fact. Present research studies confirm the experience of many; at this time no cure has been established for alcoholism — nor for myopia or hypertension. Effective treatment is available for remission and control of what is now considered a chronic, progressive disease.

Analysis. Hopelessness negates expectation for improvement and also excuses all parties from participating in efforts designed for such a goal. Hopelessness is a license for maintaining the status quo; it blocks energy that might otherwise be engaged in alteration of troublesome behavior patterns, both those of the victim and of those around him. A family might respond to this message of hopelessness by withholding emotional support. The "victim" in turn, might withhold self, disengaging from proffered supports and accepting the perceived consignment to eventual failure. The community is sanctioned to withhold both financial and moral support of treatment programs.

Myth II: Alcoholics Are Irresponsible.

Attitude. Includes exasperation, amusement, anger, fear.

Fact. Alcoholics are individuals with individual perceptions of responsibility. Some people, who are also alcoholics, effectively function in highly responsible positions. Others, also alcoholic, experience successive disasters as a consequence of their drinking. Ethanol progressively distorts finer thought processes, interferes with memory, can be physiologically addictive and fosters emotional dependence.

Analysis. Responsibility civilizes autonomy. A label of irresponsibility cancels any expectation of independent, conscientious, trustworthy, dependable behavior. It per-

mits dependency and capricious, asocial response from the labeled and also permits distrust and appropriately controlling behaviors from the labelers. The adult who is "irresponsibly alcoholic," is treated as a wayward — or evil — child by family and community. Endured with hostility even while shielded from the cause-effect consequences of his own behavior, this individual is encouraged to regress to — or stagnate in — a child-like state.

Myth III: The Problem Is the Alcoholic's, Only.

Attitude. Includes denial, inattention, futility.

Fact. Alcohol is associated with half of automobile deaths; its usage correlates with suicide, homicide, child abuse, pedestrian accidents, mental hospital admissions, drownings, household fires and domestic violence (Mitchell, 1976). We are all involved with the problem drinker.

Analysis. Permission for withdrawal of support and involvement is at the heart of this myth. If the problem area is circumscribed apart from the personal boundaries of family and community, it can be appropriately ignored. For the alcohol abuser, this permits a fantasy that the whole of the pain experienced in the situation is his own, and suggests an unreal discontinuity in the family system's emotional and behavioral linkages. For the family, the myth discourages their group and individual efforts to modify their distressing situation. Although the emotions are less charged, a similar discontinuity, equally false, is portrayed to the community. The implicit message, once more, is of excusable noninvolvement.

Myth IV: Alcoholics are Skid Row Derelicts.

Attitude. Includes fear, self-doubt, anxiety, disgust.

Fact. Less than 5% of problem drinkers have worked their way into a skid row existence. The remaining 95% represent employed, or employable, individuals. Statistics have identified 18% of professionals, 30% of businessmen and 38% of technical workers as heavy drinkers (Rosenberg, 1971, pp. 25–35).

Analysis. Considerable comfort and emotional safety accompany this stereotype. By distancing and obscuring the problem through its assignment to a well-defined and socially stigmatized sub-group, its threat is seemingly contained. Since skid row is usually a considerable geographic distance from most of the community and family members, it conveys an emotional distance as well. Within their circumscribed territory, skid rowers are conspicuous. If they represent alcohol abuse, equally severe alcohol problems in the traditionally "safe" areas of the community seem inoffensive by contrast.

Myth V: Drinking Is Something One Shouldn't Talk About.

Attitude. Includes confusion, fear, embarassment, guilt.

Fact. The health hazards of alcohol abuse are little different than those associated with diabetes, venereal disease, emphysema or tuberculosis. Health workers expect—and are expected—to offer information and guidance in health-related matters. Family members, too, are generally concerned with the health of their members. Usual efforts to maintain group health and stability have widespread acceptability.

Analysis. When alcohol misuse is seen as a moral dilemma, a hopeless downward spiral or, at times, a partnership in collusion, this myth of secrecy reflects the perception and redirects its conflicting emotions. Reluctant to publicly point a stigmatizing finger, that is to suggest a problem of alcoholism, the significant other can conjure up excuses for heavy lunchtime drinking, lack of coordination behind the steering wheel or verbal abuse at the dinner table. For silence, one more face of denial, seems to effectively remove the responsibility for intervention and its attendant vulnerabilities. While it may shield the onlooker from involvement, silence also persuades the alcohol abuser that "this little problem" is discrete, of no consequence to others.

Myth VI: Alcohol: Good Old Joy Juice.

Attitude. Includes patronizing, defensiveness, denial.

Fact. Alcohol is a potent drug. It affects every human body system and has an affinity for nerve tissue. It is a depressant, sedat-

ing the central nervous system and impairing motor coordination. An ounce of ethanol—one typical drink—can be metabolized, on the average, every hour. A 0.05% blood alcohol, equivalent to two drinks, is associated with loosened thought and judgment. At 0.20%, the individual is obviously intoxicated and at blood level 0.30%, he may be unconscious (Alcohol & Alcoholism, 1972, p. 4). Various drug interactions are a particular challenge; alcohol multiplies the effectiveness of analgesics (including both aspirin and morphine) as well as antidepressants, barbiturates, antidiabetics and vasodilators; it has an additive effect with muscle relaxants and inhibits anticoagulants (*Alcohol Interactions*, 1974, pp. 1–10).

Analysis. Calculated underestimation of ethanol's potency gives permission for experimentation in its usage. The innocuous label discourages restraint on the part of the drinker and encourages constraint on the part of others. Forbearance is suggested, whether it be for a pre-teen, "acting grown-up," a senior citizen's "recreational drinking," or a young mother "taking a morning nip to settle her nerves." The myth artfully avoids reality and promotes family, community and self-deception.

Myth VII: Can't Do Anything Before the Drinker "Bottoms Out."

Attitude. Helplessness, inadequacy, anger are included.

Fact. "Bottom out" is a subjective state recognized in retrospect. The point where the downward drinking course is reversed becomes the bottom. Therapeutic interventions have initiated and supported change at every stage of alcohol abuse. As with all chronic conditions, the reversal process may require persistent repetition.

Analysis. This myth neatly packages a fail-safe promise. If interventions are launched, and fail, the failure is covered by this myth. If no interventions are launched, this, too, is covered with the rationalization that the nadir was not yet achieved. Laissez-faire is the implicit message. In any health situation, motivated clients seem benign while resistance threatens professional esteem. Yet, the vigorous medical outreach that characterizes low compliance health areas of hypertension and respiratory disease is conspicuously absent in alcohol abuse. When an acute situation of alcoholism is thrust upon family — or community — awareness, categorical interventions are made: supervised detoxification, X-rays as needed, supportive nutritional therapy. Within this framework of routinized interventions, the observers' manner may be guarded, wary; is this episode a bottoming out? Will there be a request — a motivation — for change? Without the abuser's clear plea for help, the care given may be mechanical, task-oriented, designed more to satisfy the measure of professional competence than that of human need.

Myth VIII: Draw Your Own Myth.

Attitude. Includes complex interaction of personal and cultural response.

Fact. There are countless myths that govern our reactions to alcohol abuse and abusers. Artifacts from an outgrown past, many are shared, some are uniquely individual. They all defy — or distort — essential facts and then flourish in the fantasy.

Analysis. The stereotyped response accompanies the myth and gives it significance. The myth-linked attitude of the drinker intercepts that of the family, they interact on their impersonal level, deflected from the human reality they obscure. The ensuing impersonal distortion of drinker contacts the impersonal distortion of observer and the pseudo-reality is further reinforced for both parties.

CONCLUSION

The myths that obstruct our relationships and understandings can yield to factual information and honest analysis. When a truism surfaces, check it; when an "instant attitude" intrudes, consider it fairly. As this style of open inquiry becomes base line behavior for health workers, so will it be reflected by clients, their families and communities. The "tough love" or realistic humanism it entails, facilitates adaptive growth. Whether somatic complaint or emotional distress initiates detection of a problem centered with alcohol abuse, this reality-tempered concern is designed for effectiveness.

The process of communication, detection, analysis and evaluation of alcohol-related myths is started in this chapter. Each contact between health worker and family member is an opportunity for extension and refinement of the process. The myths of alcohol abuse are susceptible to change. While new mythology is possible, the present social environment of more open inquiry offers an unparalleled opportunity for its substitution by reality and positive growth. As a family's interaction style moves beyond the clutter of ancient myths, it can become responsive to individual needs rather than reactive to stereotypes. In this kind of atmosphere, difficulties can be negotiated with honesty; successes can be recognized and shared. Health and personal benefits for the family as a system and for the individuals involved are immeasurable. As with the cost of alcohol abuse, the benefits of understanding influence us all.

BIBLIOGRAPHY

Alcohol & Alcoholism: Problems, Programs & Progress. Washington, D.C.: National Institute of Mental Health, DHEW Pub. No. (HSM) 72-9127. 1972.

Alcohol Interactions. Philadelphia: Smith Kline & French Laboratories, 1974.

Alcoholism in the United States. In *Statistical Bulletin.* Vol. 55. New York: Metropolitan Life Insurance Co., July 1974.

Baker, S., Robertson, L., and O'Neill, B. Fatal pedestrian collisions. *Am. J. Pub. Hth.,* Vol. 64, No. 4, April, 1974.

Becker, C. E. Diagnosis, treatment, rationale, pharmacological agents. Unpublished. (Address: San Rafael, California, Feb. 24, 1977).

Beebe, J. E., III. Evaluation and treatment of the drinking patient. In *Psychiatric Treatment, Crisis/Clinic/Consultation.* Rosenbaum and Beebe (Eds.). New York: McGraw-Hill Book Co., 1975.

Dietz, P. and Baker, S. Drowning, epidemiology and prevention. *Am. J. Public Health,* 64: (4) 1974.

Hollis, W. S. Fire Deaths and Drinking. In *Alcohol Health and Research World.* Maryland: National Institute on Alcohol Abuse and Alcoholism, DHEW Pub. No. (ADM) 75-157, 1974.

Mitchell, C. E. Assessment of alcohol abuse. *Nurs. Outlook* 24 (8), 1976.

Mitchell, C. E. Community health nurses and community mental health. In *Community Health Nursing: Patterns and Practice.* Archer and Fleshman (Eds.). North Scituate, Mass.: Duxbury Press, 1975.

N.I.A.A.A. Information & Feature Service. U.S. National Institute of Alcohol and Alcoholism. No. 22, March 30, 1976.

N.I.A.A.A. Information & Feature Service. No. 26,

July 29, 1976.

N.I.A.A.A. Information & Feature Service. No. 28, October 6, 1976.

Older problem drinkers. In *Alcohol Health and Research World.* National Institute on Alcohol Abuse and Alcoholism, DHEW Pub. No. (ADM) 75-157, 1975.

Rosenberg, S. (Ed.) *Alcohol and Health.* Washington, D.C.: National Institute on Alcohol Abuse and Alcoholism, DHEW Pub. No. (ADM) 74-68, 1971.

The economic cost of alcohol misuse. In *Alcohol Health and Research World.* National Institute on Alcohol Abuse and Alcoholism, DHEW Pub. No. (ADM) 75-157, Winter 1974/75.

Chapter 17

family-focused intervention

SHERILYN CARPENTER

There has been a fair amount written about the nurse therapist working with the intact family in a family therapy setting. This is usually not the condition under which the nurse works with families. The nurse has the opportunity and does work in circumstances taxing her creativity, intuition, emotions, reasoning powers and problem-solving ability. Contact with a family in any setting presents a great challenge to branch out into new, unexplored areas. Feedback and exploration from peers and supervisors is an essential component of the nurse's experience in family-related situations. The nurse's impact can be great. The interrelatedness of the family is very complicated and seen as critical to the emotional well-being of its individuals.

The family-related settings in which nurses find themselves include homes of functional and dysfunctional families, nursery schools, community mental health centers, convalescent hospitals, acute hospitals, service centers and family planning and other clinics.

The role of the nurse can and should evolve to include consideration of the entire family. At a Head Start program in a rural area a nurse identified a 5-year-old child as having serious medical problems. She made a home visit to get medical and develop-

mental history. The child had not been seen by a doctor since birth. The nurse explained there was reason for concern and asked for consent to seek resources for a medical exam. Specialized resources were scarce in the area. When she returned in what she considered a reasonable length of time, the father confronted her about the scarcity of information she had given. A high level of concern had been aroused by her visit. She then realized the impact of her initial visit on the total family and the necessity of talking with them about their feelings.

The nurse is in a unique position. She spends large amounts of time with families as they go through the normal crises of their life cycle. Every crisis or change has the potential for growth or dysfunctional adaptation. She can anticipate problems needing interventional or facilitate growth resulting in a better quality of family life. Consider the impact of the birth of the first child, postpartum depression, death of an elderly spouse or crises around illness and debilitation. Nurses also spend sustained time with families who are under stress due to sociocultural factors such as race and socioeconomic circumstances, and who may never have significant contact with mental health professionals.

We feel that the nurse can and often

does provide therapeutic interventions at crucial points in a family's life, but she has not been prepared to conceptualize or evaluate her interventions in the context of the family system.

This chapter will endeavor to help her formulate interventions keeping the family in mind, to evaluate families for appropriate referral and to coordinate her work with family therapists. Hopefully we will pique the interest of those nurses who might want to receive further training to provide family therapy specifically.

HISTORY

In the 1950's a part of the research on schizophrenia by such eminent psychiatrists as Don Jackson, Nathan Ackerman, Theodore Lidz, Boszormenyi-Nagy and Gregory Bateson focused on the relationship of the schizophrenic and family members. Out of this research Bateson, Jackson and Haley developed the theory of the Double Bind in Communication (Haley, 1959, pp. 357–374) which we will discuss later. This is a basic element in many dysfunctional families.

About the same time the Child Guidance Movement also pioneered treating the entire family by breaking the tradition of seeing only the individual. Starting with collateral interviews with family members, primarily the parents, they moved toward occasional family conferences. The next logical step was treatment of the family unit.

John E. Bell, starting in early 1950's, was one of the first therapists to use family therapy as the sole means of treatment (Bell, 1975).

DEFINITION OF FAMILY

There are many definitions of family. A family is a group usually comprised of two parents and children, of immediate kindred, living in one house and usually descended from a common progenitor. Some important functions of the family include providing for the physical and emotional needs of the adults as well as the children, rearing of the young, and providing the opportunity for continued close relationships. It is looked upon as a primary resource for all its members. Virginia Satir adds to these the following functions of . . . cooperation

economically by division of labor, transmission of culture, emancipation of young adults, a provision for eventual care of the parents . . . (Satir, 1967, p. 21). This definition points to a time element with progression through developmental stages.

Typical families go through a process called "The Family Life Cycle," a theory presented by Duvall (1967). She says, "families grow through predictable stages of development that can be understood in terms of development of the individual family members and of the family as a whole" (Duvall, 1967, p. v). Within this theory there are two basic ideas. One is that families expand and then contract in size as they progress through the cycle. A family is first developed when two people come together and it expands further as children are added. Contraction takes place as children leave the home. During each of the eight stages of expansion and contraction there are certain developmental tasks which must be carried out for the biological, social and emotional survival of the family. These include physical maintenance, allocation of resources, division of labor, socialization of family members, reproduction, recruitment and release of family members, maintenance of order, placement of members in the larger society, maintenance of motivation and morale.

The tasks are addressed in eight phases as described by Duvall (1967, p. 9) (see Table 1).

Another definition recognizes the family as a unit, an entity, a system, a small social group (Hill, 1965). It is this definition that has contributed most to the current field of family therapy. It recognizes the power of the family—the whole is greater than the sum of its parts, the effect of cooperative action of the unit is greater than independent action of its members. This definition recognizes the vulnerability of the family since the unit is weakened by stress of one of its members. This concept is expanded when we talk about homeostasis.

THEORIES AND CONCEPTS

Some of the basic concepts and theories of family therapy have been drawn from other fields—homeostasis from physiology, communication from language arts, roles

TABLE 1. EIGHT STAGES OF FAMILY DEVELOPMENT

Phase	Family Phase	Family Description
I	Beginning Family	Married couple without children
II	Childbearing Family	Oldest child up to 30 months
III	Families of PreSchool Children	Oldest 30 months to 6 years
IV	Families of School Children	Oldest 6 to 13 years
V	Families with Teenagers	Oldest 13 to 20 years
VI	Families as Launching Centers	First child gone to last leaving
VII	Families in the Middle Years	Empty nest to retirement
VIII	Aging Families	Retirement to death of both spouses

from sociology, and family life cycles from human development. As stated earlier, we will describe a family, then relate concepts to the functioning of this family. The concepts to be discussed and related to the Thomas family are homeostasis, communication, family rules, family myths and roles.

Evelyn Thomas was referred to a mental health clinic by her physician. She had complained of pains in her chest. Physical examination was negative and the doctor became aware of multiple family problems.

Mr. Thomas was unemployed, depressed and becoming increasingly discouraged. He alternated between taking over homemaking responsibilities and just sitting for long periods of time. As he became more active in his parenting role, unresolved conflicts between him and the children became more pronounced. Mrs. Thomas felt that her special time with the children was being infringed upon. The two quarreled constantly.

In addition, there were financial worries. The oldest son was getting ready to move out on his own. Recently, following a death in the family, their mentally retarded nephew had come to live with them.

Mrs. Thomas showed the most distress as a result of all these changes in her family.

Homeostasis

In looking at a family as a unit, "homeostasis implies the relative constancy of the internal environment, a constancy, however, which is maintained by a continuous interplay of dynamic forces" (Jackson, 1968, pp. 1–2).

With a change in Mr. Thomas' life this created an imbalance in the family. Mr. Thomas, after losing his job spent more time at home. His wife tried to relate to him in some old ways and became overwhelmed with his dependency and demands for attention. Before this time, there had been no need to deal with his demands on a long term basis because he was at work. Now she needed to set limits on her time and renegotiate child-rearing roles. She was referred to an assertiveness training group to help her express her thoughts more clearly.

Like most of the women in the group she went through upheaval in her marital relationship after she could more clearly express what she wanted and had developed more self-esteem. Her change of self-concept and communication upset the balance in the marital relationship because her husband had a complementary way of responding to the old forms of interaction. It became obvious that the extent to which her husband was able to participate in establishing a new homeostasis determined the growth in the relationship. Changes in the wife necessitated changes in the husband. At the beginning he was motivated to maintain the original homeostasis and force her back into her old forms of relating. The couple was referred for marital counselling.

Communication

Family interaction is always communicative. It is, therefore, understandable that communication as a concept, a theory and a tool for therapy is a common thread throughout the literature. Its importance to any discussion of family therapy is paramount. For example, the double-bind theory developed by Jackson and Haley and considered a primary cause of mental illness is a communication process. The double-bind is the communicative process wherein one receives, over a prolonged period of time, two contradictory messages or messages wherein words and actions are incongruent and wherein one is conditioned not to ask for clarification (Satir, 1967, p. 36). This happens within the family setting and, in the case of children, an added detrimental aspect is that they cannot leave and avoid the problematic interaction of confusing environment. A goal of family therapy is to help the family improve and/or develop new communication. Rosemary Henrion (1974, pp. 10–13) provides a good framework for the nurses' use of communication in working with families.

Virginia Satir, who sees communication problems as the root of family problems, has developed her approach around teaching families to communicate better. For further explanation of this central work refer to *Conjoint Family Therapy* (Satir, 1967).

Communication is a very complex process. Messages are composed of four parts: the sender, the message, the receiver, and the context (Haley, 1959, pp. 357–374) and there can be breakdown in several or any one of these components.

Communication is also nonverbal. People touch; they make nonverbal sounds such as finger tapping or key jangling; they make vocal sounds such as sighing. Appearance, facial expressions, posture and gestures, proximation (arrangement of self in space) are ways of communicating. Acting out or acting up is a way of communicating.

Families develop their own private communication system. Frequently the nonverbal is preferred or used interchangeably with verbal. Sometimes nonverbal represents a breakdown in verbal communication (as in spankings). Nonverbal communication is not always conscious; it is sometimes "mutually contradictory" to verbal communication.

It is important for the nurse to first understand a family's unique and private communication and then teach, by her own example, to request clarification, to check out, and to actively listen. The specifics about such skills are spelled out in *Parent Effectiveness Training* (Gordon, 1970) and *The Dynamic Family* (Luthman and Kirschenbaum, 1974).

Families as a unit as well as the individuals who comprise the family want to be heard and the realization that they are being heard can in itself reduce anxiety, fears or anger which are blocking the problem-solving process and make room for positive feelings. It is essential for the nurse either in the context of family therapy or in any setting to have specific training in communication skills.

Both Mr. and Mrs. Thomas used time with the nurse to ventilate their anxieties, fears and anger, providing the relief needed to start problem-solving. With the nurse as a model and aided by Mrs. Thomas' experience in Assertive Training, the couple sought clearer communication. They stopped trying to read each other's mind and making assumptions and therefore stopped manipulating interactions to get what they wanted.

Mr. Thomas' long-standing habit of lecturing the children became more intolerable now that he was home so much. The children became resentful and his lectures interfered with the day-to-day more effective communication Mrs. Thomas had with the children. Mr. Thomas gained insight about his one-way communication and its effect on his relationship with the children.

Family Rules

Families are rule-governed systems (Jackson, 1965, pp. 1–19). The rules can be inferred by observing for repetitive behavior. Family rules have five unique characteristics according to Riskin, as quoted in Ford and Herrick (1974, pp. 61–69):
1. Family rules are seldom explicit.
2. They are abstractions which may be inferred from behavior.
3. They are repetitive and redundant.
4. The family rules have rules themselves.
5. The family rules have autonomy and tend to perpetuate themselves.

There are larger and smaller rules. The larger rules "express a philosophy, contain a definition, and refer to a theoretical idea or a goal. They have character and style." (Ford and Herrick, 1974, p. 62) These are what are referred to as family life styles. Five are enumerated by Ford and Herrick (1974, pp. 62–67):
1. Children come first.
2. Two against the world.
3. Share and share alike.
4. Every man for himself.
5. Until death do us part.

The long-standing rule governing the Thomas family system was that the children always come first. Not enough attention had been given to individual needs or to the establishment of a positive marital relationship.

Mrs. Thomas continued to put energy into the increasing demands of the children, developing physical symptoms under the added stress of her husband's despair. And Mr. Thomas, in keeping with the rule, did not express his needs directly, but instead resorted to manipulative behavior.

At the same time the children expected the same full attention they had always received. They resented their cousin, who had special needs, and their mother's time with their father, and they acted-out to regain the attention to which they were accustomed.

Family rules should be openly explored, so family members can become aware of the influences of these rules on their behavior.

By bringing out the Thomas' rule of the children always coming first, both parents realized they had cut off support they could give each other.

There are also smaller rules which have to do with the operation or mechanics of the system, such as how one communicates, expression of feelings, and ideas of right or wrong.

Family Myths

Also influencing life style are family myths. These myths involve the family's belief system and in turn determine feelings and behavior (Glick and Kessler, 1974, p. 30). Rigid adherence to the myths is dysfunctional. Luthman and Kirschenbaum (1974, p. 157) talk about the family survival myth, patterns of survival upon which dysfunctional families operate. The survival patterns are made up of disturbed interaction and communication patterns, covert rules, and symptomatology. The family supports the myth that each member must play a certain role in order for the family to survive.

Another myth frequently encountered with families is "Who is boss?" This is aptly demonstrated in the Thomas family.

Everyone agreed dad was head of the household. Working and commuting, he was away from home for long periods of time and the myth was sustained. However, unemployed and home all day, it became apparent that his parenting and decision-making skills were not as good as his wife's. While grocery shopping, for example, Mrs. Thomas would hold back, allowing him to make poor choices with their limited money and become resentful. The children resented his interference; they were accustomed to dealing with their mother on a day-to-day basis.

Roles

In family units, some roles are culturally defined such as bread winner, child rearer. Informal roles are developed by the family itself such as peacemaker, faultfinder, the troublemaker, the sick one, the strong one, the clown, etc.

Glick discusses role conflict that arises when there is a disagreement about who sets the rules, who tries to enforce them and what the rules are specifically (Glick and Kessler, 1974, p. 30). It is interesting that many of the shared agreements about who does what are not discussed.

When there has been a role modification, homeostasis is disrupted. The family must face the problem squarely or role distortion will result (Spiegel, 1971, p. 375). Role distortion occurs when a family member feels forced into a role he doesn't want or has not had time to integrate. Intrapsychic or physical symptoms can occur. In the Thomas family, loss of his breadwinner role depressed Mr. Thomas. He became immobilized and was not motivated to find another job. Mrs. Thomas now had to relinquish her homemaker role and take a part-time job with his tacit agreement. She developed physical symptoms.

The children's informal roles were modified. The youngest now had to share his role as "baby" with his cousin. The role of the oldest boy, accustomed to helping mom with daily responsibility for his younger siblings diminished. He reacted with quarreling and faultfinding.

Conflicts around culturally defined roles, not demonstrated by the Thomas family but important to nurses in Community Mental Health, result when two cultures are integrated into a family. An example would be the marriage of an Anglo-American woman, culturally conditioned to expect a partnership relationship in marriage, and a Mexican-American man expecting to be patriarch of the family.

Conflicts also arise when family units integrate into different cultures. Children, primarily through school experiences, tend to acculturate more rapidly, often rejecting the traditional roles of their parents.

The Thomas family had established a homeostasis which was comfortable despite the rigidity of their rules and roles. But their physical and emotional contact was not of a quality or quantity to sustain them at a time of crisis. Also, the crisis forced them to problem-solve together and rely on each other. Through learning to express individual needs, asserting themselves, reevaluating family life style and learning new patterns of communication, they were able to achieve a greater degree of intimacy and contact within the marriage and the family.

ASSESSMENT

Assessment from the beginning of contact with a client or family is essential. It is a continuous process and, in the case of families, is best shared with them to make intervention relevant.

Sobol does an excellent job of spelling out a community health format taking into consideration health problems and practices, physical environment, living conditions, cultural background, and family support systems, including community resources and the extended family. We refer the reader to this work for further elaboration (Sobol and Robischon, 1975).

A good assessment also takes into account the more intangible aspects of family life such as Parad and Caplan's concept of family life-style. They define family life-style as a reasonably stable patterning of family organization or lack of it. Assessment includes family value system, ideas, attitudes, and beliefs which consciously or unconsciously bind the family together; it includes patterning of roles and family communications (Parad and Caplan, 1965, p. 57).

The problem-solving mechanisms unique to each family should be identified (Parad and Caplan, 1965, p. 58). This will enable the nurse to assess the family's ability to cope with stress and the expense to the family, such as in child neglect or exploitation. Children may be asked to care for younger brothers and sisters at the expense of their own social development.

The need-response pattern, the way the family "perceives, respects, and satisfies basic needs of the individual" (Parad and Caplan, 1965, p. 60) should be assessed. Quality of family life also depends on the use of leisure time and social activities.

The family's relationship to the nurse can be an indicator of the family's view of itself in relation to the rest of the world as well as its attitude toward agency and professional help. Fagan (1970) points out that a nurse making home visits is in a unique position of being seen as a helpful resource for the family. She is viewed as approachable and available.

Families vary from what is considered typical or ideal. There are childless families, single parent families, substitute families, and families that have adopted alternate life styles, like communal living. The uniqueness of these families can pose special problems, but that uniqueness itself does not make the family dysfunctional.

THE IDENTIFIED PATIENT WITHIN A FAMILY

Nurses come in contact with individuals with medical and emotional problems. It is wise to view the condition within the family context. Two perspectives are: how families create symptomatalogy and the effect of illness on a family.

Virginia Satir's concept of the "identified patient" aptly describes the first aspect. The identified patient is that family member having symptoms as a direct result of family interaction. He is obviously affected by the pained marital relationship and most subjected to dysfunctional parenting. "a) His symptoms are an 'SOS' about his parents' pain and the resulting family imbalance. b) His symptoms are a message that he is distorting his own growth as a result of trying to alleviate and absorb his parents' pain." (Satir, 1967, p. 2).

When the nurse sees the identified patient as a victim of his family, it is easy to over-identify with and over-protect him, over-looking the facts as Satir points out that "(1) Patients are equally adept at victimizing other members in return, (2) patients help to perpetuate their role as the sick, different or blamed one." (Satir, 1967, p. 3).

Jackson (1965, p. 2) and others noted very significant things about the schizophrenic in relation to his family as they attempted to treat the "Identified Patient" (IP) only: "a) Other family members interfered with, tried to become part of, or sabotaged the individual treatment of the 'sick' member, as though the family had a stake in his sickness. b) Hospitalized or incarcerated patient often got worse or regressed after a visit from family members, as though family interaction had a direct bearing on his symptoms. c) Other family members got worse as the patient got better, as though sickness in one of the family members was essential to the family's way of operating."

Debilitation of children in middle-class American families can cause excessive parental guilt. We are future-oriented and put great stock in our youth. Our orientation toward mastery of our environment forces us to focus on overcoming nature and in turn curing all problems. Debilitation implies waste or lack of worth because the child's process of "becoming" has been stopped. Parents often feel overwhelming depression when they realize their child won't grow to take a responsible role in society (Spiegel, 1971). This leaves the parents in a caretaker role for the rest of their lives.

In the case of the young schizophrenic, many professionals and paraprofessionals put a great deal of emphasis on how the IP is hurting and victimized. This tends to add to a parent's already low self-esteem or defensiveness. Alienation of the family serves only to make the IP's progress rockier. He is already in the system and finds it even harder to separate than the average teenager who leaves home with relatively few ambivalent feelings (Whitaker et al., 1961). Ackerman (1966) is another resource on this subject.

Working with families who have a member with a chronic illness often requires a change of orientation. The medical model focuses on cure which is unrealistic and therefore demoralizing for the nurse. Practice with emphasis on good care and promotion of the best quality of life for that family should be our ultimate goal.

CRISIS

Crisis work with families fits both models of family therapy and crisis intervention. It focuses on communication and problem-solving; the therapist is usually more active and at times directive. The treatment is short term in nature. As in crisis intervention, in general, the minimal goal is to restore the family to pre-crisis level of function and the maximal goal is to help the family grow beyond their pre-crisis level.

Family crises can be situational in nature, such as premature births, physical illness, death and divorce. For a more complete description of the grieving process refer to Erich Lindemann (1965). It is important for the nurse to be aware of this process as she gives support. Many times that is all that is needed.

The crisis can also be maturational as in the assertion of independence of an adolescent. Eliot (1955) and Hill (1965) describe crisis in a family as having five possibilities: 1) dismemberment (i.e., death, hospitalization, war separation); 2) accession (adoption, pregnancy, aged parent comes into home); 3) demoralization (nonsupport, infidelity); 4) demoralization with dismemberment (runaway, desertion); and 5) demoralization with accession (illegitimacy).

The more serious crises are those that have a demoralizing factor. Identifying the source of stress is important and generally in a healthy family external stress will strengthen family ties and internal stress will weaken. As devastating as it may be, loss of the family's home by fire may not have as drastic an effect on the emotional well-being of its members as continual fighting and threats of separation of the parents.

How the family handles the crisis will depend on the nature of the crisis, the state of organization or disorganization, resources of the family, and family's previous experience with crisis.

GROWTH PERSPECTIVES

Instead of looking at families from the perspective of illness and psychiatric pathology we would like the nurse to consider the growth model. Luthman and Kirschenbaum (1974) discuss individuals in a family growing emotionally even during adulthood. Sometimes the growth stops and people show signs of suffering as in depressive symptomatology. Another positive feature is the theory of positive intent (Luthman and Kirschenbaum, 1974, p. 5). Every behavior is based on the intent to grow even though the behavior appears destructive. With this in mind it makes it easier to gain rapport. Sometimes nurses get locked into seeing things only as pathology. Refer to Luthman and Kirschenbaum (1974) for further explanation.

Keeping the growth model in mind the nurse can give a family many tools to enhance family life. She can communicate clearly and clarify family communication giving family members tools to express themselves.

Loss and grieving have been discussed repeatedly as one type of change. Just by being aware of the changes in emotions a person experiences, the nurse will be more apt to explore comfortably such feelings as anger to facilitate grieving.

SELF-AWARENESS

All of us come to our profession with our own set of values, our own myths and rules and roles established in our family of origin. Work in the helping professions demands self-awareness and ability to maintain objectivity and make full use of our empathic qualities. This balance is critical when we meet with families so closely akin to our own that objectivity is hindered; or when we work with families whose culture and life styles are so different that our empathic skills are taxed. Family therapists never lose their vulnerability to these problems. Some family members may activate unresolved conflicts we have or rekindle hurtful areas. Our own therapy and self-awareness groups are helpful. Supervision and consultation are essential. Making good use of consultation and supervision often requires discipline.

CONCLUSIONS

We have come to realize that in most cases it is not possible to treat just the individual. Families are very much affected by and influence the outcome of any treatment plan. Nor can we ignore families in light of the emphasis on prevention and early intervention. This demands that the nurse be aware of the dynamics involved in family life and consider the family from the onset. The following implications follow:

1. The nurse must improve her own skills and knowledge in family-focused interventions.
2. She should be able o assess family dysfunctioning in order to make appropriate referrals and coordinate with family therapists.
3. She should be aware of the many opportunities to enhance family life.

BIBLIOGRAPHY

Ackerman, N. The return to reality. In *Treating the Troubled Family*. New York: Basic Books, 1966.

Bell, J. E. *Family Therapy*. New York: Jason Aronson, 1975.

Duvall, E. *Family Development*. 3rd ed. Philadelphia: J. B. Lippincott Co., 1967, pp. v, 9.

Eliot, T. Handling family strains and shocks. In Becher, H. and Hill, R. (Eds.), *Family Marriage and Parenthood*. Boston: Heath, and Co., 1955.

Fagan, C. *Family-Centered Nursing in Community Psychiatry: Treatment in the Home*. Philadelphia: F. A. Davis, 1970.

Ford, F., and Herrick, J. Family rules: Family life styles. *Am. J. Orthopsychiatry.* 44: 61–69, 1974.

Glick, I., and Kessler, D. *Marital and Family Therapy*. New York: Grune and Stratton, 1974, pp. 16, 30.

Gordon, T. *Parent Effectiveness Training*. New York: Peter H. Wyden, Inc., 1970.

Haley, J. The family of the schizophrenic: A model system. *J. Nerv. Ment. Dis.* 129: 357–374, 1959.

Henrion, R. Family nurse therapist: A model of communication. *J. Psychiatr. Nurs. Mental Health Serv.* 12: 10–13, 1974.

Hill, R. Generic features of families under stress. In Parad, H. J. (Ed.). *Crisis Intervention: Selected Readings*. New York: Family Service Associations of America, 1965.

Jackson, D. The study of the family. *Fam. Proc.* 4: 1–

19, 1965.

Jackson, D. (Ed.) *Communication, Family and Marriage*. Palo Alto: Science and Behavior Books, Inc., 1968, pp. 1–2.

Lindemann, E. Symptomatology and management of acute grief. In Parad, H. J. (Ed.), *Crisis Intervention: Selected Readings*. New York: Family Service Associations of America, 1965.

Luthman, S., and Kirschenbaum, M. Intervention techniques (interactional level). In *The Dynamic Family*. Palo Alto: Science and Behavior Books, Inc., 1974, pp. 5, 157.

Parad, H., and Caplan, G. A framework for studying families in crisis. In Parad, H. (Ed.), *Crisis Intervention: Selected Readings*. New York: Family Service Associations of America, 1965, pp. 57, 58, 60.

Satir, V. *Conjoint Family Therapy*, rev. ed., Palo Alto: Science and Behavior Books, Inc., 1967, pp. 2, 3, 21, 36.

Sobol, E., and Robischon, P. *Family Nursing: A Study Guide*, 2nd ed. St. Louis: C. V. Mosby Co., 1975.

Spiegel, J. Cultural Strains, Family Role Patterns and Intrapsychic Conflicts. In Howells, J. (Ed.), *Theory and Practice of Family Psychiatry*. New York: Brunner-Mazel, Inc., 1971, p. 375.

Spiegel, J. *Transactions: Interplay Between Individual, Family and Society*. (Ch. 5.) New York: Science House, 1971.

Whitaker, C. et al. Countertransference in the treatment of schizophrenia. In Boszormenyi-Nagy, I., and Framo, J. (Eds.), *Intensive Family Therapy*. New York: Harper and Row, 1961.

Chapter 18

helping adolescents in a group home setting

BARBARA R. DUNLAP

When compelled to remove a child from his home, the professional so charged with the task has relatively few choices for action open to him. Constrained by financial and existing facility limitations, the professional seeks to place the child by hopefully substituting one family for another. The rising employment of women, decreasing capability of the mobile nuclear family to cope with children in face of financial or psychosocial crises, and an insufficient supply of family-type substitutes has decreased the likelihood of foster care. Thus, foster care of culturally disadvantaged, emotionally impoverished, disturbed and delinquent children has been gradually replaced over the last 25 years by group or residential care as the preferred mode of placement.

Literature in recent years has begun to show that neither separation from parents, multiple mothering nor long term residence in group settings is necessarily harmful to the emotional and physical development of children. Additional experiments in group care of children in Israel and Eastern Europe have found those in their care healthy in body and mind, and strongly identified with the values of their setting (Wolins, 1974, p. 3). But this move toward group care has not been an easy transition. It is

no simple matter to move away from tradition, especially when the tradition (the family) is seen as psychodynamically and economically functional. Increasingly, it has been recognized that not being able to live with one's family is a considerable emotional insult, no matter why it is necessary (Bettelheim, 1974, p. 102). Extrafamilial settings are suspect though essential. "The family is seen and acknowledged as the natural, as the proper locus for the socializing of children, others are obviously unnatural, improper and at best inadequate and possibly unacceptable." (Wolins, 1974, p. 118) Yet, it remains that some families are unable to care for the needs of their children, for whatever reasons, and those children involved must be cared for in different settings.

Child care institutions, and more recently, halfway house and rehabilitation institutions have moved toward duplicating the externals and character of family living in the organization of their setting. There exists a wide range of models, from a cottage-type institution, to the group home and extended family. Each unit has as many children as would be found in a family—six to eight—with house or cottage child care workers serving as authority figures and as

137

providers. For adolescents, group care seems to be the most effective and successful method of providing for the total physical and emotional needs of the emerging young adult.

For the adolescent in group care, the family is replaced by the group or therapeutic milieu in teaching him to become a somebody rather than a something. Actually, the group and family are interrelated, for family incapacity and group success serve to unlock the usually well guarded gates of the adolescent. The group, as did the family, has the responsibility to be responsive to the needs of its members in every stage of growth. Aside from food and shelter, this means providing opportunities for the acquisition of knowledge and skill in role performance, an atmosphere that provides respect for fluctuations in growth, for failure and tears, and an appreciation for the present (Wolins, 1974, p. 8).

It is generally agreed that "the basic motive of the organism is a drive toward health, and if it is free to move, it must progress in healthy directions." (Combs et al., 1971, p. 75) The problem for those involved with adolescents in group care is how to create the conditions for freedom, those which will set free their striving for fulfillment. When successful at creating those conditions that free, "the individual's own basic drive for actualization and fulfillment can be counted on to move them in those directions." (Combs et al., 1971, p. 75) If these conditions are created, the group can become a way-station where members can pause, take a long look at where they have been and an even harder look at where they may go.

Before an adolescent can begin to care about what the milieu has to offer him, others have to prove that they genuinely care about him, that he is a good person, and that he can obtain a better future than he has had in the past. Thus, the development of trust is what sets the stage and tips the scale in favor of the adolescent's being able to positively utilize the milieu. The adolescent in group care is often seriously impaired in his ability to learn from adults, who have been experienced in the past as unpredictable sources of both support and rejection.

Building a trusting relationship takes time, and involves much testing of limits, rules and regulations to see whether adults are true to their dialogue. In testing the limits of a relationship, the adolescent tries to see whether adults are genuine in what they say and feel toward him. Adults may be tested to see whether they are comfortable with their own emotions. How can someone who expresses affection but not anger be trusted? Rules, expectations and disciplinary measures will be tested for consistency, for flexibility; and more importantly for the strengths and weaknesses of adults—how open they are with who they are and what they feel and believe.

To trust means to open one's self to changes in how one sees oneself and one's relationships. Adolescents in group care typically have distorted self-concepts; their behavior and feelings are a product of how they see themselves and the situation they are in, and it tends to be self-perpetuating. H. S. Sullivan (1953) perceived a potential in individuals to selectively ignore present aspects of their relationships with others. Attributed to early anxiety experiences, opportunities for growth in current relationships are distorted, often with little differentiation between reality and fantasy and expectation. This is often the case with the adolescent, who fits aspects of current relationships into the scenery of the past. It is the role of the adults in the group setting to help the adolescent learn to see himself in another light, to respect himself. The adolescent needs to unlearn old expectations and experience the present in relationships.

Developing trust and redefining one's self-concept is a process in which change comes slowly. Failure to respect the slowness of change can destroy the very things that those involved in a group setting seek. It is necessary to believe in one's efforts as worthwhile and to remain patient, for evidence of change comes slower than the change itself. "The importance of the helper is never entirely without meaning unless the helper makes it so. Life is not reversible. One cannot unexperience what has happened to him. Any meaningful experience or series of experiences may not be sufficient to produce the changes we hope for.

But they are always significant." (Combs et al., 1974, p. 59)

The purpose in the group milieu is furthered by several guidelines, as suggested by Hobbs (1966). First, the teaching of competence can pave the way for self respect and respect by others. This is especially applicable to academic skills, where failure is often a well rooted expectancy. To tolerate the tension and frustration of working toward knowledge and concepts without becoming discouraged or anxious is especially hard for the adolescent who has come to believe himself to be dumb or below average. To push past the "I can't do it" attitude requires encouragement, an unconditional acceptance of him where he is, and an undoubting belief that tasks previously failed at can be achieved. Failure is more often a result of others' expectations rather than actual ability.

Learning to see oneself as able and resourceful comes in part from dialogue with real problems. On paper, an exercise in fractions may appear irrelevant and frustrating, but when applied in the kitchen as in doubling or halving a favorite recipe, fractions become real and something to be discovered. Reading and vocabulary are no longer boring when watching an old silent movie or when looking at the comics, and spelling is important when composing a letter. Wanting to explore a task or problem requires a certain curiosity about the world around us. Too often a frustrating unsuccessful school career will all but destroy an individual's innate need to explore, understand and master. Adults can be significant in helping a turned-off adolescent get turned-on to what is going on around him. Planting and raising a garden, sprouting an avocado seed, watching a cat in the birthing process, setting up a bird feeder, experimenting in the kitchen can all be roundabout learning experiences. Leisure time hobbies and activities should be shared when possible as part of the daily routine, for example by tinkering with the house car, crocheting when watching TV, repotting a plant, building a bookcase, playing an instrument, leading a yoga session. When the adults are turned-on and interested, their enthusiasm can infect all those around.

You can't really teach curiosity, it must be demonstrated.

Competence comes also from a sense of responsibility toward oneself and others, and responsibility is learned from being given responsibility. "It is never learned from having them withheld. Like anything else, it is learned from being given the opportunity to take the consequences of one's own acts in an atmosphere of safety." (Combs et al., 1971, p. 117). Being in charge of a week's cooking in the home (or for the group) may be a disaster the first time around. But as long as mistakes are accepted as something to be learned from and not condemned, the message conveyed will be, "It's OK to fail. I still believe you to be able and responsible." Learning to deal with failure, picking oneself up and trying again is the core of responsibility.

Second, cognitive control over behavior can be taught. Learning to manage one's own life often stems from learning to talk things over, not necessarily with the intent of acquiring insight, but self-control. Symptoms, especially self- or other-destructive ones, should and can be controlled. Behavior that interferes with an adolescent's receiving the security, affection and discipline he needs, alters normal development. Expectations by adults as to what is acceptable and nonacceptable behavior should give preference to exploring the dynamics of detrimental behaviors.

In a group home situation where there are an average of six to eight individuals under one roof, it is inevitable that at one time or another somebody's personal boundaries will be invaded. A blaring stereo, a borrowed and then lost article of clothing, a cake eaten without having had a piece are common trigger points for angry outbursts. Members have to learn to live with one another, and as in society, have to learn to control outbursts toward one another. In dealing with anger or any other feeling in the present tense, there is no place for analyzing or discussing what occurred in utero. It is all too easy to blame present behavior on past injustices. Members should be held responsible for their behavior at all times. Pleas of being emotionally upset, discriminated against by society or abused by parents are too often cop-out pleas for behavior.

It is important to emphasize to the adolescent member that the anger per se is normal and fine; what needs to be dealt with is what is done with the feeling. Learning to direct feelings appropriately is a multitrial process, and often begins by learning the difference between swinging one's fist and what happens when it hits another's nose. Glasser (1975) cites a parallel process of learning to fill one's needs without depriving someone else of his needs. Symptoms or self-defeating behaviors are described as unrealistic irresponsible ways to fill needs and usually destroy what they are meant to accomplish. Self- or other-defeating behaviors may be based in part on an individual's past, but they are primarily a result of what he is or is not doing in the present and represent an inability to face reality. That is where the focus must lie, for "because no one lives a life where his needs are always fulfilled, it is impossible not to find a wealth of buried conflicts which, being similar to present difficulties, seem to explain a person's inability to fill his needs now." (Glasser, 1975, p. 67)

The key is not insight, but an awareness of what the adolescent is doing now. Adults must not feed into self-defeating behaviors by permitting or expecting them. If a child is expected to fail, he most likely will. If a member is permitted to withdraw from the group because it is the only way he knows to deal with his feelings toward the group, then the withdrawal will never cease, neither will the anger. Limits of acceptable and expected behavior must be made explicit and also consequences for crossing those boundaries. Though consequences may range from being grounded to writing an essay, to have meaning, they must reflect consistency, the behavior involved and the particular individual. Action on behavior should be taken with a concern for the adolescent's ability to function in the community, the message being concern for behavior, not personality.

Third, feelings should be nurtured. It is through the expression of feeling that one learns to own his whole self. Learning to recognize, accept, appropriately direct feelings, puts a person in charge of his life. People can deal with their life problems if they know what they are, not necessarily why they exist. A person is then free to define himself and this freedom depends on an awareness of the here and now. Dealing with life's vicissitudes, feelings and problems becomes a growth process, not a corrective process (Marram, 1973, p. 114).

Feelings need not only be recognized, but also directed toward appropriate sources. "When feelings are expressed indirectly and diffusely, there is little release or satisfaction and the feelings continue to grow inside." (Moustakas, 1959, p. 27) Resentment or anger toward another group member, houseparent or teacher sours easily into long-standing grudges if not expressed as immediately as possible.

It is difficult to direct uncomfortable feelings toward someone whose love one doesn't want to lose. For one who has known little affection, tender feelings may be the most difficult. Anger seems to be the allaround stickler to express, to direct and to feel OK about. Many of those in group care have sat on their anger for so long, they are often afraid of what will happen when it is expressed. Perhaps it will rage out of control; or loved ones will think less of them for it; or it will blow their calm and controlled image. Anger is energy, and like other emotions, must go somewhere. Too often it is turned inward; as mankind's most primitive emotion, anger can be the most disabling when neglected.

Learning to funnel anger or any other feeling into constructive behavior takes time and practice. The group by its very nature will provide numerous opportunities for exploring and directing one's feelings, but only if the emotional climate is an accepting one and the adults are immediate and appropriate with their feelings. At first it can be an uncomfortable process, with feelings emerging as diffuse and misdirected. With encouragement and feedback, positive and negative feelings can be separated toward particular people and put more in line with actual situations.

Sometimes other outlets for emotional

energy are necessary and should be included in the schema of the milieu. Appropriate outlets must be differentiated from those that are not. It's OK to shout praise to the Lord, as long as it's not in the middle of a busy intersection. Any activity that expends physical energy can help to release tension, frustration and anger; a run on the beach, jogging in the park, a game of tag or basketball. Learning to tap one's creativity can also be a release for emotional energy — keeping a journal, candle making, carpentry, finger painting, learning a new craft. Discovering that emotional energy can be an asset is often dependent on the kinds of experiences included in the environment and how open the adults are with how they deal with their emotions.

The last point concerns the importance of the group. As an arena for human relatedness, it can become a source of motivation and peer control. When a group is functioning well, it is hard for a member to break the unity by behaving in a disturbing way. When the group is not functioning well, the frictions can also be learned from and dealt with in a constructive manner.

The group can provide an abundance of here and now resources for practical support (advice, help with environmental situations) and emotional support (sympathy, encouragement, companionship, respect, recreation). The group can become the ultimate basis of security and esteem for its members; it can fill members' needs for closeness and intimacy and allow them to experience the pleasures of friendship and affection. When functioning, a group can work collectively on its concerns while allowing members to work on their individual concerns. The group experience can be a "slice of life"; a sampling of reality and what it is like to live with other individuals.

In that learning is a social process, the group can provide the props for achieving important learnings. Most of what we come to grasp is a consequence of some kind of interaction with others. Having others to identify with is important to the learning process, "not only because it provides interaction and stimulation, but also because it makes it possible for persons to explore more widely and to be more creative and less hesitant in their approach to life itself." (Combs et al., 1974, p. 234) The group can provide valuable sources of feedback and evaluation for one another. It can also exert a healthy pressure to keep one's act together; a pressure that can far exceed any adult influence.

Each member, including the adults, form a spoke in a wheel which can provide an atmosphere where members feel secure and where there is an allaround validation of one's self-esteem. When the wheel is not turning smoothly, it is time to assess how and what it is that is getting in the way of the group's functioning. Airing gripes, grudges, resentments and unrealistic expectations of one another in community meetings can help redirect misplaced emotional energy and provide a practical exercise in group problem solving. As in a family, when there is tension and discord in the group, no one is exempt from feeling it. The group can be led to accept responsibility for its own well-being by asking not "why" but "what can be done." A group cannot improve its functioning without self-awareness; through feedback and confrontation, members can expose for observation and comment by all, sources of tension, stress and strain. One of the most freeing experiences for members is the realization that conflicts can be worked through, that the power lies in their hands and that the goodies to be obtained from each other are self-determining.

As has been pointed out, we learn by example, as a result of interaction with significant others. If the adults/houseparents/counselors are honest, appropriate and authentic in their behavior, they will tend to ellicit the same from those around them. Rigid and stereotyped responses are often greeted by adolescents with anger, resentment, testing and acting-out. A group situation is no place to play "shrink", for technique, including reflection, silence, interpretation, seems to function as a defense against the immature being, and it is doubtless valuable for that reason. Furthermore, it is a safe and harmless way to interact and hence has value for that purpose." (Jourard,

1971, p.148) Working with a young person caught in the midst of evolution and often turmoil is a human experience, and true encounter can occur only if one is in touch with one's own humanness.

BIBLIOGRAPHY

Bettelheim, B. *A Home for the Heart*. New York: Bantam Books, 1974.

Combs, A., Avila, D., and Purkey, W. *Helping Relationships: Basic Concepts for the Helping Professions*. Boston: Allyn and Bacon, Inc., 1971.

Glasser, W. *Reality Therapy*. New York: Harper & Row, Inc., 1975.

Hobbs, N. Helping disturbed children: Psychological and ecological strategies. In Combs, A., Avila, D., and Purkey, W. *Helping Relationships: Basic Concepts for the Helping Professions*. Boston: Allyn & Bacon, Inc., 1971.

Jourard, S. *The Transparent Self*. New York: Van Nostrand Reinhold Co., 1971.

Marram, G. *The Group Approach in Nursing Practice*. St. Louis: C.V. Mosby Co., 1973.

Moustakas, C. *Psychotherapy with Children*. New York: Ballantine Books, Inc., 1959.

Sullivan, H. S. *Conceptions of Modern Psychiatry*. New York: W.W. Norton & Co., Inc., 1953.

Wolins, M. (Ed), *Successful Group Care*. Chicago: Aldine Publishing Co., 1974.

Chapter **19**

child abuse: a shared responsibility

MILDRED ANDREINI

The nurse is only one of many professionals who must accept responsibility for the protection of children who may be the victims of abuse or neglect. Critical to the nurse's effective role in the identification, assessment, treatment and prevention of child abuse and neglect are a knowledge base of the dynamics of child abuse and neglect, skill in related nursing practice and an awareness of personal feelings and attitudes regarding the maltreatment of children.

Among the matters tied closely to our concept of child abuse and neglect are our personal views of the role and perhaps sovereignty of the family, our experience and attitudes toward child rearing, our ideas about discipline and corporal punishment and our understanding of child development.

Child abuse and neglect are symptoms of the presence of multiple difficulties in families and in parents as individuals. Studies and experience indicate that maltreatment of children occurs in a variety of circumstances with causes based in the parents' past, the nature of the family, the marital relationship, and environmental stresses which impinge on the family.

Recent figures released by the Depart-

ment of Health, Education, and Welfare indicate that more than a million children in this country are subjected to physical abuse or neglect every year (Delinquency Rehabilitation Report, 1976). Douglas Besharov, Director of the National Center for the Prevention and Treatment of Child Abuse and Neglect, Department of Health, Education, and Welfare, is quoted as saying that more than 2,000 American children die each year from causes associated with abuse or neglect. Children from infancy through the late teens are victims of abuse or neglect. While much of the emphasis has been placed on the young child who is injured by his parents or guardian, documentation of serious physical and sexual abuse of adolescents has alerted us to the fact that abuse and neglect of children is not limited to children under age 5 years. It has been estimated that 25% to 28% of abusive incidents involve children between 12 and 18 years of age (Delinquency Rehabilitation Report, 1976).

This chapter is based on my experience as coordinator of the Anchorage Child Abuse Board, a multidisciplinary diagnostic team that provides multiprofessional consultation on child abuse and neglect, offers community education and training and administers a Parent Aide Program which utilizes volunteer lay therapists to help abusive and neglectful parents.

HISTORICAL PERSPECTIVE

Child abuse and neglect are not new phenomena. Infanticide and torture of young children have been practiced by both primitive and civilized societies for centuries. Children have been beaten, maimed and often killed in attempts to discipline them, to educate them and to exploit them. Lloyd DeMause's (1975) historical perspective of these despicable practices is interesting as well as awesome.

Abusive and neglectful treatment of children have been indicative of the low status of children. Society has generally supported the concept of children as property or objects belonging to their parents with few rights of their own. These attitudes are reflected in the case of Mary Ellen, a child who was rescued from a seriously abusive adoptive home by the Society for the Prevention of Cruelty to Animals in 1875. At that time, there was no law under which any agency could interfere to protect children who were being subjected to torture or maltreatment by their parents or guardians. The incident with Mary Ellen prompted establishment of the Society for the Prevention of Cruelty to Children in New York City.

While numerous private and public agencies have existed in this country since the beginning of this century, it has only been in the last 15 to 20 years that an understanding of both the diagnostic aspects and the treatment issues of child abuse and neglect has been developed through research and study. It is interesting to note that as early as the 1920's, Dr. John Caffey, a pediatric radiologist was conducting radiologic study of bone changes and other signs of injury to children. In a report made in 1946, Dr. Caffey suggested that bone changes frequently seen on radiologic examination were the result of trauma, probably nonaccidental trauma inflicted upon children by their parents or guardians (Caffey, 1972).

Dr. C. Henry Kempe, Professor and Chairman of the Department of Pediatrics, University of Colorado Medical Center, began the trend toward medical, sociological and new legal approaches to child abuse and neglect in the early 1960's when he coined the phrase "the battered child." Dr. Kempe had the opportunity at the University of Colorado Medical Center to examine and study many children and their families and he found that nonaccidental injuries and neglect of children's physical and emotional needs occurred at an alarmingly high frequency. Dr. Kempe and an associate, Dr. Ray E. Helfer, documented and described the battered child syndrome in *The Battered Child* in 1968. They considered the issues of identification of families prone to abuse their children, therapeutic approaches, legal aspects of the problem and community responsibility to protect children in a subsequent book, *Helping the Battered Child and His Family*. The research and study by Drs. Kempe and Helfer as well as a number of other professionals from a variety of disciplines led to a broadened awareness of the widespread maltreatment of children in the United States and the recognition that parents can be helped.

DEFINITION OF CHILD ABUSE AND NEGLECT

In January 1974, federal legislation was passed which established the National Center on Child Abuse and Neglect; appropriated monies for research, program demonstration and development of services; and defined child abuse and neglect as " . . . the physical or mental injury, sexual abuse, negligent treatment, or maltreatment of a child under the age of eighteen by a person who is responsible for the child's welfare under circumstances which indicate that the child's health or welfare is harmed or threatened thereby. . . . " (Public Law 93–247, 93rd Congress, S.1191. January 31, 1974.) Many state statutes define child abuse and neglect for reporting and litigation purposes as comprehensively as the federal law and all states have passed legislation which includes at least a minimal definition and procedures for reporting.

ROLE OF THE NURSE

The nurse has several important roles in child abuse and neglect cases. In addition to case finding and reporting suspected child abuse and neglect to the designated agency, the nurse's role extends to the treatment phase including ongoing follow-up, coordination of services and collaboration with other disciplines in both case evaluation and management.

The role of the nurse in child abuse and neglect has often been limited to case finding and reporting suspected cases to a designated state or private agency. Nurses, like other professional and lay persons, have reacted and responded to obvious child abuse or neglect with both fear and horror, have at times simply ignored the obvious signs, or have placed the responsibility for protecting maltreated children with official state agencies or "someone else." Therefore, it is imperative for the nurse, whether in an institution, school, or community setting, to develop awareness and skills in the recognition of the problem of child abuse and neglect; to understand the process by which children are protected and parents are helped; and to take part in the responsibility for delivery of services, both on an individual and a community basis.

The identification of child abuse and neglect presents numerous problems to both professional and lay persons due to the feelings, assumptions, and connotations associated with a label such as "child abuser" or "neglectful parent." A careful inventory of feelings and attitudes regarding child abuse and neglect as well as the role of the family is imperative before the nurse can proceed effectively in helping abused and neglected children and their parents through early recognition and intervention.

Medical diagnosis of abuse has been documented for several decades on the basis of both radiological assessment and the nature of injuries (Caffey, 1972; Helfer and Kempe, 1972). Research and work with families during the past 20 years has also revealed a number of indicators of the potentially abusive family. The key to identification as well as treatment lies in a thorough assessment of the family through observation, careful interviewing, a sensitivity to the complexity of each case and an openness to the full, sometimes conflicting, range of the available evidence about abuse or neglect.

Many abusive parents were reared in such a way that they failed to receive a "mothering imprint," that is, they were emotionally deprived and perhaps physically abused by their parents. In addition, many abusive parents are lonely, isolated individuals who are unable to trust or use others; have a spouse who is so passive that he or she cannot "give," and have unrealistic expectations from their child(ren). Other factors which may contribute to abusive or neglectful behavior include immaturity and an inability to accept responsibility; lack of knowledge of forms of discipline other than physical punishment; a significant vulnerability to criticism, disinterest, or abandonment and environmental stresses (poor housing, unemployment, absence of extended family) which tap the strengths of parents beyond the point of their ability to cope.

The abused child may exhibit minor to severe injuries for which the history is at variance with the physical assessment. The child may also appear either malnourished or simply pale, passive, apathetic and unresponsive. Other signs of the child who may have been abused or neglected are agressive behavior, unusual fearfulness, or the child who "takes over" and begins to care for or comfort the parent. The child who is seen as "different" by his parent may be a target for abuse or neglect. The child who fails to respond to his parent in an expected manner or one who really is different (retarded, hyperactive, birth defect) could be identified as such a child.

The nurse is mandated by law in most states to report suspected and identified child abuse or neglect to a designated public law enforcement and/or social service agency. In most states, the public agency has legal responsibility to investigate reports of suspected child abuse and neglect and may coordinate ongoing children's protective services including court proceedings if needed. The nurse's responsibility does not necessarily end with the report to the official agency. The nurse may continue as a key person in children's protective services by providing individual counseling, parent teaching, anticipatory guidance relating to growth and development and parenting, a lifeline to parents, liaison between the agencies and professional persons offering services to the family, or as a member of a multidisciplinary child-protective team.

TREATMENT

Both the routine and the unique aspects of working with abusing and neglectful families have emerged within the experience with the Anchorage Child Abuse Board over the past 3 years. In many respects family assessment, therapeutic planning, parent education and liaison in work with these families are similar to families exhibiting other types of medical or psychosocial problems. Perhaps the most unique aspect of abusive or neglectful families is their extreme vulnerability to criticism and fear of rejection. Therefore, it is imperative that the approach to the emotional and psychological aspects of these families be individually planned and implemented with great sensitivity.

It has been found that as few as 10% of identified abusive and neglectful families may be classified as seriously mentally ill or psychotic. More frequently, the parents are repeating a pattern of child rearing they learned as children, or the family is succumbing to an extreme sociological or environmental stress situation.

Areas that a nurse-therapist may address in working with abusing or neglectful parents include individual counseling and therapy, marriage counseling or family therapy. The decision regarding the treatment modality as well as the problems addressed is specific to each family. Parents who are reasonably courageous and who express themselves well verbally are often able to work well and demonstrate considerable growth in group therapy. Some parents are unable to utilize group or individual therapy due to their extreme fear of criticism and rejection. A complete psychological assessment or psychiatric evaluation is prerequisite to the appropriate development of a therapeutic plan for the abusive or neglectful family.

Whether professional therapy or counseling is provided by a psychiatrist, psychologist, nurse-therapist or other health professional, several factors must be considered. Many, if not all, abusive and neglectful parents are emotionally immature. The acceptance of responsibility is almost an impossibility for them and problem-solving is frequently beyond their capability. It has been found by the Anchorage program that families have as much difficulty dealing with relatively minor problem areas such as obtaining transportation to pre-school or arranging the time to visit with a child who is placed in foster care, as they do the major breaks in family routine such as loss of a job or serious illness.

Many abusive and neglectful parents are repeating a pattern of child-rearing which they learned as children. Extreme physical punishment was used in an attempt to discipline, control and educate them. One of the most difficult areas in which to work with abusive parents is in changing behavior regarding child-rearing patterns. A frequent statement from parents, is, "My father whipped me and I turned out all right."

Another factor inherent in the abusive parent is extremely low self-esteem which is the result of failure to receive as a child, emotional nurturing or validation as a worthwhile person. The abusive parent's low estimate of value as an individual prohibits social integration into the community, prevents development of an effective emotionally intimate relationship with a spouse or mate, and impedes parenting capabilities. To the parent with a low self-estimate, a child's normal crying or fussing at an inopportune time may be perceived as criticism and affirmation of the parent's worthlessness.

Most abusive parents have not had a chance at any time in their lives to have dependency needs gratified. One finds frequently that there has rarely been an important person, whether it be parent, extended relative, or other significant person upon whom the parent could unconditionally depend. It is common to learn from a parent during interviews that he or she was "ignored" as a child or in many cases, beaten or exploited physically or sexually.

An approach which has been found to be successful in meeting the dependency needs of abusive and neglectful parents is the use of the lay therapist, or parent aide, a concept that was developed in Denver in the late 1960's by Dr. Kempe and his associates. Stated simply, the task of the lay therapist is to provide an opportunity in which the abusive parent may establish dependency, make some changes in behavior, and move toward independence. An important task of the lay therapist is to provide a lifeline for the abusive parent. We know that in addition to failing to receive a mothering imprint, possible marital difficulties, as well as unrealistic expectations from his or her child or children, the environmental and sociological stresses upon the family may greatly contribute to abusive or neglectful behavior.

Serving as a lifeline, the parent aide, or lay therapist, becomes an entree to the community, a liaison, an individual with whom the parent may develop a trusting relationship and reach out to in times of stress. Abusive parents may utilize lay therapists as a role model, or in simply making his or her way through everyday activities which until this time have simply been too threatening to carry out. Such simple tasks as meeting one's next door neighbor may in fact be very threatening for the abusive or neglectful parent. The parent aide becomes a very appropriate noncritical person in learning this simple task. It is interesting to note that low self-estimate and isolation based on fear of rejection are exhibited rather consistently by shades kept drawn at all times or an unlisted phone number. The reparenting or dependency gratification needs of an abusive parent have in the past been met by several different types of persons. Social workers in certain instances have been able to provide this nurturing, supportive kind of relationship over a long period of time, as have certain health and other social service professional persons.

However, the reality of health and social service systems today is that a few professional persons have time to spend many hours a week with each client. Thus, the parent aide becomes the extension of the professional team, meeting a very special need in the abusive parent, and yet supporting the work of the professional team.

The parent aide/parent relationship is characterized by frequent home visits, times during which the parent can explore feelings, concerns, fears and hopes with the parent aide. The relationship is established over a long period of time, usually from 8 to 24 months. The parent aide is a nonofficial, nonauthoritarian, noncritical individual who serves as a trusting friend as well as a supporting and nurturing figure. Dependency on the parent aide for emotional support is encouraged early in the relationship. The parent is encouraged to call the parent aide during times of stress, to utilize the parent aide as one who can share negative feelings as well as joys. Dependency is encouraged without strings attached. Gradually, through the nonwavering trusting relationship, the parent is encouraged to develop some independent skills, whether it be reaching out to other significant persons in the community for either help or friendship or whether it be coping with a complicated social service or health delivery system.

The primary focus of the parent aide therapy is emotional support and the development of a trusting relationship. Once that has been established the parent aide can move toward fulfilling a broader role and meeting a wider range of needs including assisting the parent in coping with the environmental stress which may be contributing to the abusive or neglectful situation. The primary environmental stress factors that can precipitate or complicate an abusive or neglectful situation include lack of food, no shelter or inadequate housing, unemployment, limited income or poor budgeting of financial resources and lack of transportation. In addition, both the absence of extended family or the pressure from extended family members who demand attention and support from young parents but offer nothing in return can exacerbate abuse or neglect in a high risk situation. In Anchorage, experience indicates that the high cost of living, the distance between the state and the rest of the nation, extreme weather conditions and a general scarcity of both goods and services are factors in creating increased stress upon families.

The parent aide is often an important helping person in both meeting the dependency needs of abusive or neglectful parents and in assisting parents in coping with environmental crises, but the parent aide must at all times be considered a member of a therapeutic team, not a substitute for other forms of help. Families do very well with a variety of combinations of helping team members. A multidisciplinary approach has been identified as the most effective way to help abusive and neglectful families.

RELATIONSHIP OF THE NURSE TO THE PARENT AIDES

In the role of nurse-coordinator of the parent aide program, involvement with the parent aides occurs in several areas. In collaboration with professionals from other disciplines, the nurse-coordinator participates in the selection of the parent aides through interviews and individual assessment. Factors investigated in the parent aide assessment process include the way he was reared, i.e., was a "mothering imprint" received? If the individual is a parent, how does he view his children? How does the individual cope with crisis? Does the prospective aide have a lifeline, recreational activities and a supportive relationship with another adult? Can the individual reach around an abused child to meet the dependency needs of an abusive parent? A thorough screening process is imperative to an effective lay therapist program. In the Anchorage program, each potential parent aide is interviewed twice and two professional persons conduct each interview. The nurse-coordinator participates in one interview with each prospective parent aide. The data gathered during the screening process are used not only to screen inappropriate individuals from the program, but to more effectively train, assign and supervise parent aides in their work with a family.

In the Anchorage program, the nurse-coordinator conducts the parent aide training, incorporating presentations by a public health nurse on child growth and development, by a psychiatric social worker in the psychodynamics of child abuse and by a pediatrician on the diagnosis and medical treatment of the abused or neglected child. The training program for the parent aides utilizes group process to impart theoretical and practical information about child abuse, to improve communication skills, to explore the parent aides' feelings about child abuse and neglect and to investigate community resources that are brought together to cre-ate a multidisciplinary team approach to helping the abused child and his family. Care is taken to expand qualities inherent in the parent aide such as the ability to listen in an accepting way and the ability to be nonjudgmental.

Supervision for the parent aides is provided by the nurse-coordinator at weekly 2-hour group sessions. Supervision provided within a group setting is conducive to a nonthreatening exploration of the parent aides' feelings regarding their supportive role in the abusing family. It has been found that Parent Aides require support, frequent clarification of their role in the overall treatment plan for the family, and ongoing assistance with active listening techniques. Continuing focus on communication theory is also utilized in assisting the parent aide to help the abusing parents to whom they are assigned.

In facilitating a team approach to helping abusive families, the nurse-coordinator integrates the work of the parent aide with the professional persons who are working with a family. In the Anchorage program this coordination is achieved in part by nurse-coordinator contact with persons working with each family and partially through periodic case review before the Anchorage Child Abuse Board consultation team.

Thus, the relationship of the nurse to parent aides is seen to include selection, training, supervision, coordination and the provision of emotional support that enables the parent aide to function successfully with families.

CONCLUSION

The nurse, regardless of work setting, may be the first professional person to identify child abuse or neglect. Whether the family is actually abusive or neglectful or potentially at risk to be so, it is important to realize that most parents will accept intervention to assist in improving their relationship with their children. Immaturity, denial and a pattern of punitive child-rearing practices may appear to be enormous roadblocks to both parents and helping persons, but honesty, objectivity, and a willingness to "hang in there" by both helper and parents can result in a better understanding of the physical and emotional needs of children, an improved self-concept in parents, and a parent-child relationship in which parents feel confident and successful and children receive the nurturing support and limits they need. Nurses thus fulfill a critical role in the prevention and treatment of child abuse.

BIBLIOGRAPHY

Caffey, J. The first annual Neuhauser presidential address of the Society for Pediatric Radiology. *The Am. J. Roentgenol.* 114: 217–228, 1972.

Children Today. U.S. Department of Health, Education, and Welfare, Office of Human Development, Office of Child Development, Children's Bureau. DHEW Publication No. (OHD) 76-30014, May-June 1975.

DeFrancis, V. *Community Cooperation For Better Child Protection*. Denver, Colorado: The American Humane Association, Children's Division, P.O. Box 1266.

Delinquency Rehabilitation Report, February 1976. Department of Health, Education, and Welfare by the American Humane Association.

DeMause, L. Our forebears made childhood a nightmare. *Psychol. Today* 8: 85, 1975.

Gil, D. G. *Violence Against Children*. Cambridge, Massachusetts: Harvard University Press, 1970.

Goldstein, J., Freud, A., and Solnit, A. J. *Beyond the Best Interests of the Child*. New York: The Free Press, Macmillan Publishing Co., Inc., 1973.

Helfer, R. E. *The Diagnostic Process and Treatment Programs*. DHEW Publication No. (OHD) 75-69, Washington, D.C.: U.S. Government Printing Office, 1975.

Helfer, R. E., and Kempe, C. H. (Eds.), *The Battered Child*. Chicago: University of Chicago Press, 1968.

Helfer, R. E., and Kempe, C. H. (Eds.), *Helping the Battered Child and His Family*. Philadelphia: J.B. Lippincott Co., 1972.

Hopkins, J. The nurse and the abused child. *Nurs. Clin. North Am.* 5 (4), 1970.

Leonard, M. F., Rhymes, J. P., and Solnit, A. J. Failure to thrive in infants: A family problem. *Am. J. Dis. Child.* 111: 600, 1966.

Satir, V. *Conjoint Family Therapy*. Palo Alto, Calif. Science and Behavior Books, Inc., 1967.

Steele, B. F. *Working with Abusive Parents from a Psychiatric Point of View*. DHEW Publication No. (OHD) 75-70, Washington, D.C.: U.S. Government Printing Office, 1975.

Young, L. *Wednesday's Children*. New York: McGraw-Hill Book Co., 1964.

Chapter 20

psychiatric nursing in rural areas

JEANETTE JUSTICE

True or false? People who live in small towns and rural areas of America are the happiest?

Looking at one aspect of this question in broad general terms, rural America has been noted for its declining and aging population, where a considerable number of people live below the poverty level. Per capita incomes are significantly below those of urban residents, as are educational expenditures. More than half of its people live in substandard housing, many without adequate plumbing. On the other hand, behavior specialists have found that most people who live in rural areas prefer country living. According to the findings of university studies, the answer is true. Small town and rural lifestyles tend to coincide with closer ties with fellow human beings, more meaningful relationships, lasting friendships and a feeling of belonging.

The proportion of the country not included in standard metropolitan areas includes over 54 million persons, who are often located in relatively isolated areas, ranging from farming villages to a simple wide place in the road. Within such small towns and rural communities old values are highly regarded. Attitudes of the citizens reflect a primary identification with home, family, school and work. While the advent of television has extended some of the expectations of rural residents, there remains a uniqueness which differentiates rural from urban inhabitants. Unlike the city, the small town is like an extended family, with a vast reservoir of community responsibility toward problems of individuals. Rural lifestyles continue to have an element of helpful neighborliness and a sense of community, usually without the fragmentation common to urban life.

Few places in the United States have been left untouched by the mental health movement of the 1960's. Psychologists and social workers, those who have been most influencial in promoting the point of view of the humanistic theorists, are generally in key positions in planning for the delivery of community mental health services. Rural areas are very often the recipients of clinics and outreach programs coordinated by mental health teams struggling to establish a formal structure within the community. Mental Health, as a separate discipline, generally deals with crisis intervention.

In the crowded metropolitan areas, multidimensional services are provided. Mental health programs have been initiated to aid emotionally troubled clients in divorce adjustment, interpersonal conflicts, sexuality, grief, loneliness, alcoholism and drug abuse. The limited nature of such services in rural areas may seem discouragingly inadequate to mental health planners.

The humanistic concept applied in crisis care depends upon the philosophy that the uncertainties of modern life keep the individual from finding a core identity, so that he is unable to locate himself in relationship to beliefs and values. Modern therapy tries to respond to persons who are "lost." How successfully such concepts can be extended in order to serve rural residents depends upon the recognition that different cultures have different definitions of mental health. Most rural communities plan frequent entertainments which serve as opportunities for mutual sharing of experiences. Community dances, for instance, have a natural purpose, in addition to the obvious one of pleasure. At a dance even the elders, unbending, dancing to yesterday's beat, or sitting on long wooden benches, sipping booze from paper cups, are sustained within the certainties of the community. They are gay and repetitious, laughing loudly at the fantasies spun in the dense air of the hall, friends in boots and miniskirts, remembering Pearl Harbor. Generally, whole families are there, the children picking up role cues, testing reality, learning to dance with grown-ups and each other. And people like Roger, leaning against the beautiful women to say, "As soon as spring comes, I'm gonna' ride my Harley clean across America—I'll stop by and pick you up." Mass therapy? You bet. The dancing is as therapeutic as the music. Personnel practicing in isolated areas need to explore beyond the boundaries of professional ideologies.

The psychiatric nurse practicing in a rural setting should evaluate the situation realistically. Community resources are often of an informal nature and not readily apparent to the newcomer. Ujhely (1969), in focusing on the role of the nurse in community mental health, suggests that the nurse must be able to establish herself by reaching out into the community, communicating what she thinks and feels. This presupposes that the nurse has discovered the behavioral system of the particular area. Reaching-out, so that

mental health programs can be established, involves an acquaintance with the community's structure and needs, and often an exchange of information with local agencies. The psychiatric nurse, new to a rural or small town setting, may have to make some personal adjustments in order to be successful in her role. There is the story of an intelligent, urban psychiatric nurse practitioner, faced with an exciting employment opportunity as the only nurse in community care and treatment in a small rural county. Puzzled that her clinic was not being utilized as she had anticipated from previous experience in the city, she tried to "get a group started" at the local high school. She wore her hair in pigtails, saying "let's relate." But her program was frustrated by school officials for a number of reasons, not the least of which was parental concern. Next, she publicized the beginning of a therapeutic dance program, hoping to help individuals express emotional needs, and perhaps incidentally to establish herself as a care-giver. All of her planning was short-lived. She had not discovered that there is a generalized resistance to the idea of having personal emotional problems. There was a gap between her expectations for adolescents in the high school and the expectations for adolescents in that community. Furthermore, children feel stigmatized by mental health problems. Nurses have some importance as a professional, and any intervention needs to be understood by the community. Often, it is the process that is important.

Crisis intervention cannot move into rural areas unless the practitioner, as well as the team of mental health professionals, can plan to build upon other programs already in progress. It is crucial to mobilize community resources. Aid is usually available to support people in emotional turmoil; this aid is primarily through the physician-patient relationship because there is frequently a displacement of emotional to somatic complaints. Remedial assistance is also available from social agencies including schools, welfare and probation departments and often through a combination of these agencies.

Knowing that there is a collective store of information, the psychiatric nurse moving into the rural scene will need to solicit peer support from other professional nurses. A collaborative relationship with nurses in the community's hospital is essential if indifference toward mental health services is to be avoided. There is enormous hostility to people who use a different approach. There is the story of the out-of-uniform psychiatric nurse who smoked cigars and refused to share any information with the nurses on the floor when she was called in for consultation. She was quite capable in arranging referrals for the mentally sick patients, but her area of expertise was "highly confidential." The opportunity for closer cooperation, and thus colleague acceptance, was impossible. Had this nurse realized that the primary medical care team is the keystone of community psychiatry, her difficulties in relating might have been alleviated. Liaison services in the form of programs for sharing information with nursing personnel are invaluable. Programs to define or discuss crisis intervention, counselling, or how the psychiatric nurse functions in short term and long term follow-up, tips on how to help the mentally ill when giving direct patient care – all of these would have established the psychiatric nurse's identity as well as a positive relationship with her peers.

Statistics from the National Institute of Mental Health suggest that there are many areas where an influx of persons discharged from state mental hospitals has resulted in the inability of community services to keep up with the needs of ex-patients. Once a mental health department discharges a patient, he becomes the responsibility of social service departments and community mental health programs. Frequently, because of the emphasis on crisis care, mental health programs are not structured to deal with the individual needs of the chronic client. Even group therapy is seldom provided, and the inability to supply even minimal therapy has increasingly become a national issue. Of course, not all discharged chronic patients need to go on welfare. Most are hospitalized for a short time and then return to home and family and perhaps a job with the help of community programs.

One very successful psychiatric nurse in California conducts regularly scheduled group sessions with ex-patients in a rural outreach clinic. Her career specialty had been in surgery, until reversing her occupational interest to mental health. One reason for her success is a vivid personality, and another may be found in the well recognized directive and methodical, perhaps compulsive style of the surgical nurse. This is used most effectively in dealing with the confused and the "crisis-prone" individuals who attend her clinic. Because these individuals are not a part of the community, they usually lack a network of emotional support. The nurse can provide individual guidance on a continuing basis. She is often responsible for seeing that her clients are taking medications as ordered, making sure that there are no side-effects and often adjusting dosages from time to time as indicated.

Caplan (1974) recognized that communities are made up of informal care-givers, people to whom others turn in time of crisis, and simply helpful people comprising a vast web. It is a person-to-person support system that mental health professionals are often unaware of. The community support system, in the model offered by Caplan, keeps a collective memory bank for the person in crisis and can offer a realistic judgment of current behavior. In rural areas, where rather rigid values are held, this informal system is a potent force. Informal care-givers are available to offer sympathy and advice.

What community does not have persons who are marginally crazy like Charlie? Charlie has the trash concession, and survives despite his difficulty with writing and figuring because his customers make out their own receipts. It is an exercise in mutual trust. Sometimes Charlie throws things at his wife and then feels guilty and depressed. The care-givers, his customers, are available to say, "You're still the same person. Nevertheless, this is right, and that is wrong." When he buys his wife a gift, the storekeeper, who probably went through school with Charlie, takes the appropriate change from Charlie's purse. Psychiatric care has never been considered for Charlie, perhaps because he is not "lost" in the existential sense, but knows who he is. The same system of neighborliness that sustains Charlie also sustains the local physician.

For example, when oral polio vaccine became available, one local doctor took his public health "crew" to every bar and bowling alley and picnic site in the county, and because he knew the people, and was known and trusted, 90% of the population was vaccinated. And when "Doc's" son was killed in Vietnam, it was a community grief experience, in which he himself needed to support others.

Caplan offers examples such as the corner druggist and the village hairdresser, informal care-givers who provide sympathetic judgment and advice to the individual who may be miserable or temporarily confused. Such care-givers are essential in assisting a person who is grappling with some current situation by helping him judge himself appropriately. The prevailing attitude is, "We'll go on loving you no matter what has happened to you."

If a support system is to work well, mental health professionals are cautioned that they may be strangers, and may act destructively by validating the client's current misperception of himself. Certain phases in a person's life history are crucial to ways of working out what is perhaps a temporary upset. Informal care-givers, Caplan explains, "support the individual within the network of his identity."

In one instance, a psychiatrist, new to rural mental health services, mistakenly exclaimed, "I see people walking around this village who have a desperate need for psychiatric care, and they're not receiving it!" He had not discovered that in rural areas, where people are well-known to one another and desirous of maintaining friendly and respectable relationships, there is a higher tolerance for and acceptance of bizarre behavior.

Was the psychiatrist referring to Clara, living in the same house all of her 80 years, who walks in the graveyard in order to tell the dead people all the latest news? She is still active in community affairs, and her mind is sharp. Perhaps the psychiatrist was referring to Vernon, captain of the election precinct for as long as anyone can remember, who shouts, "The polls is open," to a deserted street, and spends the long election day spinning tales from a memory filled with fact and fantasy. The poll watchers, Vernon's neighbors, are there at closing time, to

make sure the tally is correct. Jennie is a recluse, living at the end of a rutted dirt road. She keeps her gun handy to assure her privacy. She leaves the grocery list in the mail box when her government check is due, and hides from the mail lady. But the mail lady makes sure she gets her order. If anything were to happen to Jeannie, people would know. People like Paul would know. Paul works in town, so he travels the country road every day, and he watches out for his neighbors. In fact, most rural residents are watchers, and if anything appears out of the ordinary, it is noticed and talked about. Often Paul will stop to visit, bringing flowers from his garden or an interesting rock he has found, and like Clara, he too carries all the latest news. Many eccentricities are accepted in small communities, and there is indeed a collective storehouse of information developed and imparted as a source that gives meaning to life.

If we link people with mutual support systems, what is the role of the professional in rural America? The local physician often capably supports patients through emotional crisis, as do tranquilizing and antidepressant drugs prescribed. General practitioners have a long tradition of working with and through local community agencies on behalf of their patients. Help for the mentally disturbed and their families can be arranged through churches and voluntary and social organizations. The primary responsibility of the mental health team is to listen, to discover the community on its own terms, without superimposing previous biases or frames of reference. The psychiatric nurse, as a member of a rural mental health team, should be aware of the differences between rural and urban areas. It is necessary to recognize that rural areas present another cultural dimension with a mutual self-help system. Population orientation is needed. First, identify the need for mental health services and then use the available facilities to satisfy the needs of the population. The opportunities for closer cooperation between doctors, public health nurses and social workers should lead to a great improvement in the care of mentally sick persons in the community.

Public health nurses recognize that regardless of the mental health services administered by others, many mental and emotional components of the clients they serve constitute a public health problem. Often, the public health nurse is the primary contact and is able to prevent referral of the person to specialist in psychiatric services. For instance, she is available to listen to the woman in mid-life crisis crying, "I need someone to talk to, like you. . . . I know I probably need therapy, but I can't go to Mental Health. Why, it'd be all over town if I went there!" Sometimes it is the office nurse who listens and who cares in crisis situations like that of the mother whose adolescent son was referred in good faith by the sheriff, after smoking marijuana. "That psychiatrist down there at Mental Health told my boy he should move away and be on his own! His dad needs him on the ranch. How can we manage without him?"

Is the public health nurse, or the office nurse, competent to act as a consultant in such situations? It is well-known that people are more susceptible to help when they are involved in crisis in their lives. By the same token, not everyone needs psychotherapy, when simpler methods of counselling will do. These nurses, public health and office nurses, may be considered a part of the community in which they function, and they are able to support the individual by interpreting problems with appropriate feedback cues. Therefore, unless dialogue is initiated early-on with peers, the psychiatric nurse may be excluded as a care-giver.

The psychiatric nurse is in a unique position to supplement the support system in rural areas. She is competent to understand client behavior, and she can offer reassurance or advice as a part of her therapeutic role. The nurse can share with other care-givers some of her specialized knowledge, a precious commodity in rural areas. She can supplement the system from a broad background of experience and education. The only way to do this, and to establish a viable identity, is to reach out into the community.

BIBLIOGRAPHY

Aguilera, D. C., and Messick, J. M. *Crisis Intervention*. St. Louis: C.V. Mosby Company, 1974.

Bayer, M. Psychiatric nursing care in a community hospital. *RN* 71–82, 1974.

Bulbulyan, A., et al. Nurses in a community mental health center. *Am. J. Nurs.* 69: 328–331, 1969.

Bush, M. T., et al. The meaning of mental health: A report of two ethnocentric studies. *Nurs. Res.* 24: 130–138, 1975.

Caplan, G. *Support Systems and Community Mental Health*. New York: Behavioral Publications, 1974.

Feldman, S. Administration in mental health: Issues, problems, and prospects. *Bull. Pan Am. Health Organ.* 60: 212–220, 1975.

Keys, J., and Hoffling, C. K. *Basic Psychiatric Concepts in Nursing*. Philadelphia: J. B. Lippincott Co., 1974.

Kuenzi, S., and Fenton, M. V. Crisis intervention in acute care areas. *Am. J. Nurs.* 830–834, 1975.

Larson, M. L. From psychiatric to psychosocial nursing. *Nurs. Outlook* 21: pp 520–528.

Ujhely, Gertrude B., "The Nurse in Community Psychiatry", *Am. J. Nurs.* May 1969, pp 1001–1005.

3

The Application of Psychiatric Nursing Concepts

Chapter 21

a functional model for emotional care

D. JEAN WOOD

Through all phases of nursing education, including continuing education and graduate level, nurses have been taught that the patient is a person and that the patient's emotional as well as physical and spiritual needs are significant to patient care. However, nurses are not successfully taught how to operationalize emotional care with real patients in real health care settings. Nurses have the information that their patients have and will demonstrate emotional needs but the nurses do not have clear ideas about what ought to do about these needs. The author has been practicing, teaching and consulting about psychiatric-mental health nursing for more than 20 years. In her consultation with nurses in general care settings about meeting patients' emotional needs she has discovered that:

— nurses do not believe that they are taught a conception of human emotional needs that can be effectively applied by *all* nurses with *all* patients;
— nurses do not consistently or effectively utilize information from patients about their needs and their expectations of emotional care;
— nurses do not hold themselves as accountable for the outcomes of emotional care as they do for the outcomes of physical care.

Nurses *are* concerned about the gap that exists between their personal and professional commitment to effective emotional care and what goes on between them and patients every day. Student and practicing nurses want a model for providing emotional care that will bridge the gap between the patient's needs and their own good intentions. Input from nurses stimulated the author to propose a model which clearly says what can be done with any patient/ client to meet his basic emotional needs. This model has been implemented by students and practicing nurses in a wide variety of patient care settings and their positive feedback has provided the impetus for this chapter.

CHARACTERISTICS OF A FUNCTIONAL MODEL FOR EMOTIONAL CARE

Emotions are, by definition, internal feeling states. As such, they are not available for very objective analysis — not until we become much more knowledgeable and skillful about psychological research. We know much more about physical states of being because we have been able to define them and measure them so much more specifically. We have no psychological research that tells us what the emotions are and how they function with the same degree of specificity that we know the respiratory and circulatory systems and their functioning. Over the years, many differing ideas have been developed about emotional needs and how to meet them. At the present time we have very limited ability to demonstrate the "rightness" or "wrongness" of the one set of ideas or another. While this lack of certainty about human needs can be (and has been) an obstacle to developing clear guidelines for action, it also can be seen as an opportunity to use the data from our nursing experience to clarify human needs. Nurses are in the unique and enviable position of having direct access to large numbers of people in various life-stress situations from birth to death. In fact, we are responsible for taking care of them. What an excellent opportunity we have to get information about human emotional needs and how to meet them. All we have to do is ask!

Clearly, a functional model for identifying and meeting our patients' emotional needs should be patient-centered: it should consider the patient/client the primary source of information. Although we have subscribed to a patient-centered approach to nursing care for some time, we have not effectively or consistently involved patients in planning for and evaluating our care. We do not have the final word about what all people are like; therefore, we need our patients to tell us what *they* are like. Our capacity to predict what people's needs are under varying circumstances is very limited—so limited that we should constantly be collecting information from our patients and sorting it out to keep us from taking their needs for granted.

Since there is no "right" conception of human emotional needs and how to meet them, we are free to use ideas that are most helpful to us in guiding our practice. Nursing is concerned with the present and future well-being of patients with various socioeconomic, ethnic, age and diagnostic groupings. Therefore, our model of emotional care needs to be *flexible and operational*. That is, it should readily apply to us, too. It should be that basic and that functional.

Lastly, a functional model of emotional care should be *outcome-oriented* so that we can use it, test it and revise it as we go along.

Every nurse should be able to provide satisfactory or better emotional care. Therefore, nurses need a model of emotional care that says what satisfactory or better outcomes are, how to attain them and how to evaluate them. Patients can help us become more knowledgeable about the outcomes of care, the means to attain satisfactory outcomes and how to judge the quality of outcomes.

A *patient-centered, flexible, operational and outcome-oriented* model of emotional care will *not* meet all needs for all people in all situations. However, it *will* meet several basic and significant needs for all people in all situations. The existence or importance of other emotional needs is not denied. However, if we can assure that all nurses clearly understand how to identify and plan to meet basic needs, patients will be well served. In the following material several basic emotional needs are identified and guidelines are set forth for assessing and meeting these needs and evaluating the outcomes of our care.

IMPLEMENTING A FUNCTIONAL MODEL FOR EMOTIONAL CARE

Everyone has the following basic needs that affect how they feel about themselves and their environment: 1) the need for information, 2) the need for attention/recognition and 3) the need for emotional support or caring. It is through assessing and meeting these needs that we provide basic emotional care for our patients.

1. The Need for Information

Human beings are unique in their problem-solving capacities. Access to reliable information makes it possible for us to use our capacities more effectively to identify priorities and choose among possible courses of action. Often, health care providers assume that they know what information is useful for patients to have and they limit access to other information. Patients have a right to have information from nurses about:
—the health care setting (hospital, clinic, etc.) its personnel, policies and procedures,
—their specific health care concerns, and
—the management or treatment of their health care concerns.
The amount and kind of information people

can take in and use at any one time will vary. Therefore, informational needs should be checked regularly and varieties of means for providing information should be made available.

Example

In hospital X, nurses and other health care providers developed a comprehensive approach to preoperative teaching because of their awareness of their patients needs. Patients with regularly scheduled surgery are admitted at a predetermined time so that planned preoperative teaching can be carried out by nurses who have time to assure that their patients informational needs are met. Patients see a slide-tape program and then have an opportunity to discuss any question with a nurse. In addition, a pamphlet has been developed with basic information about common procedures and common experiences of surgical patients. This pamphlet is given to patients and they are encouraged to let the nurses know if they want further information. The surgeon and the anesthetist also meet with the patient to provide information about what can be expected pre- and postoperatively.

It has been demonstrated that a planned approach to preoperative teaching reduces patient's anxieties about surgery and increases their cooperation with postsurgical programs of turning, coughing and exercise. The need for information about surgical procedures may be clear; however, patients have a right to information about any intervention with which they are unfamiliar. The following are ways nurses can assess and meet their patients' needs for information.

1. Nurses can ask patients and their significant others what information *they* want. Although basic information about the procedures of the hospital or clinic may have been given, patients may want it to be repeated, clarified or elaborated on. They may not have heard it, were afraid to ask more about it, or did not think of their need at the time. Questions such as, "Is there anything you want to know about——?" "Do you have any questions?" and permissions such as "Please let me (or some other designated person) know if you have any questions," affirm the patient's right to information and the importance of meeting informational needs.

2. Nurses can plan to offer information about commonly occurring procedures verbally, in writing or by audio-visual means. Increasingly, informational packages are being developed by nurses and other health care providers to provide basic information about common health care procedures or situations such as admission and discharge routines, diagnostic procedures, medical or surgical treatments, labor and delivery circumstances, etc. While pamphlets or other means of delivering information are very useful, we would still want to know what additional information a patient might need.

3. Nurses can find out whether the information given meets the need or if more or different information is needed. Patients can help us evaluate the outcomes of our care if we will plan to ask them whether the information we offered was useful to them and made any difference in how they felt or how they saw their situation.

2. The Need for Attention/Recognition

We all have a need for an unspecified amount of personal notice from others—a need for others to take heed of and respond to the person that we are. In a busy health care setting, this basic need may be neglected as staff members concern themselves with meeting high priority physical needs and with meeting the needs of "squeaky wheels"—the patients who are willing to call attention to themselves. Just as we develop routines for attending to basic physical needs for food, water and rest, we need to develop routines for assuring that we meet basic emotional needs. Without a planned approach, we react to the need situation that demands our attention and ignore the others.

Example

The nursing staff in a long term care center asked a nursing consultant to advise them about how to deal with several problem patients who were disruptive to the center's routine because of their demanding, attention-seeking and agitated behavior. In the course of discussing and planning for these patients' needs, it became clear that the center's staff had no planned approach to providing regular attention for their patients. Since the staff was interested in doing this, a planning session was scheduled. They "brainstormed" all of the possible ways they could provide attention and then selected the following to become aspects of their care taking routines:

—birthdays and special holidays would be noted with a notice on bulletin boards, and these days would include planned group and/or individual activities, an opportunity to select a special meal item and a decorated cake for the evening meal;

—during visiting hours, at least one staff member would be assigned to circulate and provide attention to those patients who did not have visitors;

—patient care assignments would be structured so that patients would have the same nursing staff member for at least three consecutive days to facilitate individualization of care;

—opportunities for patients to give attention to each other would be identified and supported.

The quality of health care is affected by how much time and attention is given to patients. Nurses can improve the quality of their care by assessing and meeting their patients' needs for attention in the following ways.

1. Nurses can let patients know by words and behavior that they consider them to be unique individuals. By looking people in the eye when we speak to them, calling them by the name they wish to be called and listening to what they say, we acknowledge them as individuals in their own right.

2. Nurses can individualize the care they give. We can ask patients what they would like taken into consideration in their care; we may not be able to individualize every aspect of care, but neither should we individualize none. Every caretaking situation should be examined for the opportunities it presents for individual notice or attention, and all nurses should be concerned about the amount of individualization they can provide in their care.

3. Nurses can find out from patients how much of someone's undivided attention they want and can plan with them to see that the patients have what can possibly be provided. Anticipatory planning regarding attention would reassure many patients that their needs would be met. In the author's experience, planning for time and attention

has readily resolved problems with "difficult" patients.

4. Nurses can ask patients if what was done made any difference in the way they felt or how they viewed their situation.

3. The Need for Emotional Support Or Caring

Although we cannot be very specific about the nature and function of human feelings/emotions, we know all people experience them. This fact should be acknowledged as should the fact of emotional stress. Physical illness, disability or disruption can readily provoke fear, anger and/or sadness as emotional responses. These feelings or emotions can be experienced as very intense and stressful. All people have the need for ease from emotional stress and will automatically act in some way to relieve or minimize their perception of stress. These internally generated coping actions should be supplemented by comfort measures, which others can provide to ease perceptions of emotional stress. Nursing is a helping relationship, and meeting needs for emotional support is the essence of helping others.

Example

The 25-year-old Mr. Y was admitted to a large urban hospital for evaluation of a cough and bloody sputum. He had moved to a nearby community 6 months previously to take a job in a small parts factory and had recently been laid-off. His wife visits and hears the news of his diagnosis with him: terminal carcinoma of the lung. He is pale, stunned and trembling; she is crying loudly, wringing her hands and moving about in an agitated manner. The unit is very busy, but the charge nurse takes the time to ask someone to sit with Mr. Y while she takes his wife to a nearby conference room. She lets Mrs. Y cry, quietly sitting beside her and holding her hand. Then as Mrs. Y begins to calm, the head nurse asks who she can contact to be of support until Mr. and Mrs. Y are able to think about what they need to do next. The chaplain is contacted and agrees to spend an hour or so with the couple. Social services are also contacted, and they agree to assist the couple to contact relatives and begin to think about their financial and other support needs. The nursing staff decide to involve both Mr. and Mrs. Y in planning for his care while he remains in the hospital so that they can be given as much support as possible during this time period.

Crisis situations such as the one described clearly call for us to provide support. However, the need for support or caring is an ever present emotional need in us all, and nurses can assess and meet this need in their patients in the following ways.

1. Nurses can acknowledge emotional states they perceive in others—comments such as, "You look unhappy," "You seem dissatisfied," "You look angry," acknowledge that others are experiencing feelings and how they appear to us. The comments give others an opportunity to confirm or deny their emotions in the face of someone's interest. This exchange gives the nurse an opportunity to get more information about the other's emotional state.

2. Nurses can seek information about others' emotional states. Emotions are not well defined by psychologists and they are less well defined by the average person. Therefore, open-ended and more general questioning allows others to tell us in their own terms what they are experiencing. Questions such as, "How are things with you right now?" "How did your visit go?" "How have things gone since I saw you last?" etc., permit the other person to select what concerns him most and tell us about it in his own words.

3. Nurses can find out when people want support. We can ask, "What would be helpful to you at this time?" or "Would it be helpful if X were done to make you feel more at ease?"

4. Nurses can find out what people usually do to ease stressful situations—what their "support system" is. Who usually helps them during times of stress and what is comforting? Their usual comfort measures may or may not be available to them and they will need others that they or we will provide.

5. Nurses can facilitate people's use of their support systems. That is, we can make it easier for people to comfort themselves and/or get comfort from others as they are accustomed to do. We can assist them to link themselves with family, friends, ministers, etc.—people whom they see as sources of support.

6. Nurses can *provide* support. Comforting measures such as a word or two, a touch, or our presence and undivided attention are especially helpful when another's usual support system is unavailable or not adequate to the stress they are experiencing. These support measures are generally undervalued by health care providers. It does not take special training to demonstrate caring and concern to others.

7. Nurses can problem solve with and for others about stressful situations and how to resolve them. If we acknowledge that our estimation of another's stress and that person's own will differ and that there is no "right" answer, then we are free to work toward mutually acceptable goals and outcomes. We may not be able to change the fact that a patient or client may die or be permanently disabled. Nevertheless, is there some level at which we might both feel satisfied with the outcomes of care? We must concern ourselves about what we *can* do with and for people in the time we have to spend and the constraints of the caretaking setting.

8. Nurses can ask patients/others if what we did made any difference in how they felt or how they perceived their situation.

SUMMARY

A functional model of emotional care is one that is patient-centered, is flexible, can readily be carried out, and is concerned about outcomes. It addresses basic emotional needs that are often overlooked or taken for granted: the need for information, for attention and for emotional support. In meeting these needs and the patient's physical and spiritual needs, nurses provide care for the whole person.

BIBLIOGRAPHY

Benjamin, A. *The Helping Interview.* Boston: Houghton-Mifflin Co., 1969.

Burgess, A. W., and Lazare, A. *Psychiatric Nursing in the Hospital and the Community,* 2nd ed. Englewood Cliffs, N. J.: Prentice-Hall, 1976.

Carlson, C. E. (coordinator), *Behavioral Concepts and Nursing Intervention.* Philadelphia: J. B. Lippincott Co., 1970.

James, M., and Jongeward, D. *Born To Win.* Reading, Mass.: Addison-Wesley Publishing Co., 1971.

Orlando, I. J. *The Dynamic Nurse-Patient Relationship.* New York: G. P. Putnam's Sons, 1961.

22

emotional
impact
of cancer

SR. PATRICE BURNS
(as told to Lois C. Dunlap)

One of this nation's goals for some time has been the conquering of cancer—the discovery of the cause or causes, a specific treatment and most important, a method of prevention. When this goal is reached one of the most devastating diseases man has ever had to deal with will all but be eradicated. As we work toward that end, those of us involved in the delivery of health care to such consumers must concern ourselves with all aspects of this disease—medical, social, economic and emotional with quality of care a primary priority. And in many instances this implies the need for improvement of nursing practice, especially in attempting to deal with the psychological component of the disease.

Cancer patients can be found anywhere along the continuum from wellness to illness and in all age groups from infancy to old age. They are seen in acute care or long term care facilities, as inpatients or outpatients, in the hospital, clinic or home setting. Regardless of how old this individual is, his degree of wellness or where he is encountered, his diagnosis poses a number of real threats. Quite common is the fear of death, of prolonged pain and of bodily mutilation.

The cost of care may seriously jeopardize a person financially. Cancer can disrupt a patient's normal pattern of living and bring about tremendous changes in the relationships he has had with those most meaningful to him in his life. The individual fears his loss of usefullness and becoming nonproductive and totally dependent. This can be more anxiety producing than the threat of death itself. Physical attractiveness, and thus ones self-image, is openly threatened and the patient fears that his illness with all of its negative and repulsive aspects will cause others to flee from him. Frequently, the cancer patient faces the possibility of never being able to live up to the norm which our society sets up as important—to marry, to relate successfully sexually, to have children, to succeed and to be accepted. In measuring his worth according to these standards, the cancer patient fears failure. Prolonged illness and hospitalization cause the patient to become socially displaced and isolated from life. He feels that he is no longer in control of his life and body. Furthermore he can't quite understand the external forces which have taken over this control.

The cancer patient must not only deal with these very real stresses resulting directly from the disease itself, but in addition, he must deal with all of the misconceptions about its nature, cause, cure and control, and the effects these misconceptions have on him and his life—all of which make cancer one of the greatest stress producers known to man. Along with tuberculosis and venereal disease, cancer is definitely a low status disease. Other chronic diseases with a similar prognosis do not carry the same negative connotation. It is still spoken of as "unclean" by some and secretly feared as "contagious." Cancer patients, their families and friends often see cancer as "rotting or being dirty," giving cancer an image similar to that of the leper in biblical times. Because of these perceptions cancer patients are frequently avoided by their family, friends and acquaintances. The absence of this disease being listed as the cause of death in obituary notices in local newspapers is given as one illustrated proof of the shame of dying with cancer. Husbands or wives shun physical closeness by their spouse or children. Some people mentally associate cancer with venereal disease and latent guilt feelings are sometimes aroused. Many patients will not tell their friends or family members, other than those immediate ones who know, that they have cancer. Joe, a man of 65, was a perfect example of this behavior. He had lived with a diagnosis of cancer for some time, was receiving radiation but would talk to no one nor would he acknowledge the fact that this was the diagnosis. One day he developed a myocardial occlusion. He began talking to everyone available about this new diagnosis, fully accepting it and expressing a desire to eventually die from another heart attack in preference to "another" illness. He did not fear this disease as he did his cancer.

Some of the misconceptions about cancer lie at the roots of a patient's denial of his illness. The very fact that the specific cause for cancer is still not known helps to create such false ideas and fears. They are reinforced in turn by the very real fact that many cancer patients either lose their jobs or are not considered employable—incapable of work—because of their diagnosis.

Cancer patients also find it extremely difficult if not impossible, to obtain many kinds of insurance. Because of certain technicalities, health insurance is often terminated after a period of time as a workers illness forces him to leave his place of employment and to switch from a group plan to an individual policy. Is it any wonder then that often the most educated or informed persons do not seek medical help or advice which will possibly result in a diagnosis of symptoms which are present and possibly recognized as serious. The possibility of cancer being present causes patients to deny to themselves or suppress even the idea of such a possibility. Instead they attribute their symptoms to a variety of other causes. They avoid seeing a doctor and rationalize away their behavior. Being too busy to find the time, the attitude of, "It's all in my head," and "I've been working too hard, just need a rest," are common examples. Others go from doctor to doctor seeking a more acceptable diagnosis.

IDENTITY AND BODY IMAGE

The self-concept or identity might be defined as "all the perceptions an individual has of himself—his attitudes, beliefs, thoughts, feelings, goals, fears, fantasies, what he has been, what he may become, and the worst of it all—constantly being formed by the interaction of his biologic givens, the environment in which he lives, the people with whom he relates, and his perceptions of these multiple interrelationships." (Donovan and Pierce, 1976, p. 205). The body image is the sum total of the feelings and perceptions a person has about his body. This body image seems to be one of the most central yet inflexable aspects of the self-concept. The body image is affected by feelings, attitudes, and conditioning and changes during the course of life. It begins to develop between the ages of three and five, and is most influenced by the significant others (especially the mother), environmental stimuli and the individual's own physiologic and psychologic characteristics. Most people learn to accept how they appear to themselves and others and this view is generally more or less realistic. In a culture such as ours, with its emphasis on youthful, healthy, and beautiful bodies, even the physically well frequently have difficulty facing advancing years with its threat on their idea of self. However, the cancer patient is often faced with the prospect of radical surgery that may be mutilating, changing his entire appearance. The magnitude of the surgery alone is frightening. The meaning of the loss through surgery is related to 1) the visibility of the loss, 2) the functional loss and 3) the emotional investment in, or the meaning of, the affected part regardless of the objective severity of any of these catagories (Donovan and Pierce, 1976, p. 209). When the cancer is in the head and neck area, the surgery frequently results in the loss or impairment of speech, swallowing, breathing, control of saliva, and obvious face and neck deformity—all in varying degrees. Such treatments which alter the face are responded to with terror. A beautiful face is highly valued in our society—millions of dollars are spent annually to improve the facial appearance of many. The face is the first and most obvious feature we observe in a person and the automatic response to facial ugliness is to withdraw and pull away from what we perceive as repulsive. These patients have a vital need for the loving support and acceptance of their family members—it is the responses of these people which are so important to the patient.

The colostomy patients is often repulsed by the idea of feces coming from his abdomen. His lifelong habits of cleanliness make an indelible impression on his thinking that this is "dirty." There are also the fears of "smelling" and "leaking" which are socially unacceptable. Patients can be reassured that there are appliances available which eliminate these problems. Encouraging a patient to join an "ostomy" club postoperatively is often psychologically helpful.

An individual's sexuality is highly personal and a central aspect of his identity. Almost any body part or function can have sexual meaning and any alteration in that organ or function can alter one's perception of and expression of his sexuality. Breast cancer probably represents the most common assault on sexuality. Women fear that they will be only "half a woman" after a mastectomy. These patients should be reassured that prostheses are available and that they will be able to continue in their sexual relationships as before. The most important factor in a woman's adjustment following mastectomy seems to be the response of the man with whom her sex life is most intimately involved. Helping him to express his feelings is a frequently overlooked matter. Even a hysterectomy, though not visible to others, carries for some women a serious loss making her less of a person and "incomplete" in appearance especially to men.

A patient's response to his change in physical appearance is an individual thing which gives the nurse some indication of where the patient is coming from—that is, where his greatest values lie. A 24-year-old and beautiful woman on chemotherapy fully accepted her loss of hair showing no shame at her baldness when visitors entered the room. In the next room, a woman of 79 years of age receiving the same medication was extremely upset as her hair fell out. She spent much time before a mirror fussing with her hair and carefully saved every piece she lost with the intention of matching it with a hairpiece as soon as possible. Once it was learned that the older woman had spent 40 years of her life as a beautician, it became understandable why her hair was most important to her. The younger woman had never been too concerned with her hair and, therefore, accepted the loss very readily. The nurse must listen and become aware of these individual differences, accepting the patients' response without reservation.

Depressive reactions associated with surgery for cancer frequently reflect marked changes in body form and function which have significant meaning in the individual's total adaptation to life. This disruption in function, even if temporary, becomes most disturbing when it involves valued life activities. These valued life activities are expressions of character defenses basic to the maintenance of self-respect and represent attempted solutions to important problems of childhood. An organ can play a basic role in the ability to relate to other people, and when this is lost, depression can set in. Also "when a sense of worth is predicated" on performing service for others and rigid self-denial, the sense of diminished vitality and subsequent inability to serve can result in serious depression." (Sutherland and Orbach, pp. 17–20)

Some patients refuse to look at their incisions or surgical sites and will not touch those areas. Many display helpless dependent behavior relying upon the nurse to give complete care – to irrigate, suction and change dressings. Here we see the very same mechanisms of denial and avoidance which kept the patient from seeking a diagnosis of his symptoms in the first place. The nurse plays a vital role in the patient's acceptance of his altered body image. The patient will test the nurse first, watching the nurse's eyes or body movements for signs of withdrawal or disgust. He will become confident and secure through the reassurance and support given by the nurse. Costello reports the following necessary steps in providing patient support when dealing with altered body image. The patient: accepts the importance of viewing his operative cite; touches and explores his operative cite; accepts the necessity of his learning to care for the defect; develops independence and competence in his daily care; reintegrates his new body image and adjusts to a possible lifestyle (Costello, 1974, p. 5).

PAIN

The almost universal association of excruciating pain with cancer is a false one. In reality, pain is usually a late symptom of the disease and depends upon the location of the tumor, the stimulation of pain-sensitive fibers by a variety of processes and other physiological, pathological, psychological and sociological phenomena. Some patients, even in the terminal stages have little or no pain. Even when pain does occur, various methods of treatment are available, depending on the type of malignancy and its location, and should be adequate to control pain and keep the patient as comfortable as possible. Radiation, chemotherapy and surgical procedures are all used in the appropriate conditions. Medications may be given to relieve pain by specifically counteracting the cause of pain, (steroids) or may modify the perception of

and reaction to the sensation of pain (analgesics and narcotics). Pain should really be considered as a dual phenomenon, one part being the perception of the sensation and the other the patient's reaction to it. Depression, anxiety and fear all tend to exacerbate the total pain experience and one's response to pain, in general, tends to be a highly personal thing. Also, the same patient will not react to the same pain in the same way all of the time. Medication for chronic pain in cancer should be given in increasing larger dosages until the patient is pain-free, giving the next dose before the effect of the previous one has worn off, therefore, before the patient may think it necessary and thus erasing the memory and fear of pain. One of the rights of the patient dying with cancer is the right to be free from pain (Donovan and Pierce, 1976, p. 33). It is the responsibility of the nurse to see that this right is protected.

CARE OF THE DYING

Although death is not necessarily synonomous with cancer, all cancer patients are confronted with this component of life whether their illness is curable or not. In recent years, many qualified authors have described the dying process as a psychological event in a variety of ways. The steps and stages the dying individual goes through have been clearly described (Kübler-Ross, 1969). There is no intent here to review these widely read authorities but to simply relate to some of the behavioral implications of these stages.

Death has the potential of being the loneliest experience any of us will ever have to face. However, this need not be. In some fashion, those who are dying reach out for support and companionship, even if in hidden and disguised ways. It is up to us who are caring for them to be aware of and recognize this need. If the patient is not dealt with honestly by those around him, he will feel totally alone and will become increasingly more dejected, withdrawing into himself. However, in actual practice the question of "to tell or not to tell" a patient that he is dying is really more a matter of "when and how to share what" with him. A patient will very often bring the subject up himself. His words will tell you how much information he is ready for, can understand and accept. The truth can be told in many ways. It behooves us to handle it with as much gentleness and hope in our voice as is humanly possible. Just as in principle it is wrong to deliberately plan to deceive a patient, it is likewise wrong to believe that it is essential for every patient to know that he is dying. Occasionally a patient does not want to know the truth — he does not wish to regard his illness as fatal or he wishes others to take charge of things. If our aim is to make dying easier for the patient, then it seems we should allow this patient to maintain his very necessary defense. Older patients seem to accept the inevitability of death. It is the younger patient who tends to feel that death is an intrusion on this life and premature. With a patient who denies the seriousness of his illness (or the fact that he is dying) a nurse can ask certain nonthreatening questions which will make him think about death as a possibility, rather than tearing away this defense indirectly or directly. "Is your son able to take over your role in the family?" is such a question when appropriate. These questions help the patient to discuss the reality of the situation and to realize that he actually desires to talk about the ramifications of his death. "What do you really feel is going to happen to you?" also, often gets at the crucial matter. It has been the experience of many who have worked very closely with dying patients over a period of many years to find that even those who do not ask and are not told the truth gradually become well aware of the fact that they are dying. They accept it quietly, some never wishing to discuss it openly. We must respect this desire. The nurse must not take the initiative in such cases, inflicting her values on the patient, but if the patient begins to ask leading questions it is totally wrong to hedge or to lie. It is so easy to judge the patient who is unable to face the full truth. Many patients, never openly discussing their death, seem to have a premonition of some kind, knowing almost exactly when they are going to die, often a patient who wants to spare his spouse the stress of watching him die will

see to it that she is not there by planning some activity for her which will remove her from the bedside.

Hope seems to be an essential element of working with cancer patients. For some patients it is a hope that despite everything, they will recover — that something unforeseen will happen that they may possibly have a remission, that they will live for a little longer time. For others it is not a matter of reaching out for a miracle cure but of more realistic wishes; of hopes of seeing certain friends again, of holding a grandchild, of helping one's family make plans, of getting things ready or of simply dying in a manner which will eliminate stress for loved ones. One thing to avoid is reinforcing the hope of recovery when the patient himself has finally accepted his inevitable death. The hope of the cancer patient usually grows out of facing and tackling the reality of his illness and its component of death as honestly as possible. It very often means being vulnerable and trusting in the unknown which comes as a result of one's own belief and life experiences. There are still doctors who tell a patient that he has X number of months to live, giving him a definite data for a death sentence. Needless to say this upsets patients and is in effect a prediction impossible to make. Some patients die sooner than the doctor predicts, other later. A better response to the patient would be, "You will progressively go downhill but no one can tell how long it will take. However, we will try to keep you as comfortable as possible during this time." With this promise in mind, the patient can set out to take care of the things he feels are important in preparation for his death, living each day to the fullest as much as is possible, without the constant dread of an assigned data which he is aware of as daily coming ever closer.

Patients have to work through their dying each in his own way. In helping the patient with this, no nurse or counselor should attempt to inflict her beliefs on the patient. What is more important is just being there with him, being available if he should have a desire to talk or to ask questions and preventing that feeling of being alone. It is important to visit these patients regularly even if you get indications from their behavior that they would rather you not come. Very often in such cases it is an attempt on the patients part to push you away because he wants to make the preparation easier for both himself and for you. If there is estrangement, then it is easier to die. Many nurses are uncomfortable with such behavior and make the mistake of staying away from the patient. Some patients, with much emotional unfinished business and not ready to die, respond to terminal illness with anger and resentment. Sometimes in combination with or alternating with depression, the patient often feels that fate is robbing him of goals and pursuits not quite achieved but now slipping out of reach because of his illness. Present and projected activites, which will give him a feeling of self-fulfillment must be given up. This anger is often directed toward both the medical staff and the family. In our culture there are many taboos controlling the expression of anger. This accounts for the anger very often being displaced onto God or objects in the environment. It can seldom be openly and fully expressed and so is manifested in many different kinds of behavior—irritability, demanding behavior, or silent withdrawal being most common.

Mr. B., a 48-year-old father of five, hospitalized for several weeks with terminal metastatic cancer had suddenly become mute the day of his admission. There was no organic reason for his inability to talk. He was responsive in every other way. The counselor who visited him each day would enter and take hold of his hand saying, "Hi!" making no further attempt to encourage him to speak. She observed over time that no one was talking to him about dying and that in fact, his wife would speak to her in his presence as if he wasn't there at all. She began to feel the anger he was feeling— anger about what was going on around him. One day while visiting, the counselor felt it important to let him know that she knew he was angry. She told him it was all right to feel such anger, that she and his wife knew and understood what he was going through and how difficult it was for him to talk about it. He reached up and kissed her on the cheek. With their expressed permission to have such feelings, the patient was gradually able to talk to them about his feelings and his impending death was openly discussed and prepared for as he had so desired.

With the dying patient, no one should be fearful of getting too involved. For years, nurse educators have been advocating against getting involved with patients believing that the nurse will become less effective if this happens. A transference relationship should present no problem with the dying patient—there is no need to work through or understand its meaning. As with the unnecessary fear of addiction to pain-killing medication, the patient takes both with him to his grave. There is, therefore, no need to fear the consequences of holding a dying patient's hand or of displaying any other acceptable expression of love and caring. It is through these physical expressions of care that the fear of being alone, of abandonment, is prevented and that realistic hope is maintained. Touch can be very effectively used to communicate our support, interest and concern for the patient. A firm touch on the shoulder, a pat on the cheek, a clasp of hands tells him that someone cares and that someone is there who can be depended upon. Suffering is made tolerable when someone cares and "faith in God and His care is made infinitely easier by faith in someone who has shown kindness and sympathy." (Saunders, 1976, p. 18)

THE FAMILY

In dealing with the families of cancer patients the most critical husbands or wives are very often those who have experienced difficulty in the marriage situation. The behavior appears to be a last ditch attempt to work out guilt feelings over the part in the past marital problems. They switch from doctor to doctor, each time finding fault with the care their spouses are receiving, often threatening to sue medical personnel or the hospital itself. One's initial response may be to feel negative toward such behavior. It is most important to avoid being judmental but rather to accept each family member as he is. The fears of the family members, in reality, are not much different from those of the patient—the fear that their loved one will die, will suffer prolonged pain, will be mutilated and disfigured. They have fears for themselves—fears of abandonment, of role changes, of loss of support. The nurse needs to be aware of the strengths and weaknesses of all family members involved. The treatment of a patient's illness may necessitate his separation from his family for long periods of time, reversal of family roles and large expenditures of family funds. All of these create tremendous problems and stresses on the patient's family.

All of the psychological implications of surgical procedures faced by the patient also affect the patient's spouse. The absence of a breast, the offensiveness of a colostomy, the disfigurement of radical neck and face surgery can each cause distance and an inability for husband and wife to express love and closeness. The responses of those who are emotionally close to the patient are most important to the patient—even more important than the actual severity of the defect itself. Therefore, it is important that both the patient and the spouse be helped to express their own feelings to one another. The nurse can play a vital role here. Problems relating to sexuality pose a specific but complex group of concerns. An individual's sexuality and its expression are a highly individualized thing. Its very personal meanings are multiple and complex. Cancer of the genital organs creates an assault on one's sexuality—the effect of the surgery depending on the meaning of the organ, of the disease and of the treatment to the individual person. The nurse must avoid either minimizing or overemphasizing the meaning of sex to the patient. She can also convey an acceptance of the patient's concern over loss or possible loss of sexual potency as a valid concern, suggesting possible ways to compensate for this loss.

When the patient is terminal, the relatives experience a variety of reactions which are hard to predict. Each must go through the same denial, anger, bargaining, and depression as the patients (Kübler-Ross, 1969). Usually a family member's reaction to bereavement will be more guilt-ridden and prolonged when the impending death was not faced realistically. Death-denying relatives need to be helped to face the truth and encouraged to talk about the patient and how they are coping with the stress created by his illness. Most relatives actually jump at the opportunity to unburden themselves, if need be, break down and cry when someone who cares shows an interest in listening. Many family members express deep concern that they haven't done all they could have for their loved one—another indication of guilt and a sense of failure. In order to help set realistic goals for family members and to choose appropriate interventions, it seems imperative that each person must be assessed separately in terms of needs and individual perceptions. Caring for the patient with cancer is a challenge—a challenge to provide nursing care which gives support for the patient, which offers hope for some realistic goals, and which promotes a positive outlook by the patient toward his difficulties. This is enhanced by involving the patient in his care as much as possible. The nurse realizes that although all patients may not realistically hope for cure, there is something which can be done for all cancer patients. The time for living may be drastically shortened for the patient but a quality of life which brings peace and tranquility to the patient can be achieved.

BIBLIOGRAPHY

Costello, A. M. Supporting the patient with problems relating to body image. In *Emotional Problems of Patients With Cancer: Nursing Interventions.* American Cancer Society Professional Education Publication, 1974.

Donovan, M., and Pierce, S. *Cancer Care Nursing.* New York: Appleton-Century-Crofts, 1976.

Hilkemeyer, R. *Cancer Nursing: the state of the art",* American Cancer Society Professional Education Publication, 1974, pp. 1–6.

Kübler-Ross, E. *On Death and Dying.* New York: Macmillan Publishing Co., Inc., 1969.

Saunders, C. "Care of the Dying" *Nurs. Times* 72 (26) July 1976.

Seminars in Oncology: Supportive Care of The Cancer Patient, Vol. 2, No. 4, December 1975.

Sutherland, A., and Orbach, C. Depressive reactions associated with surgery for cancer. In *The Psychological Impact of Cancer.* American Cancer Society, Professional Education Publication, pp. 17–21.

Twycross, R. G. *The Dying Patient.* London: Christian Medical Fellowship Publication, 1975.

Chapter 23

the coronary patient: psychosocial aspects

DORIS HOUSER

Care of the sick individual involves a multidisciplinary and multiorgan approach. It involves not only stabilizing the patient's respiratory, metabolic and hemodynamic status, but also his psychosocial status. Psychological and physiological care is interrelated and interdependent. Because each patient presents his own unique set of needs and reactive patterns from both a physiological and a psychosocial standpoint, the needs of the patient vary from time to time as he moves from a state of illness to a state of health. As one feels better physically, one feels better mentally; conversely, as one feels worse mentally, one feels worse physically. Various members of the health team, be they physicians, physical therapists, dietitians or social workers, all provide a variety of skills and services to restore the patient's health status. The nurse is often the only member of the health team who provides the communication and coordinating link in these varied services so that care of the "whole" patient is realized. The nurse is in a pivotal position to help the patient from both a physiological and a psychological standpoint. She is often the

first one the patient sees upon admission to the hospital, the last one he sees when discharged, and the one seen on a 24-hour basis in between. Nurses' care after discharge from the hospital through community health agencies is also vital to the patient's full recovery and return to a productive status in the community.

It is ironic that in this day of advanced medical technology and potential for restoration of physiological health consumer groups are becoming much more vocal about the poor quality of health care. It is apparent that technological devices and specialized medical care cannot provide another necessary ingredient, old fashioned "TLC." Although this need has been recognized for a long time, the psychological care of the patient and family unit during acute illness and recovery often tends to be more a stated policy than reality. Clinical specialization and the team approach to care can easily deteriorate into fragmented care if someone isn't holding the reins of the team and providing an individualized care plan based upon both physiological and psychosocial aspects of care.

169

Psychological care is too often considered a lofty concept that is time-consuming and better off left to the "experts." However, psychological care comes in many forms and is provided in many ways and by many people in the health care environment with varying degrees of professional expertise. Too often it is only the maid that takes time to listen to the patient, smile, and chat while scrubbing the floor. Psychological care means providing comfort physically and mentally, emotionally and spiritually; and where possible, rehabilitating the patient by maintaining and restoring the patient's self-esteem and sense of usefulness and well-being as a person. It may involve a lengthy counseling session or simply an attitude of "caring" expressed by a smile or a pat on the hand. Psychological care or "TLC" boils down to the "fruit of human kindness."

In the hospital environment, the patient who feels less able to cope with anything because of his physical problems, finds himself in a new, confusing and complex environment full of machinery and new people he is totally dependent upon. His basic physical needs may be met, but higher level needs for security, love and closeness may be neglected. He soon learns that he is also the center of a complex interrelationship between a group of people who also have individual needs — the hospital staff. With this group, there may be conflicts in staff's goals and care modalities for the patient and thus continuity of care suffers. How is the patient supposed to reconstruct his life if everyone on the staff differs in his approaches and care goals? The patient also realizes he has a "role" to play within this hospital system. He must be "good" or he is a "problem" and may be rejected by the staff. To be good, he must not complain or be angry; he must always be grateful and smiling. Would we expect the same if he were well and outside the hospital setting? Meanwhile, the patient has his own personal struggles within himself and in his relationship with his family due to the stress the illness has imposed on his life style. The patient may manifest various behaviors and mood swings that are difficult for both the family and the staff to handle. A hostile, angry patient may find a less than empathetic staff who may take his behavior as a personal affront. This lack of understanding is not conducive to a therapeutic environment.

Because of the nurse's significant role in the health care environment, it is important for the nurse to be acutely aware of what the patient is encountering in order to be beneficial to him. She needs to remember that ill people are going through a crisis in their lives. They have lost their health, at least momentarily, and this loss also affects their family and their situation in life at that point in time.

The literature is full of various concepts identifying the interrelationship between mental and physical health. Stress, both mental and physical, as identified by Seyle et al., and various crises in our lives affect our total well-being, our significant others, and our particular life style. A crisis is the perceived loss of something of value to the individual. This may be through death, divorce, loss of job, loss of money or loss of social status. The loss creates a gap in life's continuity and a lowering of self-confidence. Health is also a valued item and its loss can create other stresses or crises such as financial insecurity, job loss, diability or even death. Man trys to adapt or cope with these stresses or crises in a variety of ways. This whole process of adaptation to achieve a state of equilibrium has been called various things by different authors, such as the use of coping mechanisms or the grieving process. As man goes through the adaptation process, which evolves in stages, he may manifest various behaviors ranging from depression to anger to euphoria.

Since no man is an island, the way man perceives a crisis in his life and how he adapts to it is very often affected by people and other factors in his immediate environment. How a patient and his family unit have dealt with stress in the past is an influential factor in his adaptation to illness. The patient's age and the perceived severity of the illness are other factors that influence the patient's ability to psychological reconstruct his life in spite of the illness.

The whole interplay between the physical and mental internally and the environment externally is exemplified in the coronary patient. A coronary is considered an isolated event that is a manifestation of an underlying disease process, atherosclerotic heart disease. Atherosclerotic heart disease is felt to be affected by the ravages of stress over the years. Studies have identified that with high stress situations, cholesterol levels and blood clotting factors rise. The correlation between high cholesterol diets and coronaries has been altered somewhat by more recent studies which identify the significant role that stress imposed by society and life style has played in causing coronaries. Previous studies indicated that the relatively low incidence of coronaries in the Japanese population was due to the low amount of cholesterol in their diet. A new 10-year study of the Japanese population has indicated a high incidence of coronaries, comparable to that in the United States, in areas of Japan where the western culture has been adopted. Both the Japanese in these areas and those in the United States have a five times greater incidence than the Japanese in outlying areas and living according to their ancient culture. Historically, the Japanese have close knit family units and compete in groups (Slay, 1976).

Western society encourages individual competition and this heritage had bred the so-called Type A personality. This individual has an alarm clock in his chest beside the heart which ticks away as long as he is doing something defined as being of value per society's norms, but "goes off" if he relaxes or lets up on the effort. Unfortunately, the constant ticking of this Type A alarm clock may damage the heart that is trying in vain to keep up the pace. With stress of any kind, there is also an increase in catecholamine release as the body tries to compensate for the additional demands. With catecholamine release, among other things, heart rate and blood pressure increase causing added stress on the heart. This can be a factor in causing cardiac decompensation before, during, and after a coronary.

Other studies have identified the role of stress in causing coronaries: 80 to 90% of all coronary patients have had a significant loss or alteration in life style in the year preceeding the coronary; 93% of all coronary patients have STP—stress, tension and pressure (Slay, 1976). With STP in their motors, it is no wonder that these individuals always run in high gear and find shifting gears to low during recovery from a coronary so difficult.

A coronary has a massive physiological and psychological impact on a person. To most of us, the heart is not only a vital organ, but a symbol of our emotions, our strengths, our very being. The patient with a coronary may imagine he sees the buzzard of death on one hand and a life of disability on the other with no alternatives. Understandably, he and his family are in a state of anxiety and depression. The way a person perceives his condition and how he learns to adapt to his residual abilities may swing the balance toward recovery or invalidism. Studies by Klein, Wishnie and others indicate that some degree of invalidism often occurs in the absence of definable physical incapacity and that the emotional hazards of convalescence are the primary determinate of cardiac disability.

A person in a state of anxiety or conflict looks to others for a cue that will reduce his tension. An anxious person has a drive for self-evaluation and a need to be with someone in the same plight so that he may compare himself to his peers and thus create a homogenization of feelings, or a reduction in anxiety. In the hospital environment, this process of affiliation can have both a positive and a negative effect on the patient and family. Witnessing the death of a fellow patient in CCU can increase a patient's anxiety level. This situation necessitates an open, truthful, but tactful discussion with the staff so that the patient realizes that every coronary patient is different and he will not necessarily suffer the same fate. On the other hand, a roommate that is recovering satisfactorily from his coronary can elicit optimism. Hospital visitors' lounges are notorious for the false and horrifying information exchanged between family members. However, they can also be an environment of compassion, concern and shared anxiety when family members are provided a structured means of ventilating their fears and mutual support. The wise nurse keeps an eye on the visitors' lounge and maintains communication with the family unit as they strive for methods of reducing fear and anxiety.

The process of affiliation is perpetuated by giving the patient and family factual information about heart disease, his physical limitations, usual care regimen, and by giving them an attitude of hope based on the successes of other heart patients in the same plight. Gerard's and others' studies indicate that giving a person information about himself furthers understanding and decreases feelings of uncertainty. Knowledge increases the patient's cooperation with the medical care regimen, and with adequate psychological support, decreases the threat to his ego. Feelings of worth and self-esteem depend upon a person's perception of his illness and its subsequent effect on his life style. Since self-esteem is the psychological oxygen for mental health, maintaining and restoring it are essential for rehabilitation (Houser, 1973).

A cornerstone of a cardiac rehabilitation program is the patient education program. However, as Carl Rogers has said, "Just because you have said something doesn't mean it has been learned." Giving the patient factual information is only one part of the education program; the information must be relevant to his own life style. It is necessary to repeat and reinforce information for the anxious coronary patient needs time to adapt and to reconstruct his perception of the event. Early mobilization of the coronary patient has not only yielded good physiological effects, but also psychological effects. Mobilization causes a more positive perception of the event and is a means of working off anxiety.

Anxiety and a sense of uneasiness persist for some time. Three years are often needed to reach a new adaptational level in even the uncomplicated coronary patient (Slay, 1976). As a 1-year postcoronary patient stated, "I feel like I am sitting on a powder keg that can explode any minute." The advent of various cardiac rehab programs and counseling groups throughout the country for patients and families after hospitalization identifies the value of support groups in sharing problems and finding solutions in adaptation when the patient is more able physically and mentally to deal with his situation. Rehabilitation involves helping the patient look for solutions within his physical limitations and socioeconomic structure so he can enjoy a sense of well-being and usefulness to himself, his family and his community.

The interplay between the physical and the mental is ever present. The time of hospital discharge is not usually the time of full recovery. When a patient sees his physician for a follow-up evaluation and treadmill examination at approximately 6 to 8 weeks postinfarction, a new stage begins. The patient and family have a more objective assessment of his physiological status and more specific guidelines to determine his future physical activities. This allays anxiety, uneasiness, and the feeling of being in a state of limbo.

These physiological stages are closely aligned to psychological stages and behavior typically manifested. How a patient is progressing physiologically affects his perception of the seriousness of his illness. A 10-day postcoronary patient who is walking around and feeling fine has a different future outlook than another 10-day postcoronary patient who has just returned to CCU for evaluation of an incident of severe chest pain.

Although behavior follows a typical pattern of adaptation, there is not a set pattern per stage of illness or a set length of time that a patient remains in this stage. Patients may revert from one stage to another and then back to the initial stage again depending upon variables that affect his condition. The nurse must be able to alter the plan of care to meet changing needs of the patient as he moves through the stages. The nurse who gets to know the patient and his family and assesses physiological and psychosocial status, can better identify problems for resolution. As William Osler said, "It is more important to know what sort of patient has a disease than what sort of disease a patient has." (Slay, 1976)

Table 1 identifies the psychological stages, their relationship to the physiological, and some of the typical behavior patterns.

TABLE 1. PSYCHOLOGICAL STAGES FOR THE CORONARY

Physiological Stage	Time Interval	Psychological Stage	Behavior
I(CCU)	1–5 days	Threat	Denial Tension Confusion
		Impact	Denial Regression/dependency Tension Depression/withdrawal Assertion Confusion
II(Ward)	5–15 days	Recoil	Anger/hostility Regression/dependency Limited denial Depression Aggression Confusion Euphoria Guilt Tension
III(Home)	3–8 weeks	Recoil	Anger/hostility Depression/withdrawal Independence/assertion Guilt Insight Irritability
IV(Home)	8 weeks on	Recovery	Mild anxiety/tension Acceptance Independence Insight

Different authors have labeled these psychological stages differently but definition by behaviors are very similar. Granger (1974) has identified the stages as:

1. stress,
2. disorganization,
3. reconstruction.

Since "stress" is ever present to some degree, it may be preferable to identify the stage of stress more specifically. In Table 1 the psychological stages are:

1. threat,
2. impact,
3. recoil,
4. recovery (Moore, 1969).

The stages of threat and impact are comparable to Granger's stage of stress, the stage of recoil to disorganization, and the recovery stage to reconstruction. Fear is the predominant emotion that commonly manifests itself in some form of anxiety and depression. When the patient becomes ill and after he is admitted to the hospital, there is often a period of time when the diagnosis is not substantiated. Even if the diagnosis is a certainty, the patient may be denying the event. This is the period of *threat*, a feeling of impending disaster and perceived loss. He knows something is wrong, but is afraid of what it might be, thus he uses denial as his means of coping with the event. When the patient intellectually realizes he has had a coronary, the emotional reaction is one of shock and disbelief. "Why me?" This is the period of *impact*. In his struggle to internalize the crisis, he may find denial more comfortable or he may become depressed and withdrawn by the impact of this event on his life. "Will I live?" "What will I be good for?" "Will I just be a burden on my a1family?" These are all questions that run through the patient's mind. Just because you put the body to rest, doesn't slow the brain down. This is a period when an attitude of hope projected by the staff is beneficial. It is a time when the patient should be allowed the privilege of coping in his own way. Denial is not an abnormal phenomenon at this time. Without this coping mechanism, the potential for psychosis more readily exists. Crying is a useful emotional cathartic. Bottled up anxiety and despair need a means of release before the blocks of recovery can be built.

A patient who progresses well physically and is transferred to the ward unit begins the reconstruction process and struggles in his efforts to come to terms with the event. He recognizes that he is now a viable being who has a future. Before, there wasn't any point in planning for the future as there was a question if one existed. This is the period of *recoil*. The patient begins to gain insight, begins to be more assertive and independent in his behavior as a means of providing his vigor and worth. It can also be a period of anger and hostility. The questions arise: "Why me?" "What did I do to deserve this?" "Did I do something that caused it?" "Is God punishing me for some misdeeds?" The family also ask themselves these questions and as a result, both patient and family often express a profound feeling of guilt. Alternating feelings of guilt, despair, and anger within the patient and in his interpersonal relationships with the family may cause problems. The patient may take his anger and hostility out on his spouse. The anxious spouse is devastated by this behavior and either lashes back or dissolves into tears and depression. Helping the spouse to recognize the motivation for the hostile and irritable behavior of the patient during and immediately after hospitalization is helpful. It is still a difficult emotional process for the whole family unit, but the patient needs to know he has their love and support. Verbalization is a useful cathartic at this time for both the patient and his family. This is not only a means of reducing tension, but a means of eliciting positive feedback from the staff regarding the patient's perception of the coronary and its effect on his life activities.

The first few weeks after the patient is discharged from the hospital and recovering at home prior to resumption of work and other activities is often a difficult period for the whole family unit. The first few days at home are frequently a new period of depression. This may come as a surprise to the family who may think that the patient has accepted everything very well by his happy and witty behavior in the hospital. The patient is now in the quiet of his own home with constant reminders of his change in role. He no longer has to put up a front for the hospital staff so they won't regard him as a problem or perhaps delay his discharge. He is not confronted with the many stimuli in a busy hospital environment. He may be physically tired from lack of proper rest in the hospital and from the trip home from the hospital. He needs time to rest, time to reorganize his thoughts and emotions. In fact, he may want to be left alone more, a disturbing behavior for the overprotective spouse. After this initial period of depression and withdrawal, he may suddenly become independent and aggressive in his behavior in an effort to regain his role in the family unit and prove his vigor. A spouse that frets and "nags" the patient and the onslaught of well meaning friends and relatives with "all the answers" serve as burrs under the saddle. If the patient is a male he may be bored with the time on his hands and assert himself by directing household activities. The husband's intrusion on a wife's daily household routine can cause resentment and further problems. The female coronary patient may feel guilty about her inability to pick up all the household chores immediately after discharge, and the husband is equally upset when she directs him in tasks he finds awkward and distasteful. When a husband and wife have been accustomed to pursuing their daily activities separately and then suddenly find themselves together on a 24-hour basis, an adjustment is necessary.

A prescribed walking-exercise program for the patient and resumption of low energy activities in and outside the home provide an emotional outlet that maintains the sanity of all family members. This is the time when phone communication from the hospital staff is helpful in providing encouragement, reassurance and reinforcement of the care regimen.

If there are children in the home, either small or teen-aged, they feel the impact of the illness and adjustment period. Children should be kept informed so that they understand what is happening and do not react with fear and frustration. Children are remarkably understanding and helpful when the situation demands it. After the parent is discharged, it is often most gratifying for him to find that his children still look to him for advice, regard him in his previous role, and, perhaps innocently, but openly express optimism for the future.

Eight weeks after an uncomplicated coronary, the patient has regained physical and emotional stability and has accepted the effect of the event on his life and any modifications this imposes. Because this is often the turning point in the medical care regimen when the physician can more objectively evaluate the patient's physical status, long range goals can more realistically be defined. This begins the stage of *recovery;* a time for reconstruction and making realistic future plans. The patient gradually resumes his work status and role in the family and community. Providing all goes well and the patient has learned to make appropriate modifications, there is a profound and ever expanding sense of relief. There is a feeling that maybe things will work out all right after all, and a state of not just existing on hope, but seeing it become a reality. The crisis is abated and the perceived loss has been regained in some form. This does not mean that recovery is complete at any given point in time. The coronary patient realizes that he exists with a chronic pathology, a dragon that may be "sleeping," but one that can rear its ugly head at a future data. Living with that realization is a lonely and very personal cross the coronary patient must bear.

The concerns and behavior of the coronary patient throughout the normal adaptive process varies from patient to patient. Normal coping mechanisms may become maladaptive if they persist for too long a time and/or if they interfere with the patient's physical progression. Other variables also affect the adaptive process and may pose particular problems that require intervention by the staff.

Age is one variable that significantly influences the patient's perception of the event. A coronary patient in his 40's or 50's views the illness much differently than a 70 to 80-year-old. The latter age group expect health problems and are not as stunned by the event. They are also usually retired and have grown children; thus, they do not have the additional concerns of job and financial insecurity that plague a young family.

The occurrence of physiological complications that either prolong the recovery period or pose a new crisis, understandably causes regression in the psychological adaptive process. The occurrence of family problems, financial and job insecurity, the patient's previous life style, personality pattern, how he has coped with stress in the past and his concept of the sick role all can affect adaption to the illness.

The presence of a loving supportive family unit that has dealt together successfully with other crises in their lives, tends to make the adjustment easier. Strained marital and family relationships prior to the coronary may worsen after this new crisis, although in some instances, the crisis strengthens family ties.

Another big factor is the degree of attention the patient and his family receive from the staff. A positive and trusting relationship with the staff contributes to the patient's compliance with his prescribed care regimen and helps his adaptive process. It is a normal human reaction to withhold one's feelings and reveal them only in a trusting relationship. The nurse or physician who simply impart factual information to the patient about his illness and care may not be allowing the patient to release his bottled up anxiety so that he can adapt successfully. The patient senses when the staff is in a hurry with no time to really talk and interact at the gut level. Asking the patient if he has any problems or questions with one hand on the doorknob is not a means of eliciting a trusting and open relationship. It has been observed that physicians and nurses often fail to detect anxiety and fears in cardiac patients because of a veiling of cheerfulness. Direct questioning may be required to discover that these same cardiac patients are significantly frightened by their illness (Granger, 1974).

The patients' and families' perception of the illness and their subsequent adjustment are often affected by their basic information of heart disease. There may be many myths, misconceptions or misinterpretations that comprise their information base. This information base may come from many sources such as: public media, others with heart disease, past illness, friends and relatives and health personnel. Some examples of misconceptions are:
1. every heart patient is alike,
2. can't use left arm or put hands above head,
3. can't resume sex,
4. can't lay on left side,
5. can't walk upstairs.
Recognition of the patient's information base is essential prior to the educational program.

Problems in communication with the health team can also cause misunderstandings. The following statements from patients provide examples.

"If part of my heart muscle is "dead", then how can it pump?" Cellular death to the professional lacks relevance to the layman.

"Doc said I had a little heart failure; so I guess even though it is better, my ticket is written for a trip to the Almighty." Heart failure has a different connotation to the professional than the laymen.

There are many factors that affect the patient and which obviously necessitate an individualized care regimen. Although the primary focus of care for the coronary is physiological during the acute phase of illness, the psychosocial components are ever present and become the primary focus of care as the patient becomes physically stable. An important milestone is reached when the patient is discharged from the hospital, but the recovery process is not complete at that point. As pointed out by Bilodeau (1971), "The successful adjustment achieved by most patients in the hospital seems to be shaken when the patient faces the stresses of life following discharge. Worries about change in physical activity and work capability, acceptance by the family, sexual adequacy, modifications in smoking and drinking habits, and recurrent myocardial infarction with possible death may be overwhelming." The nurse's help during and posthospitalization is important if the coronary patient is to become totally rehabilitated. Nursing's basic approach is simple:
1. Give the patient time to adapt, don't push and provide emotional support.
2. Listen to the patient and his family.
3. Teach them the facts about his illness and care regimen so he has a sound base upon which to build realistic future plans.
4. Be kind and project an attitude of hope and optimism.
Nurses are providers of health care: both physical and psychosocial. Recognition of the interplay and implementing a care plan based upon not only physiological but psychosocial care concepts are necessary for quality care of the coronary patient.

BIBLIOGRAPHY

Bilodeau, C. Issues raised in a group setting by patients recovering from myocardial infarction.. *Am. J. Psychiatry* 128: 73–78, 1971.

Bragg, T. L. Psychological response to MI. *Nurs. Forum* 14: 383–395, 1975.

Granger, J. Full recovery from myocardial infarction: Psychosocial factors. *Heart and Lung* 3: 600–609, 1974.

Houser, D. Outside the coronary care unit. *Nurs. Forum* 12: 96–106, 1973.

Klein, R., Dean, A., and Wilson, L. M. The physician in postmyocardial infarction invalidism. *J.A.M.A.* 194: 123, 1965.

Lipowski, L. J. Physical illness and psychopathology. *Int. J. Psychiatry Med.* 5: 483–497, 1975.

Moore (Cantor), M. *Disaster Behavior: A Model.* Unpublished paper; College of Nursing, University of Iowa, 1969.

Seyle, H. *Stress of Live.* New York: McGraw-Hill, 1956.

Slay, C. Myocardial infarction and stress. *Nurs. Clin. North Am.* 2: 329–338, 1976.

Wishnie, H., Hackett, T. P., and Cassen, N. H. Psychological hazards of convalescence following myocardial infarction. *J.A.M.A.* 215: 1292, 1971.

Chapter **24**

emergency case of street drug overdose

DARRYL S. INABA

The contemporary drug patterns among our drug-seeking subculture has shifted dramatically over the past few decades. From the ghettos and barrios, drug abuse has currently spread to encompass all levels of society and ethnic communities.

As viewed by Dr. George R. Gay (1975), miseducation and our puritanical reliance upon law and punishment to legislate morality in medical situations had led the individual drug user to be viewed and to view himself as a criminal and not as a patient. In addition, there is the unexplainable romantic attraction of the criminal life style — the "hustling," the paraphernalia and almost semireligious ethic of this underground life style — at first exciting and invigorating to adolescents either bored or desperate. Even if this were not so, a large percentage of youths would still experiment with illegal drugs because of their ubliquitous availability and peer group pressure. The drug user is mistrustful of physicians and medical professionals in general. He is often reluctant to seek help in traditional medical facilities until his physical or psychological pain becomes unbearable or he suffers an acute drug crisis.

As the availability of psychoactive drugs increases, so does their usage in nonmedical experimentation. It is imperative for medical personnel involved with emergency department and psychiatric care to keep medically abreast of the current trends in drug abuse, thereby maintaining this problem within the framework of a medical, rather than a criminal interaction.

The dynamic patterns of drug abuse have resulted in an unending stream of new psychoactive substances, a new and ever changing vocabulary of "street language," infinite varieties of drug nicknames and finally, a multitude of medical complications. Since all of these factors vary tremendously from community to community, it has been exceedingly difficult for the emergency department staff to diagnose and treat a "street drug" overdose. Though somewhat overlapping, it is fair to classify the more common street drugs of abuse into three groups based upon their intrinsic and immediate pharmacological actions rather than their current legal, social or "street" designations. These classes are:

1. Depressants
   a. Opiate and opioid analgesics
   b. Sedative-hypnotics
   c. Alcohol
   d. Most organic solvents (glue, gasoline) and miscellaneous inhalents

2. Stimulants
   a. Amphetamines and "diet pills"
   b. Cocaine
3. Psychotogens and marihuana

A full toxicological overview of abused drugs is obviously beyond the scope of this text and has been presented elsewhere (Jaffe, 1975; Dreisbach, 1975; Inaba and Katcher, 1975). A practical toxicology review of the most commonly abused drugs each class will be presented here.

1. DEPRESSANTS

Opiates and Opioids (Heroin, Codeine, Propoxyphene)

The opiate or opioid overdose victim classically presents with Jaffe's diagnostic triad of coma, pinpoint pupils and depressed respiration (Jaffe, 1975). In addition, lower pulse rate and blood pressure along with areflexia, cyanosis and clammy pallor are seen (Gay, 1975; Jaffe, 1975; Dreisbach, 1975; Inaba and Katcher, 1975; Gay and Inaba, 1976; Smith and Wesson, 1974). Diagnostic of a pure opiate-opioid overdosage is the administration of 0.4 to 1.2 mg (1 to 3 cc) of naloxone (Narcan) in intravenous bolus. Naloxone, unlike nalorphine (Nalline) and levallorphan (Lorfan), is a specific opiate-opioid antagonist free of any major agonistic activity of its own. Continued or large doses of nalorphine and levallorphan may result in respiratory and CNS depression. Thus, naloxone can safely differentiate between the pure opiate-opioid drug overdose from the barbiturate or mixed depressant drug overdose (Inaba and Katcher, 1975; Gay and Inaba, 1976; Hasbrouch, 1971; Jasinski et al., 1967; Foldes et al., 1965).

Although naloxone is a specific opiate-opioid antagonist, effective treatment of the opiate overdosage must be initiated with the general principles of cardiopulmonary resuscitation (Gay and Inaba, 1976; Gay and Way, 1971):

1. Establish an airway:
   A. Clean patient's mouth. Mucus, blood, vomitus, gum, or tobacco may be found.
   B. With the patient in supine position, tip the head slightly back. Grasping jaw at angles of mandible and at point of chin, draw the head back, chin high, to a "sniffling-like" position, but be careful not to hyperextend. Pull the tongue forward, making sure it isn't occluding the posterior oropharynx. If oropharyngeal reflexes are absent, insert an oropharyngeal or nasopharyngeal airway; if one isn't available, hold the tongue forward with your fingers.
   C. Breathe for the patient if he or she is apneic — mouth-to-mouth, or mouth-to-nose, or use an Ambu bag if one is handy. If room air is 20% oxygen, your mouth-to-mouth respiration will get at least 15% oxygen into the patient. Make sure air is entering the lungs — that the chest (not stomach) is expanding. Listen for breath sounds with a stethoscope. Don't stop to look or call for endotracheal equipment — you are dealing with a true emergency and hesitation can spell disaster. Endotracheal intubation should be attempted only by a trained anesthesiologist or surgeon — and only when the patient has been previously properly oxygenated. You have about 2 minutes to achieve intubation. If unsuccessful, resume mouth-to-mouth, oxygenating the patient well before attempting intubation again.

2. Quickly assess the cardiovascular system:
   A. Check the pulse for rate and rhythm. Check precordial, femoral, temporal, or radial pulses. Don't be lulled into complacency by the strong full pulse of hypoxia, which may be premonitory to terminal arrhythmia and cardiac cessation. Remember: If the patient arrives with a heartbeat, you should be able to save him.
   B. Begin external cardiac massage if heartbeat is absent, placing the palms of your hands over the patient's lower sternum, depressing firmly 50 times per minute. Determine cardiac status with ECG. Institute appropriate action — defibrillation, pacing, etc.
   C. In severe cases of narcotics overdose, the patient's cardiovascular system may be so depressed that pulmonary edema develops. Intubation or tracheostomy — plus continuous positive pressure respiration — may be life-saving.

3. Continue treatment for heroin overdose:
   A. Give intravenously 2 cc (1 cc/0.4 mg) naloxone hydrochloride. This may be repeated 2 to 3 times at 2- to 3-minute intervals without fear of adverse or agonistic effect (IV works in seconds; IM administration may take 20 minutes or more to act). If the patient has "collapsed" veins, as many addicts do, try the external jugular or the femoral or inject at the base of the tongue if all else fails.

B. Stay with the patient until he is fully responsive. If he used a long-acting narcotic, such as methadone hydrochloride (Dolophine), he may lapse back into coma if continuous monitoring is not provided for several hours. With the ever expanding methadone maintenance programs in this country, providing a continuing increase in street-availability of this government-approved highly potent opioid, methadone overdoses are being seen in increasing numbers.

C. If the patient fails to respond, follow established emergency procedures to secure a route for administering IV fluids — preferably with a large bore cannula. If moderate to severe acidosis is suspected, administer sodium bicarbonate. Begin the administration of glucose-electrolyte solution. Draw blood for chemistries. Search for nonoverdose etiology — evidence of trauma, blood loss, acute infectious process and increased intracranial pressure.

D. If long-standing drug depression is suspected (for example, when a patient is discovered unattended), be on guard for atelectasis or pneumonia. In any event, hospitalization, vigorous pulmonary therapy, and aggressive antibiotic therapy are indicated.

Naloxone has also been reported to antagonize the depressant effects of pentazocine (Talwin), propoxyphene (Darvon) and other narcotic antagonists such as nalorphene and cyclazocine (Fint et al., 1966; Jasinaki, 1968). Of special interest is the occurrence of seizure activity seen with propoxyphene and meperidine toxicity (Jaffe, 1975) which may also respond to naloxone (Fint et al., 1966).

Some limitations of naloxone include: 1) A short duration (2 to 4 hours) of action relative to the opioid drugs, thus the possibility of relapse toxicity especially in methadone overdosage (Hasbrauch, 1971; Jasinaki et al., 1968; Fink et al., 1968). 2) Large doses may potentially precipitate withdrawal syndrome in an opiate addict. These precipitated withdrawal symptoms are much more severe and difficult to manage than those induced by abstinence alone (Jasinski et al., 1968).

Complicating the clinical picture of the acute heroin overdose are the various techniques employed by the "street" community in their treatment of the "OD". Of the many various "street" methods of resuscitation, two of the most commonly used and misunderstood methods are external stimulation and the intravenous administration of salt, milk or vinegar solutions.

External stimulation techniques such as sharp slapping of the body, squeezing of sensitive areas (i.e., testicles or nipples), walking the victim around, placing him in a cold shower and applying ice to the testicles may all have some possible benefit in borderline cases. Since opiates only depress the automatic regulation of respiration but not voluntary control, external stimulation of the conscious or semiconscious opioid-overdosed patient may prevent apnea (Jaffe, 1975). However, such procedures may result in an airway occluded with blood, mucus, or broken teeth, as well as broken bones and lacerations from over vigorous application. Further, methods which produce hypothermia may exacerbate the preexisting hypotension and complicate the management of the opioid-overdosed patient (Gay et al., 1972; Baden, 1972).

Intravenous salt and vinegar solutions are thought to bind heroin and nullify its depressant effects. A volume of salt equal to the amount of heroin used is diluted in tap water and injected intravenously. These powerful sclerosing agents are painful and are frequently deposited outside the vein, causing extreme pain. Thus, painful stimulation may again be of some benefit in arousing the borderline overdosed patient. Formation of painful abscesses, sclerosing of the veins, infections, and the potentiation of pulmonary edema from a strongly hypertonic salt solution severely compromise the use of these methods (Baden, 1972).

Intravenous milk is also thought to reverse a heroin overdose. However, such therapy must result in microscopic embolisms, which may account in part for the lipoid pneumonia and foreign body granulomas found in the lungs of addicts (Baden, 1972; Siegel et al., 1970).

Emetics and intravenous amphetamines are also commonly used street procedures in the management of narcotic overdose.

The force-feeding of milk and vinegar to induce vomiting is thought to stimulate the overdosed heroin addict and hasten his recovery time. Emesis may stimulate the autonomic nervous system and reverse to some extent the hypotension induced by a depressed vasomotor center. Such therapy in unconscious and semiunconscious patients probably accounts for autopsy finding of milk aspirations in the lungs of opiate-overdosed patients (Baden, 1972; Siegel et al., 1970).

The "speed reversal" or the use of intravenous amphetamines and cocaine in the treatment of heroin overdose is thought to pharmacologically antagonize the depressant drug. The use of such drugs may precipitate life-threatening convulsions that must be treated with depressant drugs, which may once again induce severe depression in the patient. Furthermore, there is a narrow margin between stimulant and depressant effects of cocaine, making it a very precarious antidote for the "street" treatment of opioid toxicity (Gay et al., 1972; Mark, 1967; Picchioni, 1971; Gay et al., 1975).

Professionals involved with the management of an acute heroin overdose must be cognizant of the fact that any one or a combination of these "street methods" may have already been employed to complicate the overall medical status of the patient.

In addition to the above, a complete clinical evaluation should include an assessment of the ever present medical complications of intravenous illicit drug usage. Most notable of these is "cotton fever" which is characterized by violent shaking tumors, chills and fever. When heroin is prepared for self-administration, cotton is used as a filter to trap adulterants; thus, some of the drug also remains trapped within the cotton as well. These crude filters are saved, and when money or drug availability is poor, water is added to the "old cottons" to extract any remaining drug for intravenous use. The cause of "cotton fever" is unknown though acute septicemia or an allergic pyrogenic reaction are most suspect. An allergic reaction may result from broken-down cotton fibers and may on rare occasions, lead to systemic shock requiring acute medical intravention. However, "cotton fever" is generally transient and subsides within 24 hours without treatment.

Bacterial endocarditis, embolism, septic and aseptic abscesses, thrombophlebitis and cellulitis have also resulted from improper sterilization of injection apparatus and poor needle techniques. In addition, the common practice of sharing "outfits" (needle and syringe) between friends has resulted in the transmission of viral hepatitis, syphilis, tetanus and even malaria. Other complications of heroin addiction include the following: pulmonary emboli (caused by materials used to "cut" or dilute heroin); pulmonary edema; frequent upper respiratory tract infections (especially pneumonia); malnutrition; and degenerative nerve changes (seen rarely and probably allergic in origin) (Gay et al., 1972; Surgical Complications, 1971; Becker, 1971; Bick et al., 1971; Dismukes et al., 1968; Lauria et al., 1967; Morrison et al., 1970; Ricter et al., 1968; Gay and Trantham, 1975).

Sedative-Hypnotics

All of the substances classified as depressants (opiate-opioid, sedative-hypnotic; alcohol and organic solvents) are capable of producing motor incordination (ataxia), stupor in which arousal is difficult and severe respiratory depression. The subclass known as the sedative-hypnotic agents represents a wide variety of chemical compounds generally used in medicine to treat anxiety and insomnia. The prototype of these agents are the barbiturate drugs. Other nonbarbiturate and benzodiazepine sedative-hypnotics along with their common trade and street names are listed in Table 1.

The major acute toxic effect of barbiturates is on respiration. The barbiturates are depressants to the medullary centers of the brain responsible for respiration. Both respiratory drive and rhythm are affected with increasing dosages of these drugs. Unlike the situation with the opioid drugs, coughing and laryngeal reflexes are not necessarily depressed along with this respiratory depression. Ultimately, acid-base imbalance, coma, respiratory arrest, and circulatory collapse result from barbiturate overdosage.

Lethal blood levels seen with long-acting barbiturates have been stated to be 10 mg% and 3 mg% for short-acting barbiturates (Jaffe, 1975). However, the lethal dose of barbiturates is highly variable with a num-

TABLE 1. SEDATIVE-HYPNOTIC DRUGS

Generic Name	Common Trade Names	Common Street Names
Barbiturates		
Secobarbital	Seconal	Reds, red devils, seccies, F-40's, mexian reds
Pentobarbital	Nembutal	Yellows, yellow jackets, yellow bullets, nebbies
Equal parts of seco and pentobarbital	Tuinal	Rainbows, tuies, double trouble
Amobarbital	Amytal	Blue heavens, blue dolls, blues
Nonbarbiturate sedative-hypnotics		
Glutethimide	Doriden	Goofballs, goofers
Methaqualone	Quaalude, Sopor, Parest, Optimil, Somnafac	Ludes, sopes, soapers
Ethchlorvynol	Placidyl	
Chloral hydrate	Noctec, Somnos, Kessodrate	Jelly beans, miki's, knock-out drops
Methyprylon	Noludar	Noodlelars
Meprobamate	Equanil, Miltown, Meprotabs	
Benzodiazepines		
Diazepam	Valium	Vals
Chlordiazepoxide	Librium, Libritabs	Libs
Flurazepam	Dalmane	
Clorazepate	Tranxene	
Oxazepam	Serax	

ber of factors affecting the susceptibility in any individual. In particular, low blood levels may be observed when other general depressants are ingested to yield additive effects but lower individual blood levels of each drug.

Unlike the opioid depressants, there is no specific antagonist to the effects of barbiturates. The standard for the treatment of acute barbiturate poisoning is outlined in a protocol known as the "Scandinavian Method" (Clemmesem and Nilsson, 1961). This method has demonstrated a mortality rate of less than 2% and calls for conservative supportive measures to manage barbiturate overdosage. Careful observance is made in maintaining an airway, breathing, heart rate, circulation and urinary flow as outlined in the previous section on the treatment of opioid overdosage. Hemodialysis can hasten the elimination of barbiturates and forced alkaline diuresis may be of value with long-acting barbiturates.

Analeptic or stimulant drugs like amphetamine, methylphenidate, and doxipram are not routinely recommended. Though these agents do stimulate the central nervous system and result in an increased respiratory rate and blood pressure, they are not specific antagonists and may increase oxygen need. The dual action of depressant and stimulant drugs in the body results in unstable and abnormal nervous activity. In addition, high doses needed to counteract barbiturate depression may lead to generalized convulsions. It is now generally accepted that the risks of using analeptic drugs in barbiturate poisoning outweigh the potential benefits (Mark, 1967; Picchioni, 1971).

Complicating the sedative-hypnotic overdose is often the problem of mixed depressant drug usage. These combinations of alcohol and/or opiates with sedative-hypnotic drugs often results in synergistic effects that are often more than additive of individual toxic effects. Thus, toxicity seen from mixed depressant drug use may be much more severe in intensity and prolonged in duration.

Though generally abused orally, occasional intravenous abuse of the short-acting barbiturates results in rapid sclerosing of venous tissue, phlebitis and extravascular abscessing. This is due to the high alkalinity and, therefore, irritation caused by barbiturate compounds (Gay, 1971).

Of utmost importance in the treatment of the sedative-hypnotic drug overdose is careful attention paid to aftercare once the patient has recovered from acute toxicity. Chronic physical dependence on all of these agents and alcohol can lead to a life-endangering withdrawal seizure activity (Jaffe, 1975; Wikler, 1968; Isbell et al., 1955). Treatment of physical addiction can be accomplished by either Wikler's pentobarbital approach (Wikler, 1968) or Smith's phenobarbital substitution (Inaba and Katcher, 1975; Smith et al., 1970).

Alcohol

The oldest depressant drug, ethyl alcohol, has been used since the beginning of recorded history and continues to be one of the most physically and emotionally debilitating of all abused drugs. It is socially acceptable within our society and has, therefore, led to much confusion as to what constitutes use, abuse and addiction to this substance. The pharmacological and social issues involved with alcoholism are thoroughly discussed in volumes of literature elsewhere. It is sufficient here to reemphasize that ethanol is sedative-hypnotic agent having high acute and chronic toxicity and high addiction liability.

Seemingly benign, ethanol overdose accounts for the majority of drug cases treated at large rock-music festivals (Gay et al., 1972). Teen-age and pre-teenage children have been treated in grade II and III coma secondary to high ethanol intake. General cardiopulmonary resuscitation procedures must be applied to such cases with special care to prevent aspiration of vomitus in a recovering victim.

Organic Solvents and Miscellaneous Inhalents

Though delegated to the lowest preferability by the "sophistication" of the drug-using subculture, availability and low costs continue to stimulate periodic experimentation of a wide variety of chemical solvents and inhalents.

The more popular organic solvents include model airplane glues, plastic cements, gasoline, brake and lighter fluids, nail polish remover, cleaning fluids, paints, thinners and varnish remover. These contain a variety of organic hydrocarbons including benzene, toluene, xylene, carbon tetrachloride, acetone, chloroform, trichloroethane, amyl acetate, naphtha, ethyl and isopropyl alcohol. Most of these are general depressants to the CNS. The chlorinated and florinated hydrocarbons also have direct toxic effects on the heart, liver and kidneys (Allen, 1966; Flowers and Horan, 1972; Kupperstein and Sussman, 1968; Know and Nelson, 1966; Powars, 1965; and Durden and Chipman, 1967).

As with all CNS depressants, these substances can produce initial stimulating effects via depression of inhibitory centers in the CNS. This is rapidly followed by CNS depression during which time the patient may exhibit euphoria, excitement, slurred speech and tinnitus. Delusions and visual hallucinations have also been reported, accompanied by mental confusion, bizarre behavior and coma. If inhalation is not interrupted, coma and death may result (Ackerly and Gibson, 1964; Easson, 1962; Winek et al., 1967, 1968). In addition, "sudden sniffing deaths" secondary to cardiac arrhythmias have been reported with the abuse of fluorinated gases used as aerosol propellants (Bass, 1970).

Treatment of an acute toxicity to organic solvents can only be supportive. Removal of the substance and proper ventilation are the mandatory first steps in the treatment of these cases.

Popular inhalents not too readily available to the drug abuse subculture are nitrous oxide ("laughing gas") and amyl nitrite ("poppers", "snappers"). Though very little toxicity has been reported on these substances, increased availability (especially of illicit amyl nitrite) may lead to a greater number of toxic reactions.

2. STIMULANTS

Amphetamines and Diet Pills

Amphetamine ("speed") abuse in the late 1970's seems to be increasing but not nearly to the peak of its popularity during the late 1960's. Methamphetamine known as "crystal" and "crank" along with Benzedrine and Dexedrine are still widely available through illicit drug manufacturers. In addition, a current popularity of Ritalin or "pellets" seems to indicate a renewed interest in stimulants by the drug-seeking subculture.

Physiological toxicity of the amphetamines and "diet pills" manifests in signs and symptoms consistent with overstimulation of the CNS. Hyperreflexia, restlessness, irritability, tremors, confusion with paranoid delirium, palpitations and cardiac arrhythmias may all progress ultimately to convulsions, coma, circulatory collapse, cerebral hemorrhage and potentially death (Innes and Nickerson, 1975).

Toxicity to amphetamine is rare under a 15-mg oral dose. Survival has been documented at doses of 400 to 500 mg while death has followed an intravenous dose of 120 mg. Chronic abuse, however, is accompanied by a huge tolerance to these drugs (Innes and Nickerson, 1975).

The psychological manifestations of acute and chronic toxicity for both amphetamines and cocaine are fairly indistinguishable from each other. Initially, anxiety, excitability, and confusion occur and may progress in severity culminating in paranoia and a true toxic psychosis (Gay et al., 1975; Innes and Nickerson, 1975; Post, 1975).

Paranoid psychosis may result after a single large dose of amphetamines and inevitably follows the chronic use of high doses. Often, visual hallucinations originate in the peripheral visual field; these may be accompanied by auditory hallucinations. In the beginning, the user may be able to attribute his paranoia to the amphetamines. He may even self-medicate his psychosis with heroin or barbiturates since it is quite common for drug abusers to treat unpleasant drug effects with other drugs. Later, as amphetamine abuse becomes more intense, he loses the "intellectual awareness" of his paranoia.

These paranoid thoughts, coupled with the physical hyperactivity brought about by the drug may predispose the subject to violence. Ellinwood (1971) has reviewed the role of amphetamine-induced paranoid

psychosis in 13 homicide cases. Violence related to amphetamine abuse was well documented in the Haight-Ashbury District in San Francisco in 1968 and 1969 (AMA Committee, 1966; Carey et al.,1968; Connell, 1966; Ellinwood, 1969, 1971. Espelin et al., 1968; Kramer, 1967, 1969; Post, 1975).

Treatment of the more severe physiological manifestations of amphetamine and cocaine requires prompt and specific support therapy as outlined by Gay et al., (1975). Acidification of the urine with ammonium chloride is also effective in increasing the urinary excretion of amphetamine.

Psychotic manifestations of acute amphetamine toxicity have been treated with chlorpromazine. Phenothiazines are also said to raise the LD-50 and reverse many of the toxic signs (Espelin, 1968). Counseling, viz., the "talk-down" therapy alone (described in the section on psychotogenic drugs) or with sedative-hypnotic drugs (e.g., diazepam) has been used effectively in the vast majority of amphetamine and cocaine psychoses treated at the Haight-Ashbury Free Medical Clinic. Even if untreated, the toxic psychosis will probably resolve over a period of several days to several weeks with abstinence. Some residual confusion, memory loss and delusional ideation have been reported following acute toxicity but all gradually resolved over a period of 6 to 12 months (Kramer, 1969).

The question of whether permanent physiological changes persist after acute and chronic amphetamine toxicity recurs frequently. Cases of intracranial hemorrhage following acute amphetamine poisoning have been reported (Goodman et al., 1970; Kane et al., 1969) as well as necrotizing angiitis (Citron, 1970) in amphetamine abusers.

Cocaine

Cocaine, also known as "coke," "snow," "blow," "girl," "jam" and "flake" (Jaffe, 1975; Gay et al., 1975), is perhaps the most euphorogenic as well as the most monumentally illegal drug of our times. Now, through the mid-1970's, there is a substantial increase in the abuse of cocaine. The toxic manifestations of cocaine are very similar to those described for amphetamines with the added toxic effects of rebound respiratory depression and direct cardiac toxicity (Gay et al., 1975).

Acute toxicity to cocaine and its synthetic analogues has been referred to classically as the "caine" reaction (Table 2). It is a classical biphasic toxicity with an early stimulatory phase, which may then be followed by a profound depression with circulatory collapse and death (Gay et al., 1975).

A prolonged or chronic use of cocaine may lead to irrational affect, a delusional state resembling paranoid schizophrenia and, not uncommonly, proneness to violence. The chronic user is plagued with lingering depression, listlessness, increasing nervousness, inability to concentrate and disturbed sleep patterns (Post, 1975).

In *all* cases, acute or chronic, the treatment of the cocaine user is symptomatic. In cases of acute toxicity, death most often occurs within 2 to 3 minutes, but may occur up to 30 minutes following ingestion/injection. Though as little as 30 mg of cocaine has resulted in death, it is estimated that the liver can detoxify a minimal lethal dose (500 mg) of this drug within 1 hour. If the acute overdose victim survives the first 3 hours, his chances of recovery are almost certainly assured. The user of illicit cocaine (due to the paranoia-provoking qualities of the drug, and because he realizes the several legal sanctions involved in the possession and/or use of this substance) seldom is seen in the offices or emergency rooms of traditional medical facilities. Most often, self-medication with a combination of alcohol, barbiturates and/or other sedative-hypnotics will be employed in an attempt to bring the user "down." If seen in a medical situation, however (after it has been fully determined that the patient is not in an exhaustion phase, and threatening imminent collapse), mild tranquilizers and/or sedative-hypnotics may be employed (in normal recognized doses). The use of Valium and chloral hydrate is probably the safest and yet most fully effective medical recourse. A very valuable hint to remember: the paranoid "coke-head" must be approached with real caution. Even casual physical "touching" should be avoided; gentle, quiet vocal reassurance should instead be employed.

The supportive treatment of the "caine reaction" has been summarized by Gay et al. (1975) and is presented below.
1. Administration of oxygen, by positive pressure and artificial respiration if necessary. First, be *assured* that an open airway is present.
2. Trendelenburg position (head down). Wrap arms and legs if necessary to increase central return of blood.

TABLE 2. THE "CAINE" REACTION[a]

Phase	Central Nervous System	Circulatory System	Respiratory System
I. Early stimulative	Excitement, apprehension; other symptoms of emotional instability. Sudden headache. Nausea, vomiting. "Twitchings" of small muscles, particularly of face, fingers.	Pulse varies probably will slow. (Usual) elevation in blood pressure may occur. Fall in blood pressure may occur. Pallor of skin.	Increased respiratory rate *and* depth.
I-a. Advanced stimulative	Convulsions (tonic and clonic −) resembles grand mal seizure.	Increase in both pulse rate *and* blood pressure	Cyanosis, dyspnea, rapid (gasping or irregular) respiration.
II. Depressive	Paralysis of muscles. Loss of reflexes. Unconsciousness. Loss of vital functions. Death.	Circulatory failure. No palpable pulse. Death.	Respiratory failure. Ashen gray cyanosis. Death.

[a] Gay et al., 1975.

3. Inject *small amounts* of short-acting barbiturates (e.g., 25 to 50 mg of Sodium Pentothal), *if* convulsions are *present*. May be repeated but *gently*. (Do *not* force general depressant effect to point of no return.) Recent work by Rappolt indicates that 1.0 to 6.0 mg of the β-blocker propranolol (Inderal) given IV in 1.0-mg increments will dramatically terminate a "cocaine OD" within 3 minutes; oral propranolol (40 mg) may be used, but onset usually coincides with the duration of action of cocaine per se, some 40 minutes (Gay et al., 1975).

4. Keep patient cool and keep crowds away. (Keep cool yourself, crowd hysteria can "gang-panic" anyone.)

5. General muscle relaxants may be given to facilitate administration of positive pressure oxygen.

6. Continuously monitor vital signs.

7. Have some ice handy for hyperpyrexia.

3. PSYCHOTOGENS AND MARIHUANA

Also referred to as psychedelics, psychotomimetics and hallucinogenic compounds, the feature distinguishing the psychotogens from other drugs of abuse is their capacity to induce states of altered perceptions, thought and feelings that can be further described as hallucinations, delusions, illusions, perceptual distortions, or in short, the "psychedelic experience." (Jaffe, 1975; Freedman, 1968, 1969; Jarvik, 1970).

Many drugs and natural products with widely varying pharmacological properties are capable of inducing a "psychedelic experience" if administered at adequate dosages in the proper setting. Thus, the differing drugs discussed here will be classified as "psychedelic" if that is their intended use by the drug-abusing population.

Some of the more common psychotogenic substances abused today will be briefly presented here.

Of all of the different psychotogenic substances, the most commonly abused and comprehensively studied continues to be LSD (lysergic acid diethylamide). The general description of an acute intoxification to LSD, its characteristics and its management, is also applicable to some other psychotogens as well. Specific differences in toxicity and treatment of other common psychotogens will be discussed later in this section.

The physiological reaction to LSD and many of the other psychotogens is distinct but resembles superficially that of anticholinergic drugs and is characterized by reflex hyperactivity; anxiety mydriasis and increased blood pressure, pulse rate, and body temperature. Piloerection, muscular weakness, tremor, sweating, nausea, stimulation of uterine smooth muscle and hyperglycemia have also been reported (Jarvik, 1970; Hoffer, 1964; Taylor et al., 1970). These physiological responses have rarely been severe enough to endanger human life and as of this date, no recorded deaths due to the direct toxicity of LSD have been reported in man. However, eight recent cases of near fatal reactions associated with coma, hyperthermia and bleeding with massive LSD overdoses have been reported (Klock et al., 1974). Also, deaths due to respiratory depression, convulsion and marked hyperthermia have been reported in different species of laboratory animals receiving massive doses of LSD (Jaffe, 1975; Jarvik, 1970; Haffer, 1964).

The clinical interaction with the LSD or "acid" abuser is in the management of the acute panic reaction more commonly known as the "bad trip" which occurs soon after taking the drug. Neuropsychiatric sequelae to such reactions have been divided into four basic categories: 1) the prolonged "bad trip," acute axiety or panic reaction; 2) post-LSD depression; 3) long term schizophrenic or psychotic reactions; and 4) the "flashback" phenomenon (Kleber, 1967).

A "bad trip" due to a psychotogenic drug is characterized by an acute anxiety reaction that may progress to a full-scale toxic psychosis. A full description of this phenomenon has been presented in many references (Greenblatt et al., 1970; Langs et al., 1968; Smart et al., 1967; Taylor et al., 1970). Smith (1970) has further classified the "bad trip" into three distinctive types:

1. Body trips. These involve distorted perceptions of the subject's body dealing with his physical appearance. A feeling of ugliness or dirtiness may be the precipitant factors in this type of experience.

2. *Environmental trips.* These include distortions of the visual field surrounding the individual. Often, frightening illusions and hallucinations develop to the point that subjects lose touch of reality and believe themselves to be going insane.

3. *Mind trips.* These involve subconscious material which surfaces into the consciousness of the individual. Identity crises and guilt feelings cause the subject to enter into feelings of depression, failure, disgust and suicidal states.

The initial management of the "bad trip" should consist of the "talk down" therapy. The therapist attempts to convince the patient that his perceptual distortions and feelings of panic are temporary effects of the drug which should dissipate as the drug is metabolized. The subjective effects of LSD, which has a half-life of 175 minutes, normally begin to clear 12 hours after ingestion. As a first step measure, verbal contact should be made with the patient in a calm, reassuring, confident manner before any medication is given. This should be done in a more peaceful setting with less noise, fewer people, and less confusion than that which normally occurs in the emergency room of a hospital. It is more important to be supportive and friendly than it is to be a clinician in the management of a "bad trip." Time should be spent asking gentle questions in an attempt to redirect the patient's thoughts toward pleasant experiences. Reassurance and reality defining is oftentimes all that is needed in the management of the "bad trip" (Garson et al., 1969; Martin, 1970; Taylor et al., 1970).

Drug therapy of this initial anxiety reaction should only be considered after the patient is found to be refractory to the above procedures or if the patient insists that he needs something to bring him back to reality. Although chlorpromazine 50 mg IM initially, followed by 100 mg p.o. has been the recommended therapy of choice in the past, exacerbation of the anxiety state, orthostatic hypotensive episodes, precipitation of postpsychotic depression, an increased incidence of the "flashback" phenomenon, and potentiation of anticholinergic psychotogenic drugs now limit the usefulness of phenothiazine drugs in the initial management of the psychotogenic "bad trip" experience. Furthermore, some clinical experience has suggested that the therapeutic effectiveness of the phenothiazines in the management of the "bad trip" may be more dependent upon the sedative qualities of these drugs rather than their antipsychotic properties (Martin, 1970; Schwarz, 1971; Shick et al., 1970; Taylor et al., 1970; Tec, 1971).

This conclusion suggests that the minor tranquilizers or the sedative-hypnotic drugs such as the benzodiazepines, chloral hydrate, or barbiturates, may be effectively used in the initial management of the "bad trip" (Levy, 1971; Schwarz, 1971; Shick et al., 1970; Taylor et al., 1970).

Complicating the diagnosis and treatment of all illicit drug ingestions and especially so with illicit psychotogenic drugs is the inconsistency of the composition of illicit drugs. Trade names, dosage forms, dosages, purity and strength of illicit drugs vary greatly from time to time, community to community and from dealer to dealer. Also, drugs with low marketing potential are frequently misrepresented for drugs with higher marketing potential. It has been determined by chemical analysis that many samples of LSD and phencyclidine have been sold as THC or tetrahydrocannabinol, the active constituent of marihuana. It would be best to initiate therapy in the overdosed drug abuser by directing management toward the symptomatology of the patient and then matching this with the history of the suspected durg ingested (Martin, 1970).

These "bad trip" panic reactions are the most common acute adverse reaction to LSD and other psychotogenic drugs. These reactions are generally temporary and last for approximately 24 hours with LSD. However, they can also become more prolonged, lasting for more than 48 hours, and sometimes progressing even further into a long-lasting toxic psychosis (Smart et al., 1967).

The "flashback" or "free trip" is a poorly understood phenomenon described as a transient, spontaneous recurrence of certain aspects of the psychotogenic drug experience following an earlier intoxication after a period of relative normalcy (Shick et al., 1970). Flashbacks occur most frequently in the individual who has had a multitude of LSD experiences, has taken other psychoactive drugs (often major tranquilizers such as chlorpromazine) or is in a period of psychological stress (Schwarz, 1967, 1971; Shick et al., 1970). This phenomenon can occur sporadically or several times a day and can last from minutes to hours, or persist for as long as a year (Louria, 1968).

Treatment of the prolonged reaction and "flashback" should follow the same guidelines as the "talk down" therapy with major emphasis placed upon reassuring the patient that he is not "brain-damaged" and that he is not "going crazy." In view of the fact that different psychoactive medications may precipitate or exacerbate the "flashback" phenomenon, medication should be conservative and offered only when the patient exhibits extreme anxiety. Shick and Smith (Shick et al., 1970) recommended the use of the minor tranquilizers or sedative-hypnotic drugs rather than major antipsychotic tranquilizers.

Other commonly abused psychotogenic drugs are:

Mescaline (3,4,5-trimethoxyphenethylamine) is the active component of the peyote cactus (*Lophophora williamsii*) which is still ingested for religious practices by the Southwestern Plains Indians (Albaugh and Anderson, 1974; Der Marderosin, 1966; Frykman, 1971). The drug is generally taken orally as dried cactus buttons, as tea or in gelatin capsules. Subjective effects are very similar to LSD and treatment of an acute anxiety reaction resulting from mescaline should be treated similarly. Oral doses of 5 mg/kg (generally 6 to 12 buttons) cause effects lasting for about 12 hours. Each button contains approximately 45 mg of mescaline. Nausea, diaphoresis and static tremors are frequently seen with therapeutic doses (300 to 500 mg) of mescaline (Jaffe, 1975).

Available "street" or illicit mescaline is very rare although it is a highly preferred agent. Of 41 samples of "street" mescaline analyzed in the San Francisco area, only two contained mescaline; the remaining samples contained LSD, PCP or no drug at all (McLaughlin, 1973; Pharm Chem Newsletter, 1973).

Psilocybin, the "Magic Mexican Mushroom," was first reported in the medical literature by Helm in 1957. Later in 1958, Hoffman and co-workers, isolated O-phosphoryl-4-hydroxy-N,N-dimethyltryptamine from Medican mushrooms. This compound which they named psilocybin, has been isolated in *psilocybe cubensis*, *P. mexicana*, *Stropharia cubensis*, and one species of the Concybe genera. Other hallucinogenic fungi have been studied: some of these contain another psychotogenic compound, bufotenine (Buck, 1961; Shulgin, 1969).

The subjective effects of psilocybin are similar to those of LSD and mescaline with a dose of 20 to 60 mg lasting from 5 to 6 hours (Lingeman, 1969). Like mescaline and THC, psilocybin is a sought after psychotogen, but very little of it is available to the illicit drug market. Of 22 psilocybin samples analyzed by Pharm Chem Laboratories in 1973, only one contained appreciable amounts of this drug (Pharm Chem Newsletter, 1973).

MDA (3,4-methylenedioxyamphetamine), a psychotogenic drug structurally similar to mescaline and STP, was first synthesized in the 1930's. Doses of up to 150 mg are said to intensify feelings, facilitate insight, increase empathy and heighten aesthetic enjoyment. However, it rarely induces hallucinations, or perceptual alterations, or causes depersonalization at this dosage (Narango et al., 1967; Shulgin, 1969).

Effects begin about 40 to 60 minutes after ingestion and generally persist for 6 to 10 hours. Marked physical exhaustion with free-floating anxiety has been reported to last up to 2 days in some cases (Jackson et al., 1970). Toxicity from MDA is somewhat more of an acute problem than it is for other psychotogens. One nearly fatal case and two severe cases of adverse physical reactions consisting of dilated pupils, tachycardia, diaphoresis, rapid labored breathing, fever, generalized piloerection and muscular spasms have been reported in six persons who had each ingested 500 mg of MDA (Richards et al., 1971). Several deaths previously reported as a result of MDA toxicity in 1973 are now known to have occurred from ingestions of PMA (para-methoxyamphetamine), a more toxic psychotogenic amphetamine (PMA, 1973).

MDA seems to be a "fad" drug with its abuse on the street related more to its unpredictable popularity than to its availability. Recently, *N*-methyl MDA derivatives have also appeared on the illicit drug market.

STP acquired its initials from the triad of serenity-tranquility-peace. This seems totally inappropriate for the expected pharmacological properties of the actual drug DOM or 2,5-dimethoxy-4methyl-amphetamine. Its psychological effects are similar to LSD and include dilated pupils, increased systolic blood pressure, and a slight increase in body temperature. Five milligrams of STP will produce hallucinogenic effects for 5 to 6 hours. Ten milligrams of the drug may have effects lasting for 16 to 20 hours. More prolonged reactions (up to 72 hours), a higher incidence of acute panic reactions, and an increase in the occurrence of the flashback phenomenon have been reported with STP. The drug has low preference in the drug abuse population (Martin, 1970; Smith, 1969, 1970; Snyder et al., 1968). More recently, the appearance of a new 4-Bromo STP derivative has been noted on the illicit drug market (Shulgin et al., 1971).

Phencyclidine or PCP, also called "Hog," "Peace Pill," "Krystal" (not to be confused with "crystal" or methamphetamine), "Ozone," "KJ," "erth," and "Angel's Dust," was originally intended to be used as a general anesthetic in man. However, the frequency and severity of CNS side effects soon limited its use to veterinary medicine (sold under the trade name of Sernyl). Its psychotogenic effect has been described as "sensory deprivation," and it appears to alter the response of the CNS to various sensory inputs. This may result in perceptual distortions and a toxic psychosis similar to the acute anxiety reaction. The biological half-life of PCP is only 30 to 60 minutes but subjective effects last longer than those produced by LSD (Dodini, 1971; Rappolt, 1976), lasting up to 48 hours and longer (Dodini, 1971; Rappolt, 1976).

PCP has the ability to induce a broad spectrum of CNS effects depending upon the dose administered. Low dosages (2 ro 5 mg) produce first mild depression then stimulation. Within a very narrow dosage range, PCP can then go from its desirable sensory-deprived state (approximately 10 to 15 mg) to full toxicity with catatonia, coma and convulsions in dosages above 20 mg. Large PCP doses have also produced seizures, respiratory depression, and cardiovascular instability (Dodini, 1971, Rappolt, 1976). Inaba and Gay have also noted combativeness-catatonia-convulsions-coma (the 4 C's) along with hypertension and laryngeal spasms in various cases of PCP overdosage treated in the Height-Ashbury Free Medical Clinic. The dramatic toxicity of this psychotogenic compound calls for immediate specfic therapy.

Treatment of an acute reaction should be along the same guidelines as the treatment of an LSD reaction. Chlorpromazine, diazepam, and intravenous sodium succinate (6 gm in 500 cc of water infused over a 5-minute period) have been successfully used to treat the subjective effects of PCP (Dodini, 1971; Liden et al., 1975; Rainey and Crowder, 1975; Reed and Kane, 1972; Rappolt, 1976; Jong et al., 1975). Currently, emergency room physicians have suggested that physostigmine salicylate (1 to 4 mg IV) is effective in reversing the CNS as well as physiological toxicity to PCP. One must be cautiously aware, however, of the cardiac depressive and convulsive properties of physostigmine.

Generally, PCP is not currently a preferred drug of abuse by the street population because of the frequency of "bad trips" associated with its use, but it is often sold as THC and mescaline to unsuspecting drug abusers (Pharm Chem Nesletter, 1973).

DMT (dimethyltryptamine) and DET (diethyltryptamine) are psychotogenic drugs with much shorter durations of action than those of other agents. Ineffective when taken orally, DMT must be smoked or inhaled into the lungs for psychotogenic effects. DMT has a 30-to 60-minute duration of action, and it also has a rapid onset: 1 minute when smoked and 2 to 5 minutes when snorted. The subjective effects of DMT approximate that of an LSD experience but are much shorter in duration. The popularity and availability of DMT as well as other tryptamine derivatives continues to remain below that of other psychotogenic drugs (Shulgin, 1969; Szara, 1961).

Marihuana, THC or delta 9-tetrahydro-cannabinol is thought to be the major component of a number of active cannibinoids contained in the marihuana plant, *Cannabis sativa*. Although its effects are more of a sedative-hypnotic nature when smoked or ingested in moderate amounts, higher doses are capable of inducing adverse reactions similar to other psychotogens. Panic reactions, simple depressive reactions, toxic psychoses, prolonged psychotic reactions, and even "flashbacks" have been documented with its use (Jaffe, 1975; Keeler, 1967; Perna, 1969; Pillard, 1970; Talbott et al., 1969; Weil, 1970). These adverse reactions are quite rare when placed in perspective of the many users of marihuana who do not develop adverse reactions.

Marihuana or hashish (dried pressed resin of cannabis) has been demonstrated to be fairly nontoxic with no long-lasting mental or physical damage when smoked moderately for even long periods of time (Grinspoon, 1969). However, this is still a matter of much controversy, since no controlled long term study has yet been done on marihuana.

When smoked, a dose of 0.5 to 2.0 gm of crude marihuana gives effects that generally dissipate in 3 to 4 hours (Jaffe, 1975; Weil, 1968).

Synthetic THC was developed in 1965. It is very difficult and expensive to manufacture and every sample of synthetic "street" THC in the Haight-Ashbury district of San Francisco was analyzed to be PCP. However, an extraction product of hashish (sold as "hash" oil or "red oil") has been analyzed to have a high concentration of THC.

Unlike other psychotogens, cannabis has sedative effects, does not produce sympathomimetic effects and does not exhibit cross tolerance with other psychotogens. Thus, some authors have suggested a separate classification for cannabis other than that of a psychotogenic agent (Jaffe, 1975).

A critical literature review of marihuana abuse would constitute volumes of pages in itself. The basic conclusion of the Commission on Marihuana and Drug Abuse (1972) is that the present penalties regarding the possession and use of cannabis far outweigh the extent of the crime and they therefore recommend an appropriate reduction in penalties.

CONCLUSION

Because of illicit manufacturing and an ever changing array of "street" terminology, the treatment of the overdosed drug abuse patient is confused and oftentimes bewildering, especially so since management of all acute drug reactions must begin with an accurate diagnosis. Many reactions, however, can be treated adequately utilizing nonpharmacological techniques such as reassurance and good supportive nursing care. Properly approached, friends who bring in an overdosed patient may be able to provide the desperately needed drug ingestion history but treatment should always begin symptomatically and by the clinical appearance of the patient. When in doubt, specific medications should be avoided unless using the diagnostic test of naloxone in the comatose patient or when the situation represents a life-threatening emergency. Most essential to the management of any comatose patient is the established practice of good cardiopulmonary resuscitation.

The emergency treatment of the overdosed drug abuser is only a first step in the management of the current drug abuse crisis. Detoxification, aftercare and rehabilitation are the key to the prevention of further drug crises. It is imperative that all health professionals be instrumental in the establishment of facilities or referrals to adequate psychosocial medical aftercare modalities for the drug abuse patient.

BIBLIOGRAPHY

Ackerly, W. C. and Gibson, G. Lighter fluid 'sniffing'. *Am. J. Psychiatry* 120: 1506, 1964.

Albaugh, B. J., and Anderson, P. O. Peyote in the treatment of alcoholism among American Indians. *Am. J. Psychiatry* 131: 1247–1250, 1974.

Allen, S. M. Glue sniffing. *Int. J. Addict.* 1: 147–149, 1966.

AMA Committee on Alcoholism and Addiction. Dependence on amphetamines and other stimulant drugs. *J.A.M.A.* 197: 1024, 1966.

Baden, M. Narcotic abuse: a medical examiner's view. *N.Y. State J. Med.* 72: 834, 1972.

Barnett, B. E. Diazepan treatment for LSD intoxication. Lancet 2: 270, 1971.

Bass. M. Sudden sniffing death. *J.A.M.A.* 212: 2075. 1970.

Becker. C. E. Medical complications of heroin addiction. *Calif. Med.*, 115: 42. 1971.

Bick. R. L.. et al. Malaria transmission among narcotic addicts. *Calif. Med.* 115: 56. 1971.

Buck. R. W. Mushroom toxins: a brief review of the literature. *N. Engl J. Med.* 265: 681. 1961.

Carey. J. T.. et al. A San Francisco bay area 'speed' scene. J. Health Soc. Behav. 9: 164. 1968.

Citron. B. P.. et al. Necrotizing angiitis associated with drug abuse. *N. Engl. J. Med.* 283: 1003. 1970.

Clemmesem. C.. and Nilsson. E. Therapeutic trends in the treatment of barbiturate poisoning. *Clin. Pharmacol. Ther.* 2: 220–229. 1961.

Commission on Marihuana and Drug Abuse. *Marihuana: a signal of misunderstanding.* Washington. D.C.: U.S. Government Printing Office. 1972.

Connell. P. H. Clinical manifestations and treatment of amphetamine type dependence. *J.A.M.A.* 196: 718–723. 1966.

Der Marderosin. A. Current status of hallucinogens. *Am. J. Pharmacol.* 138: 204. 1966.

Dismukes. W.. et al. Viral hepatitis associated with illicit parenteral use of drugs. *J.A.M.A.* 206: 1048. 1968.

Dodini. L. K. Clinical pharmacology of the 'peace pill'. *Bull. Hosp. Pharm. Drug Inform. Anal. Serv.,* U. of Calif.. San Francisco. 18: 1. 1971.

Dreisbach. R. H. *Handbook of Poisoning: Diagnosis and Treatment.* Palo Alto: Lange Medical Publications. 1975.

Durden. W. D.. and Chipman. D. W. Gasoline sniffing complicated by acute carbon tetrachloride poisoning. *Arch. Intern. Med.* 119: 371. 1967.

Easson. W. M. Gasoline addiction in children. Pediatrics 29: 250. 1962.

Ellinwood. E. H. Amphetamine psychosis. I. Description of the individuals and process. *J. Psychedelic Drugs* 2: 42. 1969.

Ellinwood. E. H. Amphetamine psychosis. II. Theoretical implications. *J. Psychedelic Drugs* 2: 52. 1969.

Ellinwood. E. H. Assault and homicide associated with amphetamine abuse. *Am. J. Psychiatry* 127: 1170. 1971.

Espelin. D. E.. et al. Amphetamine poisoning: effectiveness of chlorpromazine. *N. Engl. J. Med.* 278: 1361. 1968.

Essig. C. F. Addiction to non-barbiturate sedative and tranquilizing drugs. *Clin. Pharmacol. Ther.* 5: 344–353. 1964.

Essig. CF. Newer sedative drugs that can cause states of intoxication and dependence of barbiturate type. *J.A.M.A.* 196: 714–717. 1966.

Fink. M.. et al. Naloxone in heroin dependence. *Clin. Pharmacol. Ther.* 9: 568. 1968.

Fiut. R. E.. et al. Antagonism of convulsive and lethal effects induced by propoxyphene. *J. Pharm. Sci.* 55: 1085. 1966.

Flowers. N. C.. and Horan. L. G. Nonanoxic aerosol arrhythmias. *J.A.M.A.* 219: 33–37. 1972.

Foldes. E. F.. et al. Studies on the specificity of narcotic antagonists. *Anesthesiology* 26: 320. 1965.

Fraser. H. F.. et al. Death due to withdrawal of barbiturates. *Ann. Intern Med.* 38: 1319. 1953.

Freedman. D. X. On the use and abuse of LSD. *Arch. Gen. Psychiatry* 18: 330. 1968.

Freedman. D. X. The psychopharmacology of hallucinogenic agents. *Annu. Rev. Med.* 20: 409. 1969.

Frykman. J. H. *A New Connection.* Scrimshaw Press. San Francisco; 1971.

Garson. O. M.. et al. Studies in a patient with acute leukemia after lysergide treatment. *Br. Med. J.* 2: 800. 1969.

Gay. G. R. Intra-arterial injection of secobarbital sodium into the brachial artery: sequalae of a 'hand trip. *Anesth. Analg.* 50: 979–981. 1971.

Gay. G. R. Treatment of acute drug reactions and overdose in a free Clinic. *Nurs. Digest* 3: 32–35. 1975.

Gay. G. R.. et al. Recognizing the battered flower child. *Hosp. Physician* 8: 43. 1972.

Gay. G. R.. Eisenbaumer. R.. and Newmeyer. J. A.: A dash of MASH—the Zep and the Dead: head to head. *J. Psychedelic Drugs* 5: 193–203. 1972.

Gay. G. R.. and Inaba. D. S.: Treating acute heroin and methadone toxicity. *Anesth. Analg.* Curr. Res. 55: 607–610. 1976.

Gay. G. R.. Inaba. D. S.. Sheppard. C. W.. Newmeyer. J. A.. and Rappolt. R. T.: Cocaine: history. epidemiology. human pharmacology and treatment: A perspective on a new debut for an old girl. *Clin. Toxicol.* 8: 149–178. 1975.

Gay. G. R.. and Trantham. J. G.: Medical-surgical complications of drug abuse. *Int. Surg.* 60: 327–331. 1975.

Gay. G. R.. and Way. E. L.: Some pharmacological perspectives on the opiate narcotics with special consideration of heroin. *J. Psychedelic Drugs* 4: 31–39. 1971.

Goodman. S.. et al. Intracranial hemorrhage associated with amphetamine abuse. *J.A.M.A.* 212: 480. 1970.

Greenblatt. D. J.. et al. Adverse effects of LSD: a current perspective. *Conn. Med.* 34: 895. 1970.

Grinspoon. L. Marihuana. *Sci. Am.* 221: 17. 1969.

Hashbrouch. J. D. The antagonism of morphine anesthesia by naloxone. *Anesth. Analg.* Curr. Res. 50: 954. 1971.

Hoffer. A: LSD: a review of its present status. *Clin. Pharmacol. Ther.* 6: 183. 1964.

Inaba. D. S.. Gay. G. R.. Newmeyer. J. A.. and Whitehead. C. A.. Methaqualone abuse—'Luding out'. *J.A.M.A.* 224: 1505–1509. 1973.

Inaba. D. S.. and Katcher. B. S.: Drug Abuse. (Ch. 22). In Young. L.. and Kimble. M.A. (Eds.). *Applied Therapeutics for Clinical Pharmacist,* San Francisco: Applied Therapeutics Inc.. 1975, p. 330.

Innes. I. R.. and Nickerson. M.: Norepinephrine. epinephrine and the sympathomimetic amines. (Ch. 24). In Goodman. L.. and Gilman. A. (Eds.). *The Pharmacological Basis of Therapeutics,* 5th ed. New York: Macmillan. 1975, p. 477.

Isbell. H.. and Fraser. H. F. Addiction to analgesics and barbiturates. *Pharmacol. Rev.* 2: 355–397. 1950.

Isbell. H.. Fraser. H. F.. Wikler. A.. Belville. R. E.. and Eisenman. A. J.: An experimental study of the etiology of 'rum fit' and delirium tremens. *Q. J.*

Stud. Alcohol 16: 1–33, 1955.

Jackson, B., et al. Another abusable amphetamine. *J.A.M.A.* 211: 830, 1970.

Jaffe, J. H. Drug addiction and drug abuse. (Ch. 16), In Goodman, L., and Gilman, A. (Eds.), *The Pharmacological Basis of Therapeutics*, 5th ed. New York: Macmillan, 1975, p. 284.

Jarvik, M. E. Drugs used in the treatment of psychiatric disorders. (Ch. 12), In Goodman, L., and Gilman, A. (Eds.), *The Pharmacological Basis of Therapeutics*, 4th ed. New York: Macmillan; 1970.

Jasinski, D. R. et al. The human pharmacology and abuse potential of N-allylnoroxymorphone (naloxone). *J. Pharmacol. Exp. Ther.* 157: 420, 1967.

Jasinski, D. R., et al. Antagonism of the subjective behavioral pupillary and respiratory depressant effects of cyclazocine by naloxone. *Clin. Pharmacol. Ther.*, 9: 215, 1968.

Kane, F. J., et al. Neurological crisis following methamphetamine. *J.A.M.A.* 210: 556, 1969.

Keeler, M. H. Adverse reaction to marihuana. *Am. J. Psychiatry* 124: 128, 1967.

Kleber, H. Prolonged adverse reaction from unsupervised use of hallucinogenic drugs. *J. Nerv. Ment. Dis.* 144: 308, 1967.

Klock, J. C., Boener, U., and Becker, C. E. Coma, hyperthermia and bleeding associated with massive LSD overdose. *West. J. Med.*, 120: 183–188, 1974.

Know, J. W., and Nelson J. R. Permanent encephalopathy from toluence inhalation. *N. Engl. J. Med.* 275: 1494, 1966.

Kramer, J. C. Introduction to amphetamine abuse. *J. Psychedelic Drugs* 2: 8, 1969.

Kramer, J. C., Fischman, V. S., Littlefield, D. C. Amphetamine abuse: patterns and effects of high doses taken intravenously. *J.A.M.A.* 201: 305–309, 1967.

Kupperstein, L. R., and Sussman, R. M. A bibliography on the inhalation of glue fumes and other toxic vapors—a substance abuse practice among adolescents. *Int. J. Addict.* 3: 177–198, 1968.

Langs, R. J., et al. Lysergic acid diethylamide (LSD-25) and schizophrenic reactions. J. Nerv. Ment. Dis. 147: 163, 1968.

Levy, R. M. Diazepam for LSD intoxication. Lancet 1: 1297, 1971.

Liden, C. B., Lovejoy, F. H., and Costello, C. E. Phencyclidine—nine cases of poisoning. *J.A.M.A.* 234: 513–516, 1975.

Lingeman, R.: *Drugs from A to Z: A Dictionary*. New York: McGraw-Hill, 1969.

Louria, D: Lysergic acid diethylamine. *N. Engl. J. Med.* 278: 435, 1968.

Louria, D., et al. Major medical complications of heroin addiction. *Ann. Int. Med.* 67: 1, 1967.

Mark, L. C.: Analeptics: Changing concepts, declining status. *Am. J. Med. Sci.* 254: 296–302, 1967.

Martin, C. M.: Caring for the 'bad trip'—a review of current status of LSD. *Hawaii Med. J.* 29: 555, 1970.

McLaughlin, J. L.: Peyote. *Lloydia* 36: 1–9, 1973.

Morrison, W., et al. The acute pulmonary edema of heroin intoxication. *Radiology* 97: 347, 1970.

Narango, C., et al. Evaluations of 3,4-methylenedioxyamphetamine (MDA) as an adjunct to psychotherapy. *Med. Pharmacolog. Exper.* 17: 359, 1967.

Perna, D. Psychotogenic effect of marihuana. *J.A.M.A.* 209: 1085, 1969.

Picchioni, A. L. Clinical status and toxicology and analeptic drugs. *Am. J. Hosp. Pharm.*, 28: 201–203, 1971.

Pillard, R. Medical progress, marihuana. *N. Engl. J. Med.* 283: 294, 1970.

Pharm Chem Newsletter. Palo Alto: Pharm Chem Laboratories, 2: 2, 1973.

PMA. STASH capsules, 5: 1–3, 1973.

Post, R. M. Cocaine psychoses: a continuum model. *Am. J. Psychiatry* 132: 225–231, 1975.

Powars, D. Aplastic anemia secondary to glue sniffing. *N. Engl. J. Med.* 273: 700, 1965.

Rainey, J. M., and Crowder, M. K. Prolonged psychosis attributed to phencyclidine: report of three cases. *Am. J. Psychiatry* 132: 1076–1078, 1975.

Rappolt, R. T. (Ed.) Monograph edition on phencyclidine toxicity. *Clin. Toxicol.* 9: 473–600, 1976.

Reed, A., and Kane, A. W. Phencyclidine (PCP): another illicit psychedelic drug. *J. Psychedelic Drugs* 5: 8–12, 1972.

Richards, K. C., et al. Near fatal reaction to ingestion of the hallucinogenic drug MDA. *J.A.M.A.* 218: 1826, 1971.

Ricter, R., et al. Transverse myelitis associated with heroin addiction. *J.A.M.A.* 206: 1255, 1968.

Schwarz, C. J. Paradoxical responses to chlorpromazine after LSD. *Psychosomatics* 8: 210, 1967.

Schwarz, C. J. Phenothiazine induced psychosis after LSD. *Can. Med. Assoc. J.* 105: 241, 1971.

Shick, J., et al. Analysis of the LSD flashback. *J. Psychedelic Drugs* 3: 13, 1970.

Shulgin, A. T. Psychotomimetic agents related to the catecholamines. *J. Psychedelic Drugs* 2: 17, 1969.

Shulgin, A. T., et al. 4-Bromo-2,5-dimethoxyphenylisopropylamine a new centrally active amphetamine analog. *Pharmacology* 5: 103, 1971.

Siegel, H., et al. Continuing studies in the diagnosis and pathology of death from intravenous narcotism. *J. Forensic Sci.* 15: 179, 1970.

Smart, R., et al. Unfavorable reactions to LSD: A review and analysis of available case reports. *Can. Med. Assoc. J.* 97: 1214, 1967.

Smith, D. E. Psychotomimetic amphetamines with special reference to STP (DOM) toxicity. *J. Psychedelic Drugs* 2: 73, 1969.

Smith, D. E. Editor's note. *J. Psychedelic Drugs* 3: 5, 1970.

Smith, D. E., et al. A new method for treatment of barbiturate dependence. *J.A.M.A.* 213: 294, 1970.

Smith, D. E., and Wesson, D. R. *Diagnosis and Treatment of Adverse Reactions to Sedative-Hypnotics*. NIDA manual contract # HSM-42-73-177. Washington, D.C.: U.S. Government Printing Office # 731-930/173, 1974.

Snyder, S. H., et al. DOM (STP), a new hallucinogenic drug and DOET: Effects in normal subjects. Am. J. Psychiatry 125: 357, 1968.

Surgical complications in the drug addict. *Mod. Med.* 39: 23, 1971.

Szara, S. Hallucinogenic effects and metabolism of tryptamine derivatives in man. *Fed. Proc.* 20: 885, 1961.

Talbott, J., et al. Marihuana psychosis. *J.A.M.A.* 210: 299, 1969.

Taylor, R. L., et al. Management of 'bad trips' in an evolving drug scene. *J.A.M.A.* 213: 442, 1970.

Tec, L. Phenothiazine and biperiden in LSD reactions. *J.A.M.A.* 215: 980, 1971.

Tong, T. G., Benowitz, N. L., Becker, C. E., Forni, P. J., and Boerner, U. Phencyclidine poisoning. *J.A.M.A.* 234: 512–513, 1975.

Weil, A. Clinical and psychological effects of marihuana in man. Science 162: 1234, 1968.

Weil, A. Adverse reactions to marihuana: Classification and suggested treatment. *N. Engl. J. Med.* 282: 997, 1970.

Wikler, A. Diagnosis and treatment of drug dependence of the barbiturate type. *Am. J. Psychiatry* 125: 758, 1968.

Winek, C. L., et al. Toluene fatability from glue sniffing. *Pa. Med. J.* 71: 81, 1968.

Winek, C. L., Collom, W. D., and Wecht, C. H.: Fatal benzene exposure by glue-sniffing. *Lancet* 1: 683, 1967.

Chapter 25

pioneering in hospice nursing

ALICE DEMI

While hospice nursing has been a reality in England for many years, the hospice movement has only recently reached the United States. While many groups are working to develop hospices, there are only a few actually functioning in the United States. As these new programs develop, nurses are using their scientific knowledge, their creativity and their personal philosophy to find new, more effective ways of meeting the needs of dying patients and their families. The role of the nurse in a United States hospice is as yet relatively undefined and unstructured. Throughout the country hospice nurses are charting new courses and setting precedents that will influence hospice care in other communities.

WHAT IS A HOSPICE?

Originally a hospice was a refuge for medieval travelers going to and from the crusades. Today, hospice has evolved to mean a refuge for the dying—travelers embarking on a different kind of journey. The word hospice is closely related to the word hospitable which means: 1) given to cordial and generous reception of guests and 2) offering a pleasant or sustaining environment (Webster's Seventh New Collegiate Dictionary, 1971). The modern hospice is this and more. It is a way to help the dying and their families to live more fully and comfortably during the terminal period and to assist them in accepting and coping with the inevitable death. Hospice care does not end with the death of the loved one but continues into the bereavement period, by giving support to the survivors throughout the year following the death of a patient.

HISTORY OF HOSPICE

In the middle of the 19th century, the Irish Sisters of Charity opened the first hospice dedicated to caring for people who were dying. Mary Aikenhead, the founder of the order, selected the name hospice because she considered death to be the beginning of a journey and her nursing home to be a resting place similar to those used by the medieval pilgrims when traveling to the Holy Land (Lamerton, 1975).

At the beginning of the 20th century,

three more hospices were founded, one being St. Joseph's in London. The hospice movement then lay dormant until the 1950's when two events interacted to give impetus to the hospice movement. First, a survey by the Marie Curie Foundation revealed the need for more hospices. Second, Cicely Saunders, a physician and formerly a nurse and social worker, came to St. Joseph's Hospice with a conviction that care of the dying could be improved and set about making this a reality. She later opened St. Christopher's Hospice where she could apply more fully her creative ideas. Today England has more than 30 hospices (Lamerton, 1975).

The hospice movement only recently reached America and today there are several hospices in operation. While many hospices are in the planning stage in the United States only a few are far enough along in their development to deliver patient care. The first hospice founded in the United States was Hospice Inc., New Haven, Connecticut, which initiated its Home Care Program in March 1974 (Craven and Wald, 1975). Hospice of Marin, Marin County, California, started its pilot program in September 1975 and was licensed as a Home Health Care Agency in October 1976 (Lamers, 1976). Both of these programs provide a variety of services to the dying patient and their families primarily in the home but when indicated, services are also provided as supplemental care when a patient is in a hospital or extended care facility. Both organizations are working toward development of inpatient facilities to complete the array of services believed necessary to meet the varying needs of terminally ill patients and their families.

Some hospices such as Parkwood Community Hospital, Canoga Park, California, are focusing on inpatient care and utilizing community agencies to provide home care for their patients when this is indicated. Parkwood, a private hospital, opened its 15-bed hospice unit in October 1976 (McKell, 1976). St. Luke's Hospital (1975), New York City, has hospice patients dispersed throughout the hospital and a hospice care team assigned to meeting the special needs of these patients (St. Luke's Hospital Center).

Hospice care is not based on a particular type of organizational structure or setting but rather on a philosophy. Hospice care can be provided i an a general hospital, an extended care facility, a private home or in a specialized hospice facility. Each hospice program must consider the unique needs of their community and the available resources and then plan innovative programs that meet these needs and are economically feasible.

PHILOSOPHY OF HOSPICE CARE

Hospice care is based on the following beliefs:

1. The quality of life is more important than the quantity of life.
2. The medical and nursing care of the dying is directed toward comfort rather than cure.
3. Control of pain and alleviation of other symptoms is a major function of hospice care.
4. The unit of care is the family.
5. Medical and nursing care is available 24 hours a day wherever the patient chooses to live – home, hospital, nursing home or hospice.
6. Hospice care is a specialty area.
7. A hospice provides comprehensive health care to the dying patient utilizing an interdisciplinary approach.
8. Volunteers, both professional and nonprofessional are an integral part of the health care team.

Each of these beliefs is interrelated and cannot be isolated from the others.

Quality of Life

The belief that the quality of life is more important than the quantity of life guides the delivery of medical and nursing care. Often the goals of a health care institution are in conflict with the needs of the dying patient and his family. Hospital personnel seem to believe that life must be saved at all costs at all times, but little thought is given to the means or the purpose. It is the belief of hospice personnel that aggressive treatment of the terminally ill detracts from the quality of life. "Just as a healthy person has a right to live, a sick and old person has a right to die" (Kerppola-Sirola, 1975). Too often, health care professionals and families have seen heroics performed to save a person who is dying of metastatic cancer. Whose needs are being met as hospital personnel defibrillate, intubate, medicate, demean and depersonalize?

Death is a final fact for all. It cannot be denied but its dignity can be — by thoughtless, underfeeling, and overscientific care. Everything that is done for the dying patient should be based on the constant awareness that although death may be postponed, sometimes dramatically, the master plan cannot be altered (Day, 1966, p. 886).

The following vignettes describe the contrasting care of two elderly people as told by their surviving children. Both children, practicing physicians were profoundly affected by the care given their parent during the terminal illness.

Dr. Netsky (1976) describes the terminal illness of his 80-year-old mother whose physical and mental condition had deteriorated over several years. Prior to entering a coma, she often asked, "Why does God let me live so long?" She felt useless and a burden to her family. On entering the hospital she received numerous, extensive diagnostic tests, treatments and consultations of specialists. Nameless packs of people traipsed in and out of her room. Her son, although a regular visitor, was never consulted nor considered as to his or his mother's desire for treatments. The son could not find out who her primary physician was, and when he did, had great difficulty contacting him. Finally, a meeting was arranged and the son told the physician that he'd prefer not to prolong the agony of his dying mother. The physician listened and agreed but nothing changed. It became a nightmare of depersonalization and dehumanization as the formerly vivacious, attractive woman became an emaciated, distorted human body with a beating heart but little other evidence of humanness. They were trapped in a system of "good care." The surviving son asks:

If a life is to be saved at all costs, should we not be certain that the life is worth saving? ... Why do they ignore the wishes of the family and fail to communicate? ... Where is love and compassion? Why prolong life when it exists only as a remnant, without hope, and is undesired by the person and the family? Who made the rule that life must always be saved and at any cost? Is death a disgrace? Is it not the expected end of life? (Netsky, 1976, p. 59).

Dr. Kerppola-Sirola (1975) describes a radically different situation when her 80-year-old father was terminally ill. Her father, a retired professor of medicine, began to lose his vigor and to have pain, although his memory and judgment remained intact. On admission to the hospital he permitted only the simplest tests. All complicated, fatiguing procedures he considered unnecessary, since he judged himself as incurably ill and too old for radical treatment. He accepted pain medication and other symptomatic treatment but refused infusions, antibiotics and intensive care. Throughout his illness, he was concerned about his appearance and dressed neatly and properly. He died as he wanted with dignity and with retention of his humanness, living fully until the very end.

The old professor's fate differs from the fate offered today to most terminally ill individuals. As in the first example, the finest treatment often has the opposite effect. Physicians find it easy to do "all that is possible" but more difficult to abstain from overzealous treatment.

The specter of malpractice is a further impediment to delivery of humane care to the dying. The following conversation occurred between a hospice nurse and a physician. The nurse had just described how she functioned in the hospice home-care program.

Physician: I would never let one of my patients die at home.
Nurse: Why not?
Physician: I'd want him to have the very best in medical care, and that's only available in the hospital.
Nurse: But suppose the patient wanted to be at home and didn't want extensive treatment.
Physician: Well, I wouldn't let him die at home. I have to think of the family. I wouldn't want the family to live with the memory of the patient dying there in the home. (pause) Later they might sue.
Later in the conversation
Physician: I hope when I'm 70 years old and

in the hospital, sick and dying—I hope I have the strength to get up out of the bed and walk out and go home to die.

Nurse: Oh! So it's good enough for you, but not for your patients!

Physician: Well maybe if I had the support system that a hospice offers, I might consider it for my patients.

Obviously, for him the welfare of the patient is secondary to protection from malpractice suits. While I recognize that malpractice suits are a real concern in all areas of practice, it is unlikely that hospice care would increase the risk of a malpractice suit.

Comfort Versus Cure

When the decision is made that nothing further can be done to arrest the illness, then medical and nursing care should be directed to promoting comfort, both physical and psychological. It is not a time to stop or decrease care but rather to change the goal of care. Schmale and Patterson (1976) suggest some guidelines for comfort care.

1. Comfort care should be initiated whenever patient and family agree that all reasonable measures for control of the disease have failed.
2. The purpose of this care is to minimize discomfort without any specific or direct attention to the underlying disease.
3. The plan of care should be flexible but specific in its detail and known to all concerned with its implementation.
4. All treatment and medication will be prescribed to minimize symptoms.
   a. Drugs, procedures, fluids, etc., not clearly needed to relieve symptoms will be omitted.
   b. Measures to relieve pain and discomfort are provided as requested by the patient with no concern for addiction or habituation.
   c. Routines such as repeated physical examinations, measuring vital signs, etc. should be discontinued.
   d. Emergency measures should not be used to prevent death.

Special skill and knowledge are necessary to give comfort care.

Aeration of the lungs, mobilization of joints and muscles, and maintaining the integrity of the skin remain important focuses of nursing care activities but the emphasis is on their value in promoting comfort, rather than to affect the course of the illness. This is explained to patients as in the following examples:

"Deep breathing exercises may be tiring and make you cough but this will clear the mucus out of your lungs and you'll be able to eat more comfortably later."

"Walking will cause you some discomfort now but it will improve your circulation and help you rest and sleep better later."

"Turning and positioning you may increase your pain momentarily but it will keep your skin from breaking down (and further distorting your body image)."

Not only is the goal of nursing care different, but the manner of delivery is different also. Nursing care activities are done at the patients own pace and according to his own selected time schedule.

Control of Pain and Alleviation of Other Symptoms

The interaction of mind and body is nowhere more evident than in the cycle of pain. Pain can consume a person physically and emotionally. It then becomes the all encompassing focus of an individual's existence. A person's basic needs must be met before he has energy and interest for higher level needs. To be free of pain is a basic need, therefore a major focus of hospice nursing is to control pain. Severe chronic pain has a cyclical effect as demonstrated in the diagram (Lipman, 1974).

Physical and psychological components interact in severe chronic pain. Anxiety may be caused by anticipation of return of pain when medication is given on a p.r.n. basis but it may also be caused by events outside of the patient as in the following example.

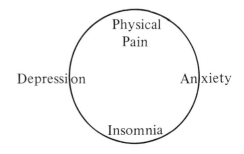

Mr. Miller was in good pain control with Brompton Mixture but had a recurrence of pain on two consecutive evenings. The nurse investigated and found that the pain occurred whenever his wife visited. A p.r.n. injection of morphine was ordered to supplement the Brompton Mixture and additional support was given to his wife. Control of pain is much more than the prescription and administration of a drug or drugs. Symptoms should be mitigated through both psychological and physiological intervention.

A modified Brompton Mixture is frequently given for control of chronic terminal pain. The mixture as used in the United States differs from that used in England primarily because diamorphine (heroin) is not legally available in this country. Modified Brompton Mixture contains: morphine, 20 mg.; ethyl alcohol, 5 cc.; simple syrup or cherry syrup, 5 cc.; with water added to form a mixture of morphine sulfate, 20 mg./20 cc. Alternative elixirs are available with varying strengths of morphine. When morphine is given orally, the dose should be increased 50% over the dose given by injection because some is metabolized. Oral administration of morphine has several advantages over subcutaneous injection; the patient can more readily self-administer the drug and it avoids the repeated trauma of injections. Brompton Mixture must be given every 4 hours round-the-clock, not p.r.n., nor only during waking hours. Patients need to be cautioned that they may experience temporary drowsiness during the first 3 days. Some physicians include cocaine in their mixture for its stimulating effect, but the majority of hospices prefer to eliminate the cocaine because of its many distressing side-effects and this cocaine-morphine mixture has not been proven to be more effective in pain control than the morphine mixture.

The method of administration of Brompton Mixture is essential for pain control. When patients are started on Brompton Mixture while on home care, the patient is contacted every 4 hours during the first 48 hours to assess pain and sedation level and adjust dosage accordingly. Most patients remain alert and comfortable with this method of pain control. Experience has shown that this method does not lead to increasing dosages. In contrast, when patients are on too low a dosage level or on p.r.n. basis, this results in inadequate pain control, dissatisfaction with the medication and/or increasing dosages often without freedom from pain or with confusion (Dimmitt, 1976; Lamerton, 1975; Saunders, 1975; Twycross, 1972, 1975).

A 56-year-old man with cancer of the pancreas was experiencing severe pain. He had been on p.r.n. doses of Schlessinger's Solution and Demerol injections, and had not obtained any relief. He was started on Brompton Mixture, 60 mg. every 4 hours, but this did not relieve the pain. Within a 24-hour period the dose was increased gradually to 120 mg. every 4 hours. At this level he achieved pain control. The next day he went to a school board meeting and defended a proposal submitted by his school. He remained pain-free and alert throughout the following 2 months of his illness. The dose of Brompton Mixture was gradually reduced until he was taking 30 mg. at the time of his death. Once the physical pain was under control, attention was given to the emotional pain. Individual counseling and family counseling led to resolution of prior conflicts and acceptance of the impending death. When the emotional distress was relieved, the amount of pain medication could be reduced. It is not enough to give the medication; throughout this man's illness the patient and family received constant support from the doctor and the nurse.

Anxiety may need to be treated with a phenothiazine tranquilizer, or depression with a tricyclic antidepressant, but in addition to the medication, other measures are indicated. A dying adolescent's pain was greatly increased by his anxiety. His therapist, a psychiatric social worker, used foot massage as an adjunct to his medication and effectively reduced the pain. Depression may be alleviated by bringing an elderly woman's pet canary to her hospital room or taking her for a ride to her favorite place, or getting in touch with her friends and telling them how much she'd enjoy a visit.

Side effects of medications must be anticipated and alleviated also. Morphine's side effect of nausea can usually be controlled by the concurrent administration of a phenothiazine. Constipation secondary to morphine can be prevented by administration of a stool softener such as Colace. The anticholinergic effects of phenothiazines may cause dry mouth and blurred vision which can be very distressing and may necessitate a reduction in the dosage of the phenothiazine.

Sometimes a minor symptom that is easily controlled can cause a patient extreme discomfort. (For more complete discussion of symptom control see R. C. Lamerton, C. Saunders and R. G. Twycross under Bibliography.) When a hospice nurse first visited Mr. Jackson, he was irritable and had difficulty concentrating. He was not in pain but he kept rubbing his nose. The nurse learned that he was recovering from herpes zoster and the itching of his nose was extremely distressing to him. The nurse obtained an order for hydrocortisone ointment. Shortly after the ointment was applied, his personality changed dramatically and he was cheerful and attentive.

Family as Unit of Care

The focus of care is on the dying patient and the family as an integral unit. The goal of hospice care is not only improved quality of life for patient and a peaceful death but also improved quality of life for the family, both before and after the death. Much can be done during the terminal illness to facilitate the healthy resolution of grief after the death.

Cathy, a 14-year-old with advanced cancer of the bone was referred to us for nursing care because her mother was emotionally unable to care for her. The mother was having frequent fits of rage and was trying to force Cathy to do things beyond the limits of her ability. The mother became psychotic and had to be hospitalized. The father was concerned about Cathy but needed to go to work; therefore, Cathy was left alone in the house, with a neighbor coming in to make her lunch and her younger brother caring for her after school. On the nurse's first visit, she found Cathy in her room, set-off from the rest of the house down a long corridor with her door tightly closed. Cathy, bedridden, emaciated and bald, lay flat on her waterbed covered with a quilt, so one could hardly see her body impression under the covers. She was withdrawn and hostile and resisted all care. She had been incontinent and was changing her own diapers; the room reeked of urine. She communicated with the outside world with an intercom. Within a few weeks, Cathy learned to reach out to others and accept love and care; the door to her room was left open; she entertained a few visitors in her room; and her mother came home from the hospital and assisted in her care. Cathy asked to go out on a picnic with her nurse and at first was reluctant to have her mother go also, but the nurse explained how the two of them could go alone on another outing—and they did. One week later Cathy died, and the mother who at first said, "I don't care *how* Cathy lives as long as she lives," went to the funeral service and walked up to the coffin and closed the lid, symbolically letting go.

If one were concerned only for the patient, it would have been easy to shut this mother out and cause her severe psychological damage. Instead, the nurse facilitated the mother's growth in her relationship with her child and thereby promoted healthy resolution of her grief.

Availability of Medical and Nursing Care

Medical and nursing care must be available to hospice patients 24 hours a day. In hospice home care programs, a nurse and a physician are always available by telephone and will make home visits whenever necessary. In addition, the patient also has the telephone number and may call his primary nurse. If the primary nurse is not available, then the nurse on call will handle the emergency. New patients frequently test to see whether the nurse and doctor will really answer their call. Once they know this service is really available, it gives them security and they do not abuse the service. Often patients put in a call to the nurse, and when the nurse calls back 15 to 30 minutes later, the patient will have already dealt effectively with the emergency. They need only reassurance from the nurse that they have taken the appropriate action.

While in many cases the patient's home is the best place for care of the terminal illness, sometimes inpatient care is necessary for the patient's benefit and sometimes for the family's. Caring for the patient at home may be too heavy a burden for the family or they may need temporary respite, or the patient may have no supportive family. Those living alone and with little community support would benefit from the warm, caring atmosphere and the comraderie of an inpatient hospice unit. Patients should be able to move with ease from home care to hospital and vice versa, with continuity of care and adherence to hospice philosophy. For these reasons, several hospices that now provide only home care are working toward development of inpatient facilities.

Hospice Care as a Specialty Area

How is hospice nursing different? While much of hospice care is simply quality nursing care, several factors combine to make hospice nursing a specialty area. These factors are the belief in the hospice philosophy, special knowledge related to comfort care, ability to communicate with the dying, the risk-taking behavior of the nurse and the support system within hospice.

Through ongoing education, hospice nurses explore their attitudes toward death and dying in order to formulate a personal philosophy of death and dying that is congruent with hospice philosophy. While intellectual and theoretical knowledge is useful, it is not sufficient in itself, Lamers (1976b) sounds a word of caution:

Unless intellectual knowledge and scientific training are balanced with experiences that will help the practitioner come into feeling contact with his own attitudes, prejudices and fears about death, the individual and the Thanatology Movement will produce less that will have lasting benefit than if affective and intellectual learning are combined.

Unless we are forced to think about death and dying, our ideas are poorly formed and preclude effective communication with the dying.

A physician unaware of his personal feelings about death and dying (by the same token) permits them to interfere with his effective treatment of patients (Arnig, 1971, p. 160).

This is true of all health professionals working with the dying. Failure to explore one's own feelings results in either of two extremes, indifference which leads to undertreatment and neglect or overconcern which leads to overtreatment.

Nurses in a hospice program must be risk-takers — that is, risk attachment knowing they will inevitably suffer loss. To be effective, the nurse must have a high sensitivity to others' pain, both physical and psychological, and conversely the nurse must have a high tolerance for pain. These are independent variables. Poets have often evidenced a high sensitivity but coupled with a low tolerance for pain, resulting in many premature deaths from suicide. Nurses tend to self-select themselves for this type of work. Those with a low pain threshold quickly recognize that they are unable to tolerate the pain induced by caring for and about the dying patient and his family. Working with the dying intensifies one's own personal unresolved feelings about death and dying.

One's own cup must be full when entering a difficult family situation. The nurse must often give and give of herself with little positive feedback and sometimes negative feedback from family members. How does the nurse cope? How can her cup be refilled? The feedback must come from other hospice staff. Sharing of experiences at weekly conferences helps the nurse gain a more realistic perspective of the situation and insight into the family dynamics. Sometimes daily telephone calls to other hospice staff are indicated. Immediate consultation with either the medical physician, the psychiatrist, or the nursing coordinator is available.

"Just as one cannot look long directly at the sun, one cannot look long directly at death." (La Rochefoucald, 1678)

Each person is encouraged to develop his own coping behavior. Some take their frustrations out on a tennis ball, others seek serenity through backpacking into the wilderness. Retreats are necessary to replenish one's personal resources. Some hospices schedule retreats periodically, so that together staff can explore intrapersonal and interpersonal issues, and religious and philosophical issues.

To be more effective, hospice nurses must feel that they are getting as much as they are giving. Dying patients have much to teach us about living; their concern to make each day count helps nurses achieve a realistic perspective. Hospice nurses practice in their own lives making each day more meaningful and living each day fully.

Hospice nurses develop special skills in communicating with the dying. Communication in relationship to death occurs verbally, nonverbally and symbolically. There is no set time to communicate about death and dying. Discussion tends to flow at unexpected times and is intertwined with the physical care. The nurse has an advantage over a therapist or counselor since she is with the patient for longer periods of time and also is there more frequently.

Verbal communication must be honest, simple, direct and consistent. If a patient asks, "Am I dying?", it is not enough to say "We're all going to die someday." The nurse needs to explore the emotion related to the question—such as, "Are you afraid of dying?" or "What concerns you the most about dying?" The nurse needs to deal with the patient at his level of emotional comprehension. Some patients will never talk openly about their impending death; others talk freely and want specific information as to how and when the dying will occur.

Fear of the unknown is a universal problem. This fear can be minimized by explaining everything that will happen, i.e.: How much pain will there be? Where will the pain be? What will be done for it? What will happen to my family? What's going to happen in the dying process? How will I know when I'm dying? The nurse needs to answer these questions simply and directly. It is no easy task to find the right words but knowing the patient well enables the nurse to give meaningful answers that promote psychological comfort.

Patients often need assistance in leave-taking—saying their goodbyes. They need to be helped to resolve family conflicts, and both patients and family need to be helped to let go. The nurse often acts as a facilitator

in family conferences and also when a patient is trying to communicate with his personal physician.

Nonverbal communication is often more meaningful than verbal. The fact that the nurse is there caring and comforting can communicate a sense of security and acceptance of the impending death. The patient is then able to relax and express himself verbally.

Symbolic communication occurs verbally, through dreams and through drawing and other art work. A 15-year-old boy with advanced lymphoma planned for months to get a dog. When the dog arrived, he became very sad and cried, "We have no right to take him away from his father,"—thereby expressing his unhappiness at being taken away from his own father. It is appropriate then to relate to the symbolism and talk about the dog and the dog's father and how they are going to adjust to their separation. Another adolescent longed to go to see the Golden Gate Bridge. On her last visit there, she remarked on the beauty of the ship sailing out of the harbor into the ocean. The nurse related to the symbolism and asked what the journey would be like for the ship. The girl described in detail a wonderful, peaceful voyage.

Comprehensive Health Care Through an Interdisciplinary Team

Hospice provides a broad range of services through an interdisciplinary team. The physical, emotional, spiritual and financial needs of the patient and his family are assessed and then services are provided according to these needs by the most appropriate health care professionals, or nonprofessionals. Usually a hospice staff consists of an administrator, medical physician, a psychiatrist, a social worker, a family therapist, a psychologist, a clergyman and nurses. Hospice works closely with other community agencies and assists patients in the mobilization of resources within the community.

Role of Volunteers

A unique feature of hospice care is the importance of volunteers, both professional and nonprofessional. The enthusiasm and dedication of volunteers is evident in all hospice activities. They are the link with the community. They interpret hospice to their friends, neighbors, relatives and community associates, and in turn inform Hospice staff of the particular needs of their community. Health professionals who are volunteers generally provide services that are consistent with their professional training and experience. Nonprofessional volunteers' services range from befriending a dying patient to hosting a public relations meeting to providing secretarial services. They may run errands for patients, go food shopping, provide transportation for medical appointments, provide child care, or take youngsters on an outing. They may donate artistic talent by taking photographs for publicity releases, or designing a brochure, or painting a picture for the inpatient unit.

The value of volunteers is two-fold — the volunteers provide much needed services to hospice and hospice provides a means for volunteers to give of themselves in a meaningful manner. Some volunteers are themselves cancer patients or have recovered from cancer; other have experienced the death of a loved one; others have a spiritual calling for this work. Each feels the need to become involved in a relevant way. Those who have recovered from grief often have a special insight and understanding that enables them to help others when they are bereaved. One of our most effective nurses experienced the sudden death of a young son. This nurse has a special skill in relating with dying children and their parents based on her own resolution of her grief.

For the future, hospice planners foresee a very active role for the volunteer on the inpatient unit. Volunteers will befriend patients, serve as hosts for visitors, assist with planning and implementing recreational and social activities, provide child care for young visitors, and assist with nursing activities. Planners are aware that some of this conflicts with existing roles and organizational patterns, but they are prepared to challenge these stereotyped roles.

TYPES OF SERVICES PROVIDED IN HOSPICE HOME CARE PROGRAMS

Hospice Home Care Programs provide five basic types of services: 1) symptom control, 2) total patient care, 3) family consultation, 4) professional consultation and 5) bereavement counseling. Patients and their families tend to move from one type of service to another. One woman referred herself for family consultation because her husband was having severe pain and was very stoic and refused to take any pain medication. He did not consider himself terminal and did not want hospice services. The wife was under much stress in coping both with his current behavior and with his impending death and the effect it would have on their children. The wife was seen individually for three sessions; then a family conference was held with the patient, his wife and their children. Subsequently the patient sought help with pain control and this evolved into total patient care. Later, after the patient's death, the wife and children were seen for bereavement counseling.

Many patients seek hospice care because of distressing symptoms such as pain and nausea. This service, symptom control, is given to supplement other care. Because of hospices' special expertise, hospice staff are often called to see a patient in a hospital or extended care facility because of the patient's lack of response to conventional treatment. If the patient's basic physical needs and his psychosocial needs are being met by those already in attendance of the patient, then hospice staff work in collaboration with these people to teach proper administration of medications and other comfort-care measures. One young woman was referred because of nausea, vomiting and dehydration. She was threatened with having to return to the hospital if the nausea and vomiting were not controlled. Hospice staff consulted with her physician, made medication suggestions, and then taught the patient and her parents to administer the medication. Frequently, patients and family do not administer medications according to the schedule prescribed. They must be taught what symptoms to observe for so that they know when to give p.r.n. medication. They need frequent, meaningful explanations of why medications must be taken as prescribed. Often, patients wait until the pain or nausea occur before taking their medication and then the medicine is less effective. Frequent home visits and telephone calls when providing symptom control are essential.

Total patient care service includes symptom control, teaching, counseling and direct physical care. A patient may receive any one or all parts of this service. When a patient receives total patient care, hospice assumes responsibility for planning and coordinating all of the patient's care, although hospice may not provide all of the care. Early in a patient's illness the focus may be on counseling and later as the patient progresses in his illness, the focus may change to direct physical care. Often in the later stages of illness a patient's emotional needs are best met by providing physical care, thus providing love and security.

Family consultation is provided when family members are having difficulty dealing with the terminal illness of a loved one. Sometimes the patient does not want care for himself. Other times the patient may live some distance away. Frequently, people call a hospice when notified of the impending death of a parent living many miles away. They need help in working through their confusion, anger and anxiety. Talking with hospice staff enables them to sort out their thoughts and feeling and thereby deal with their feelings more effectively. Family consultations may continue over a long period of time as in one family where the father had a brain tumor. He had always been very demanding and controlling of his family and had become more so since his illness. He refused hospice services but his wife saw a therapist weekly for more than 6 months. Through this support, the wife was able to give to her husband and yet set limits on his demands on her and the children.

Professional consultation is provided to health care professionals who are dealing with terminally ill individuals. The focus may be on either the patient and his family or the health care professional. Occasionally nurses in intensive care settings request assistance in dealing with their own feelings in relation to death and dying. One team conference was called because the nurses were very angry at physicians who were maintaining patients on respirators when the patients were known to have irreversible brain damage. Hospice provides nurse discussion leaders who are knowledgeable and comfortable in talking about these emotionally charged issues.

Bereavement counseling is provided to families after the death of a patient. Hospice staff usually attend the funerals and/or memorial services held for deceased patients. Because of the focus on the family as a unit, most survivors feel very strong ties to hospice. Each hospice has its own schedule for telephone calls and visits to survivors. These contacts are generally made by trained volunteers. Contacts are made frequently during the first few months of bereavement and then taper off toward the end of the 1st year. An anniversary visit is made and an evaluation of the survivors' adjustment. Individual counseling is seen as the basic service for survivors, but for some, additional support is needed. Therefore, survivor groups, such as the Widow to Widow Program (Silverman, 1969) are being developed.

IMPLEMENTATION OF PROGRAM

When a new patient is referred, an assessment visit is made by one or more members of the hospice team, usually the medical director and a nurse. They conduct a formal interview, perform a physical examination of the patient and obtain a medical and social history. All members of the family are encouraged to be involved in this initial visit. The data obtained are presented at a staff meeting, and a primary care nurse is assigned. This nurse is responsible for the overall planning and coordination of the patient's care and she follows the patient throughout his illness. Other team members, i.e., therapists, aides or homemakers, may provide care to the patient also.

In planning the patient's care the following are considered:

— Diagnosis
— Treatment plan
— Evaluation of pain and other symptoms
— Identification of patient/family strengths
— Speculation about possible areas in which the patient/family might need support
— Presence and involvement of children; their needs
— What other community resources might be needed?

—What points need to be stressed in consultation with the referring physician?

—Is pharmacy consultation indicated?

—What additional information is needed at this time (or later) to complete our understanding of this case and to aid in treatment planning?

—Does anyone in the patient/family setting seem to be in need of additional support by other members of the hospice treatment team (counseling, clergy, volunteers)?

—What problems in communication and understanding exist in this family setting that might require special attention?

—Has the patient received adequate medical/surgical care directed toward cure of the disease? If not, what else might be considered in our later consultation with the referring physician?

—How did the patient/family seem to respond to this visit?

—How did the medical director/primary care nurse respond to this visit?

Assessment visits are made in homes, hospitals and nursing homes. A close liaison between discharge planners and hospice nurses facilitates moving the patient from inpatient facility to home and vice versa.

FUTURE OF HOSPICE CARE

Two major problems that impede the growth of the hospice movement are lack of knowledge about hospice care and unavailability of funds. How can these problems be overcome? Lamers (1976b) answers:

The most reasonable approach to making hospice care available is to teach and preach the hospice philosophy; to make consumers aware; to teach the medical and ancillary professions; to teach ministers and hospital administrators; to lobby for new legislation; and to develop contracts with third party agents.

Change in the delivery of care to the dying will be slow and arduous but the results as evidenced in the improved quality of life will be well worth the effort.

BIBLIOGRAPHY

Aring, C. *The Understanding Physician*, Detroit: Wayne State University Press, 1971.

Craven, J. and Wald, F. Hospice care for dying patients. *Am. J. Nurs.* 70: 1816-1821, 1975.

Day, E. The patient with cancer and the family. *N. Engl. J. Med.* 274: 883-886, 1966.

Dimmitt, D. *Pain Management in Terminal Disease.* Unpublished. September 1976.

Kerppola-Sirola, I. The death of an old professor. *J. A. M. A.* 232: 728-729, 1975.

Lamers, W. Personal communication. October 1976a.

Lamers, W. Unpublished speech given to Santa Barbara Nurses Association. April 1976b.

Lamerton, R. C. *Care of the Dying.* London: Priority Press Limited, 1973.

Lamerton, R. C. The need for hospices. *Nurs. Times* 21: 105-108, 1975.

Lamerton, R. C. Drugs for the dying. Reprinted from *St. Bartholomew's Hosp. J.* November 1974.

La Rochefoucald, F. *Reflections.* 1678.

Lipman, A. *Drug Therapy in Terminally Ill Patients*, presented at Ninth Annual Midyear Clinical Meeting American Society of Hospital Pharmacists, December 10, 1974.

McKell, D. Personal communication. December 1976.

Netsky, M. Dying in a system of 'good care': Case report and analysis. *The Pharos of Alpha Omega Alpha* 39: 57-61, 1976.

Silverman, P. The widow to widow program. *Ment. Hyg.* 53: 333-339, 1969.

Saunders, C. *The Management of Terminal Illness.* London: Hospital Medicine Publications, 1967.

Saunders, C. The need for in-patient care for the patient with terminal illness. *Middlesex Hosp. J.* 72 (3), 1973.

Saunders, C. The challenge of terminal care. In Symington, T., and Carter, R. (Eds.), *Scientific Foundations of Oncology.* London: William Heinemann Medical Books, 1975.

Saunders, C. The care of the dying. *Nurs. Times* 72: 3-24, 1976.

Schmale, A. and Patterson, B. *Comfort Care Only: Treatment Guidelines for the Terminal Patient*, presented at University of Rochester Cancer Center, April 19, 1976.

St. Lukes Hospital Center. *Hospice Pilot Project*, Unpublished report, November 1975.

Twycross, R. G. Principles and practice for the relief of pain in terminal cancer, reprinted from *Update*, July 1972.

Twycross, R. G. Diseases of the central nervous system: Relief of terminal pain. *Br. Med. J.* 4: 212-214, 1975.

Webster's Seventh New Collegiate Dictionary. Springfield, Mass.: G. and C. Merriam Co., 1971.

Chapter 26

assessing the older psychiatric patient

ELEANOR L. METZ

Since the extent of mental disorders in old age is considerable (15% of the older population) (Butler and Lewis, 1973, p. 46), it is imperative that nurses be highly knowledgeable regarding the bio-psychosocial characteristics of their aged patients, the more common mental disorders of the later years and the methods of therapy that have been found to be most efficacious.

By virtue of their constant attendance on the patient, nurses, nurses aides, psychiatric technicians and other paraprofessionals are the members of the nursing team who will have the most opportunity to collect the data so vital to the initiation of the nuring process and the nursing care plan.

Evaluation of psychiatric symptoms in elderly patients who enter the realm of health care requires an understanding of the person's entire life situation—his physical status, personality, family history, racial background, income, housing, social status, educational level (Butler and Lewis, 1973, pp. 3–4).

PREPARATION FOR GERIATRIC NURSING

Until recently, there was little taught in the basic curriculums of the health sciences regarding the special needs of the older person. This is not surprising, as it has been only since 1900 that the life span has been significantly increased and that larger numbers of the elderly are becoming patients. They now constitute the chief age group that health professionals serve.

The older one gets the more liable he is to mental disorder (Pitt, 1974, p.1). Not only do the elderly suffer mental aberrations due to degenerative physical causes, but they sustain heavy psychosocial losses as well. Later life is a time of psychologic crises even in the presence of the most favorable socioeconomic and cultural circumstances (Rossman, 1971). Environmental strains added to physical insults take a high toll of the elderly psychologically.

LEGISLATION AND EDUCATION

Recent legislation that has been passed in some states requires inclusion of geriatric content and clinical practice in the basic nursing curriculum (State of California, 1976). Standards for Geriatric Nursing written by the American Nurses Association will serve as guidelines for practice and peer review.

Geriatrics refers to that branch of medicine which deals with the diseases of old age. Psychogeriatrics is the study of the mental diseases of old age. It is unfortunate that the law does not require inclusion of gerontology as well as geriatrics in the basic curriculum. Gerontology reviews the process of aging and the problems of older people. If the health professional and paraprofessional hope to be therapeutic in the psychiatric role, some effort must be made to incorporate the holistic approach into patient assessment. This presupposes that the nurse conserves what is well about the patient and enables the individual to "keep together" his own unique integrity (Levine, 969, p. 94).

An exclusive focus on the medical-psychiatric model tends to foster a negative view of the elderly. Intrapsychic phenomena, mechanisms of defense, developmental theory, the structure of grief and the dynamics of dependency are some of the key areas of knowledge everyone should have when working with older people in the mental health context (Butler and Lewis, 1973, p. 136).

PRIMARY PREVENTION, TASKS OF THE OLDER PERSON

Nurses need to realize some of the adjustments the healthy elderly are called upon to make. Much has been written in the literature recently about positive development in the later years. There is a vast difference between functional, experiential, and chronological age. Each person approaches his later years in a highly individualistic fashion. According to one writer, there are three overriding tasks each person faces in the years after the seventh decade. They are:
1. Ego differentiation versus work role preoccupation
2. Ego transcendence versus ego preoccupation
3. Body transcendence versus body preoccupation

Another writer uses a simpler classification of tasks including receptive tasks, expressive tasks and dynamic tasks (Burnside, 1976, pp. 70–72).

Receptive Tasks

These tasks include coping with losses related to reduced physical, mental, social and cultural capacities. Nurses are often in an ideal position to help the aged compensate for such losses. Helping persons to adjust to depending upon others is a delicate undertaking. Providing a stimulating environment and promoting social interaction are other ways the nurses can intervene.

Expressive Tasks

The elderly need to be able to enjoy the years that are left. Religion is one of the chief avenues for coping with dependency, loss and death. Leaving a legacy to those who follow provides comfort to many older persons. Engaging in the political arena and in community affairs helps to sustain continuity with reality. Participating in some creative new activity may bring instant renewal to a dispirited older person. Intellectual pursuits may fit the life style of other seniors. Nurses can help their clients to enjoy their fantasies and dreams and to pursue new roles and hobbies.

Dynamic Tasks

The dynamic task of aging is to be able to die in a dignified manner. Physical dying needs to be preceded by psychological acceptance of death. Nurses can assist patients and families in resolving many of the interpersonal events that impede the acceptance of death. Anticipatory grief must be permitted with opportunities provided for open discussion of the process of letting go.

Tasks relating to the middle years and to the sixth decade are quite different from these tasks of later maturity. If the patient has not resolved the earlier tasks, he will have an even harder time facing the tasks of the final years.

ATTITUDES OF CARETAKERS

Research has shown that attitudes toward the elderly are most favorable in primitive societies and decrease with increasing modernization to the point of generally negative views in industrialized Western nations (McTavish, 1971, p. 91). Thus, the health professional may bear a negative stereotype about older people before encountering them in practice. On the other hand, the nursing student can come to the learning situation with a positive feeling about the elderly based on her own life experiences only to have it changed through the negative attitudes of nursing instructors, doctors and staff. Before the nurse can effectively and objectively assess her older patients, she needs to level with herself and examine her own feelings about the aging process and the losses which may occur to her in later life, especially her own death.

INTERVIEWING

Interviewing is one of the chief methods used in psychiatry to obtain data about patients, just as it is in other clinical specialties. Observation is also important as well as just listening. All can take place simultaneously as the nurse seeks to learn about her older patients. As sensory losses are more likely to be present in the aging, the interviewer's placement of self is important. Older people respond more readily when they can look directly at the interviewer. If the aged person has better hearing in one ear than in the other, the nurse may need to sit nearest the good ear rather than in the face-to-face position. It is usually necessary to check with the patient to determine how loudly to speak. One needs to test how far one can invade the territory of the patient before proceedings. If he suffers visual impairment, closeness may be necessary. If the patient turns his head, becomes restless, or looks at the television program and not at the nurse, one must modify the psychological distance accordingly (Burnside, 1973, pp. 3-4). Staring at the ceiling while listening intently may indicate hallucinating. Rapid and slurred speech bordering on the unintelligible is often encountered. Ways must be found to alleviate anxiety on the part of the patient. Speaking clearly and proceeding at aslower space can often remedy this. The interview may have to be terminated if the patient blocks completely. The technique of several brief interviews may work better with some patients than one longer, sustained interview. The longer a relationship goes on, usually, the more trust is obtained. Testing on the part

of the older person goes on constantly just as it does with patients of other ages.

Respect for the older person must be conveyed however he presents himself. Consideration of his physical energy and attention span will be necessary. The nurse must determine his comprehension ability. Often a memory loss will not seem evident until the nurse compres dates given in the history. Checking with the staff and other patients increases the reliability of data obtained. The chart can always be consulted after the interview is completed.

A conversational format rather than an interrogational approach seems to cause less anxiety when interviewing the elderly. Often, they suffer from communication deprivation and enjoy talking with the nurse. Refocusing and asking a pertinent question or two will enable the nurse to obtain the information she desires. Interviewing the elderly requires perserverance, patience and gentleness on the part of the nurse.

In addition to interviewing the patient, the nurse can observe the home situation where possible and talk to the family members and/or neighbors. This is especially important if the patient is an unreliable source. The public health nurse is often the first professional who picks up psychiatric overtones in elderly living in the community. A unique opportunity to effect crisis intervention is frequently presented. The offering of timely and judicial supports, problem-solving methods and the initiation of new coping mechanisms can enable the older person to stay in his home. Overintervention can often deny the patient the opportunity for growth. The potential of the older individual should never be underestimated (Burnside, 1976, pp. 270-271). Telephone outreach therapy can be conducted following crisis intervention to assist the older person to continue to manage at home.

Pertinent findings from the doctor' examination of the patient and observation of the patient's interaction with other patients should also be considered by the nurse in collecting her data base. The observations of other staff members should be incorporated.

The causes of mental illness are so multiple that it may often be difficult to set priorities in nursing care of the psychiatric patient. Often the so-called "senile" patient does not have chronic organic brain disease due to cerebral arteriosclerosis or senile brain disease but is the victim of a reversible brain pathology. Congestive heart failure, malnutrition, dehydration and anemia, infection, drugs and toxic brain substances, head trauma, tumors, alcoholism, diabetes, liver failure, uremia, etc. all can cause symptoms mimicking chronic brain syndrome.

In addition to the mental disorders due to physical causes, there are those disorders due to functional causes whose origins lie in the emotions, and these are legion. Depression, paranoid states, and neuroses are the main functional disorders encountered. It has been stated that the incidence of chronic disease is high in the elderly. The majority of people having chronic physical illness also have associated emotional reactions. Add to illness the environmental stresses of poverty, isolation, lowered social status and self-esteem, which operate among many of the elderly, and one realizes that the true proportion of psychiatric need among older people has not been fully documented (Butler and Lewis, 1973, p. 46).

Psychiatrists, social workers, psychologists, mental health teams and other therapists do not see many old people; when they do, the purposes are usually diagnostic with a view to disposition (Butler and Lewis, 1973, p.23).

Nurses and their paraprofessional staffs comprise the professional group most likely to have charge of the psychiatric patient following disposition. They must formulate a plan of treatment based on the patient's hierarchy of needs just as with any other patient. If they have an attitude of hope and a belief that therapy can make a difference, they will be able to effect an improvement in their patients. Even the brain-damaged elderly can gain form therapy as Goldfarb (Butler and Lewis, 1973, p. 232), has emphasized in his dependent relationships with elderly patients.

ONE-TO-ONE THERAPY

Patients can gain from a one-to-one therapeutic relationship with the nurse. The acceptance of one's own and only life cycle in the last stage of life as described by Erikson (1950, p. 232), can be facilitated by the caring intervention of a nurse. Loneliness can dehumanize a person especially if he has no love of self and has never learned to love. The following case illustrates this:

Ruth was a quiet white-faced woman who lay very still with her eyes closed. She felt she would never return home, and no one ever came to see her. The nurse detected her loneliness, stopping by her cubicle frequently to talk to her. The patient often stated that she needed someone to talk to just to be sure she was still alive. One day she burst out, "I don't know what I'd do without you." Over time she reviewed the events of her childhood and began to laugh occasionally.

Besides one-to-one therapy, couple therapy and family therapy can assist the elderly in resolving emotional problems, in putting their lives in order, and even in changing and growing. Evidence shows that greater availability of psychotherapy on an outpatient basis would reduce chronicity and disability in psychiatric states and reduce the need for medical care (Butler and Lewis, 1973, p. 236).

GROUP THERAPY

The geriatric nurse must be knowlegeable and skillful in group dynamics in addition to being able to communicate on a one-to-one basis. Group therapy has been more widely used in work with the elderly than individual psychotherapy. It has proved especially helpful during times of transition to a new situation such as leaving the home for institutional care. Patients and families can work through this crisis with the help of a sensitive nurse group leader. Discharge may not be possible, and group work can alleviate interpersonal problems and help enrich the quality of existence for all concerned.

There are very few guidelines for group work with the aged, and nurses have been left to test out the efficacy of this therapy pretty much on their own (Burnside, 1976, p. 184). They have discovered that the older person often engages in both silent and verbal reminiscence with increasing frequency in an effort to integrate his view of self. For some, the psychic trauma of multiple losses must be resolved, and past experiences that have existed behind closed doors must be explored and placed in the proper perspective. Others review pleasurable events from a previous era in a way that can promote the attainment of the developmental task of achieving integrity. Nurses have learned that by sharing these reminiscences in group experiences, the aged can use each other for verification of their perceptions. Loneliness and isolation can be alleviated, and resocialization with a sense of some control over the life situation may be accomplished. Such groups often can prevent further withdrawal, once the patient perceives the validity of his life and becomes incorporated into a congenial group of peers (Burnside, 1976, p. 215).

Many different techniques of group therapy have been utilized in work with older persons by nurses and other caretakers in addition to reminiscing. Reality orientation can be a way of making contact with persons suffering from memory loss, confusion or disorientation. It should be used at all times by everyone who has contact with the elderly person. It consists of repetition of basic information about the person and his environment—his name, the place, the time of day, day of the week and date, the next meal and time of the bath, etc. Formal classes should be conducted at the same time everyday by the person closest to the patient, but the informal use of informational input 24 hours a day is the key to success of this technique (Barnes et al., 1973, p. 515). The geriatric nurse in psychiatric settings might teach the ward personnel how to conduct the program and supervise its implementation. Consistent input can be truly helpful.

Mr. A. was unable to remember where he came from and began to cry on admission. While he was being undressed by his wife, Mr. P., the ward attendant, offered to assist Mrs. A. and introduced himself by name to both Mr. and Mrs. A. He then told the patient the name of the hospital, the ward number and his cubicle number. He went on to relate the time dinner would be served, placed a calendar by Mr. A.'s bedside and reminded him it was Sunday, October 11th. By the next Sunday when Mrs. A. visited her husband, she found Mr. A. in a cheerful mood. Furthermore, he was able to tell her the day and date as he marked it off on his bedside calendar.

Once the elderly person is more oriented to his surroundings, remotivation can take place in a group. Remotivation should be followed by opportunities to participate in meaningful activities such as occupational therapy, recreational therapy, and vocational and social outlets.

When forming a group, it is important to select the members with the treatment goal in view. Members should be interviewed individually, and a verbal contract which clarifies the goals, time, place, confidentiality and the number of members in the group should be made. Heavy psychic demands are made upon the nurse leader. It is difficult to stimulate members while maintaining control, security and protection. It may take a longer time for the elderly to establish trust with a group leader than it does in younger groups. Co-leaders can support one another in group work with the aged and can share observations and responsibilities. The leader must deal with diminished vision, hearing and mobility. Long silences must be tolerated. The use of self is very important. Frequent use of touch is a powerful form of therapy. The room must be quiet with a comfortable temperaure and space to move about in. Props are useful in creating interest. Food, drink, pets, perfume, cigars and objects of the past such as an old flat iron or an ice cream freezer will stimulate memories. Music can evoke the past as well as the present. Singing and dancing can even be employed if the patients are sufficiently mobile (Burnside, 1976, pp. 197–213).

"Nurses who work as group leaders must be aware of possible reactions of staff and consider their rapport with the staff to be just as important as with their patient group." (Burnside, 1976, 236) There should be provision for on-going treatment if the nurse leader must terminate. Along with group therapy, the use of environmental therapy and the therapeutic community concept can afford additional options in the psychiatric treatment of the elderly.

Nurses must be able to evaluate the success of their interventions in order to determine how to modify their nursing care plans. The intense participation and activity required of them makes it difficult for them to give attention to analysis of scientific details. Direct feedback from patients can often give cues as to the effectiveness of interventions.

"Miss O: 'Mrs. C why do you keep coming back if you get nothing from the meetings?' Mrs. C: Well, I do find it helpful to hear others talk about their problems.'" (Burnside, 1973, p. 193)

Observations of changes in the patient's behavior in group therapy can give evidence of successful nursing measures:

"After being on time at the first two sessions, Mr. JI arrived approximately thirty minutes late for the next three. Since he never offered a valid excuse for his tardiness, I thought he might have been seeking attention from the group, which noticed his late arrival. To intervene in this situation, I frequently acknowledged his presence and effort to attend meetings. I also made an effort to use his first name in order to give him personal recognition. I often said that he was missed in the group when he did not come, and that I hoped he would attend the meeting earlier next time. Whenever Mr. JI passed me in the hall, I purposely spoke with him for several minutes. The personal attention given Mr. JI seemed effective, because he was on time for subsequent group meetings." (Burnside, 1973, p. 193)

Ways in which patients interact with others outside of the therapeutic milieu can be helpful in evaluating therapy:

"Although the group was smaller, and its duration was shorter than I had anticipated, group therapy appeared to be a catalyst for several patients to begin to identify their feelings, evaluate their behavior patterns, and share their feelings with others. These patients were able to resume social contacts and engage in outside activities. The consistent emphasis of 'physical symptoms are real and distressing, but often represent an expression of how you feel emotionally' was successful. The use of physical complaints decreased, and the patients were able to talk directly about the feelings they were experiencing. Referral agencies, families, and the attending physician were contacted as needed to establish channels of communication, obtain information, and provide data.

This resulted in improved continuity of care." (Burnside, 1973, p. 148)

Nurses should look for signs of increased self-esteem, restored trust, ego strength and problem-solving ability, voluntary socialization, an increase in initiative and motivation, as well as improved sensorium and orientation in the patients they treat. Setbacks are to be expected in patients with multiple diagnoses. Realistic short term goals bring about more expected results. Patients may need to practice denial and rationalization in order to bear with their losses. Some may need to cling in a dependent manner. Confrontation does not always work.

One must be prepared for discouragement and disappointment at times. Support from each other is essential to the staff in all settings. Psychiatric work with the aged is spilling out into the community into day care centers, multipurpose senior centers and day hospitals. Every effort is being made to increase community facilities so that the elderly person can remain at home. Wherever possible, he should be encouraged to participate in decisions made regarding his care. Nurses have a unique opportunity to be patient advocates as well as therapeutic practitioners in the field of geriatric nursing.

BIBLIOGRAPHY

Barnes, E. K., Sack, A., and Shore, H. Guidelines to treatment approaches. Gerontologist, Winter 1973.

Burnside, I. M. (Ed.), *Psychosocial Nursing Care of the Aged.* (New York: McGraw-Hill Book Co., 1973.

Burnside, I. M. (Ed.), *Nursing and the Aged* New York: McGraw-Hill Book Co., 1976.

Butler, R. N., and Lewis, M. I. *Aging and Mental Health.* St. Louis: The C.V. Mosby Co., 1973.

Erickson, E. *Childhood and Society.* New York: W.W. Norton & Co., Inc. 1950, p.232.

Levine, M. E. The pursuit of wholeness. *Am. J. Nurs.* 69: 93–98, 1969.

McTavish, D. G. Perceptions of old people: A review of research methodolgies and findings. *Gerontologist* Winter 1971, Part II, pp. 90–101.

Pitt, B. *Psychogeriatrics.* London: Churchill Livingstone, 1974.

Rossman, I. *Clinical Geriatrics.* Philadelphia: J. B. Lippincott Co., 1971, pp 341, 439.

State of California. Department of Consumer Affairs, "Laws Relating to Nursing Education Licensure-Practice," Title 15, Ch. 14, Reg. 1433 Course of Instruction, Reg. c(1), July 1976.

Chapter 27

emotional care of the hospitalized child

LYNN SAVEDRA

A 2-year-old is hospitalized with bronchiolitis. He sits in his crib silent, sober and unresponsive to the friendly overtures of nurses and other members of the health team. He clutches a battered teddy as he anxiously watches the door through which his mother disappeared. Toys supplied by the nurse are invitingly near but unused. Across the hall, a 4-year-old screams in protest as she gets an injection. She cries for her mother. Soon, however, with the help of her nurse she becomes engrossed with paper and crayons. A third child, hospitalized with asthma, eagerly helps pass fluids. He is no stranger to the unit and once the breathing crisis is over is friendly, cooperative and a favorite of all.

These are the children for whom the pediatric nurse cares. If the child is to successfully cope with the stress of hospitalization not only must treatments and routine procedures be administered with skill, but the emotional needs must be considered, assessed and included in a comprehensive plan of care. This chapter will discuss the commonly observed reactions of children to hospitalization, factors influencing these re-actions and the emotional care needed by the child and his family.

REACTIONS TO HOSPITALIZATION

Reactions to hospitalization vary from child to child and for a given child at different points in his hospital experience. While the degree of response differs and is dependent on a wide range of factors, the following behaviors may be expected.

Protest in the form of crying, screaming and verbalizations is one of the most common reactions to hospitalization and the resulting insults to the body. While crying may be, and often is, in response to internal discomfort or imposed threat, it is for the young child a mechanism for expressing his feelings about the total experience. Mark, a 20-month-old with eczema, cried almost continuously when initially hospitalized. Any care initiated by nurses whether stressful or soothing elicited calls for mother. His behavior was typical of that described by Robertson (1958) in his classic research on the response of the young child to hospitalization. Crying and screaming may, however, be directly related to a painful or frightening situation. The screams of a severely burned child during care of the wound are predictable. Five-year-old Julie, hospitalized with 20% second and third degree burn screamed uncontrollably when placed in a whirlpool bath. She tried to lift herself from the tub but was unable to do so. For the older child who has mastered the use of language, protest more often is verbalized. "You're mean. I hate you!", may be hurled at the nurse who in the process of caring inflicts pain and discomfort. Protest behaviors while difficult to tolerate are a positive sign that the child is able to express the distress he is experiencing.

For the hospitalized toddler who remains for a time without mother active protest changes to despair. The child becomes quiet and unresponsive often passively accepting care given to him. He may seek comfort from his thumb, a loved toy or blanket. Tension relief may be sought by body-rocking, masturbation, and fingering and touching other body parts. Although physical care presents no real problems the nurse must recognize the state of acute mourning for mother that elicits this behavior. While mother is desparately needed and wanted by the toddler, he may respond to her arrival with tears, rejecting her attentions.

This behavior was exhibited by Jennifer, resulting in increased anxiety and uncertainty in her young mother. Withdrawal, part of the usual sequence of behaviors found in the hospitalized toddler, may be noted at any age. An infant may exhibit listlessness and lethargy apparently unrelated to pathology. The older child may also withdraw, limiting interaction with the world around him. Jane, a severely burned 8-year-old who was isolated in a single bed room, following skin grafting surgery would ask for the shades to be drawn, the lights to be turned off and the door to be shut. Once, imitating the 8 p.m. nightly loud speaker announcement, she told a visitor, "Visiting hours are now over." The time was 7 p.m.

Denial is a term used to designate the third stage of the toddler's response to hospitalization. Protest and despair give way to apparent recovery. The withdrawn, tearful child becomes responsive, cooperative and accepting of his situation. His appetite improves. He readily goes from one nurse to another. No longer do tears mark his mother's arrivals and departures. He may in fact appear to be unconcerned about whether or not she visits. This behavior is most deceiving for it covers a grief so deep that he must repress his feelings about his mother. Eighteen-month-old Michael, a newly diagnosed hemophiliac, was a classic example of this behavior. As hospitalization extended into weeks as the result of a family unwilling to assume his care, his crying for mother ceased. He became a smiling child readily going to nurses, doctors, and other members of the health team. It appeared to make no difference who gave him care or attention. He greeted each new person who came to him with a beaming smile and "docta, docta." Other children and adolescents may display behavior that is denial of the seriousness of the illness, or the consequences of the illness, or even a denial of the illness itself.

As with the younger child, denial is a defense mechanism to manage the anxiety produced by the existing condition. The most obvious manifestation of denial is a statement that a known condition does not exist. Most behavior suggestive of denial is more subtle. Examples are the diabetic adolescent who refuses to adhere to a prescribed diet, the severely burned child who talks of a career as a movie star, or the young athlete facing a leg amputation who is cheerful and noncommunicative regarding fears or concerns. Fantasy so effectively used by most children can be a form of denial. In play the child structures the world as he wishes it to be. For the normal child there is a clear awareness of fantasy versus reality with no difficulty in returning to the world as it is.

Regression, more commonly seen in the young child but possible at any age, comes in response to dependency imposed by illness. A symptom of stress, regression is often a protective device. For the young child, developmental skills most recently acquired are temporarily abandoned. Sandi, recently toilet-trained, began to wet her pants giving no indication when she needed to use the bathroom. For Michael, his newly acquired habit of drinking from a cup was abandoned for the more familiar bottle. For other children, sleep patterns may be altered. Regressive behavior in the older child is evidenced by baby talk, whining, crying, thumb sucking and temper tantrums. He accepts or demands care by others. Loved toys formerly discarded may be a source of comfort. Physical contact of a comforting nature is wanted and accepted. On the evening of the day of tonsillectomies, 7-year-old Robin and 16-year-old Tom had broth, juice and ice cream placed in front of them. Their nurse left, assuming they were physically able to feed themselves. The food remained untouched. Not until a second nurse appeared, explained that pain would lessen as fluids were taken and fed the children was food eaten. Both Robin and Tom, normally independent, readily accepted being fed. One explanation for regressive behavior in the older child is that he views his illness as punishment and reverts to behaviors which previously brought pleasure. Regressive behavior may be distressing or satisfying to parents depending in part on their understanding of the mechanisms involved.

The angry verbal and physical attacks of the rebellious or hostile child are readily identified. This type of behavior is viewed by all as disruptive and difficult. There is no overlooking the fact that a problem exists. Rebellion is exhibited by refusal to comply with the program of therapy and generally noncooperative actions. The child may be sullen and silent or verbally aggressive. He is often unfriendly and antagonistic to the plan of care. Rebellion and hostility often mask a fearful, insecure and anxious child.

Reactions of children for the most part are in response to the trauma of illness and hospitalization. There is increasing recognition, however, that for some children hospitalization may be a growth experience. Feeding difficulties, sleep disturbances and enuresis may disappear. Children from disrupted families often thrive in a warm, caring hospital atmosphere. The school-age child who has experienced separation from parents and has developed a degree of independence is able to respond in a positive manner. He can be friendly and cooperative, and with support he can manage the stressful aspects of the experience. He can relate positively to the needs of other children and receives satisfaction from these interactions.

FACTORS INFLUENCING REACTIONS TO HOSPITALIZATION

A large number of factors must be considered when assessing a child's response to illness. These include his developmental level and personal characteristics, past experience, preparation for hospitalization, present experience, and the quality and quantity of parenting.

Developmental Level and Personal Characteristics

Age is a major factor influencing the child's response to hospitalization. The very young infant who has not identified his mother as a separate individual may indicate little stress if his physical and emotional needs are met by consistent, warm, caring individuals. Once a relationship with mother as a specific person has developed, at approximately 6 months of age, any separation from her is stressful. The pain of separation while most acute for the older infant and toddler is still present to a high degree throughout the preschool period. The young child feels abandoned by his parents with no certainty of their return. He may not yet have grasped the concept that an object which is out of view still exists. As the child gets older he may expect his parents to return but may be concerned that they will be unable to locate him. This fear is heightened if he is moved from one room to another without the apparent knowledge of his parents. This fear is not unique to the child for parents may be equally distressed to arrive and not find their child in the room where he had been. Inability to understand the concept of time makes usual explanations meaningless. The terms "today" and "tomorrow" are unknown quantities.

For the preschool child, fears of body mutilation emerge. Procedures involving an intrusive approach such as injections, rectal temperatures, throat cultures and enemas are particularly threatening. It is at this developmental stage that the beginning of sexual identity takes place with accompanying castration fears. Sam, age 4, scheduled for a tonsillectomy was admitted to the hospital on the day of surgery. With the presence of his mother he appeared to handle the experience with composure until the final preparation stage when according to hospital policy his nurse attempted to remove his pajama bottoms. Sam clung tenuously to the pants exerting every effort to avoid their removal. His behavior was only what might be expected for a 4-year-old who had been prepared for surgery on his throat. The young child's understanding of cause and effect is far different from that of an older child or an adult. Painful treatments, restriction of food and fluids, isolation procedures are viewed as punishment. Illness and hospitalization come as divine retribution for disobedience to parental commands or for thoughts associated with the oedipal complex. Five-year-old Jeff was heard crying, "Don't give me the shot. I'll be good," as his nurse approached with medication. Nine-year-old Larry, hospitalized on a burn unit, was heard telling his father, "If Jenny doesn't stop crying they'll put her in the tub room." The nurse who threatens the child with, "If you don't drink, I'll have to put the needle in your arm," and the parent who says, "If you're not good the doctor will give you a shot," only increase the child's belief in the concept of treatments as punishment.

The school-age child, no longer as dependent on mother, may tolerate separation from parents but feel keenly the loss of contact with peers. While fear of death has been identified in the preschool child, it becomes most prevalent in the school-age child.

The adolescent faced with the developmental task of establishing independence not only from his parents but from all adults finds the dependence engendered by illness and hospitalization a hindrance to the accomplishment of this task. He has a high concern for acceptable physical appearance and body function which are often altered by illness.

In relation to age, a child's intellectual level, personality and usual pattern of coping with new and threatening situations influence his behavior during hospitalization.

Past Experience

In assessing current behavior it is essential to consider the child's past experience relating to illness, hospitalization and separation. The nature of previous illnesses and the number and length of hospitalizations, as well as when they occurred, are influencing factors. If the child has previously been admitted to a particular unit and has warm, trusting relations with the staff, the current experience should be less threatening. Sara, age nine, hospitalized at regular intervals with asthma was a prime example. Once the respiratory crisis was resolved she might ask for her crayons and resume the play activities where she had left off on her previous visit. She knew how best to get what she wanted and no longer needed to test the nursing staff.

An often forgotten area of exploration is experiences children have had with friends or relatives who have been ill and hospitalized. The behavior of a young child is much more understandable when it is discovered that a close friend recently died while hospitalized.

Nature of the Present Experience

The nature of the present experience must also be assessed in relationship to the child's response to the hospital experience. One important aspect is related to preparation for the experience. Some situations including accidents and sudden acute illness make preparation impossible or limited. The quality and quantity of the preparation varies. A child may have been told nothing about where he is going, why he is going and what is to happen. He may have been given false or misleading information. Some children are told that they are going to the hospital but have no concept of their physical problems. Some children anticipating a tonsillectomy are told of the ice cream they will eat but not of the pain following surgery. Jack, $3^{1}/_{2}$ years old, was hospitalized for a circumcision. His mother was asked if he knew what was going to be done to him.

She shook her head and said, "No, but he will know afterwards. I couldn't bring myself to tell him." Jack returned late from the operating room; in the 20 hours he was in the hospital postrecovery, he steadily refused to void and went home with a full bladder.

Optimally the child has received an explanation that is accurate, truthful and appropriate to his level of understanding. If the child has been told several weeks before an expected hospitalization, fears and fantasies may have time to develop and multiply. If on the other hand a child old enough to comprehend what is happening has been told immediately preceding the experience, time may be inadequate for him to be emotionally prepared. The child who has been told a deliberate lie will have a difficult time believing what he is told by nurses and hospital staff.

The nature of the illness is another factor to be considered. Is it an acute illness of sudden onset or is the illness chronic, necessitating repeated hospitalizations? Is there an identifiable condition that needs correcting or does the child, as in the case of a hernia, enter the hospital feeling well only to experience the pain and distress that accompany the surgery? Illness such as a broken arm is more understandable than diabetes. The degree of anxiety is influenced by the part of the body that is affected. Conditions related to the heart, brain, genitals and eyes are particularly stressful. More important than the severity and duration of illness as a determinant of behavior are the child's concept of the illness and the fantasies aroused.

The quality and quantity of the hospital experience must be considered. Behavior frequently changes as the length of hospitalization increases. The response may be positive or negative based on a multitude of variables including the nature and type of procedures, the amount of discomfort and pain experience, the degree of sensory-motor restriction, the physical environment and interactions with the staff. A child who comes from a large family and shares a bed with siblings may respond quite differently to being isolated alone in a room than an only child who is accustomed to having a room of his own. The severely burned child who experiences pain of an intense, continuous nature may be expected to behave differently than the child who is hospitalized with otitis media.

Parents

Parents are a major factor affecting a child's psychological reaction to hospitalization. One aspect involves parent-child relationships prior to and during the hospital experience. The more disrupted the relationship the more difficulty may be expected in the child's adjustment to the hospital. Parents' attitudes toward illness and hospitalization vary. Some take illness in stride while others are immobilized by even a minor illness. Positive and negative attitudes and anxieties are readily communicated to children of all ages and markedly influence the child's emotional response to the situation. Quality of the parent-child interaction may be more important than the amount of time spent with the patient. A case in point is Mrs. Jones, whose 8-year-old daughter Jane was hospitalized 114 days with a severe burn. Home responsibilities, no readily available transportation for the 60-mile drive and inadequate finances made her visits infrequent. And yet when she did come to see Jane, the quality of her visit was such that it appeared to meet the needs of this acutely ill child. Mrs. J. sat close to the bed and concentrated her full attention on Jane. She sang songs and wrote poems that focused on her daughter. She sat and listened as her child talked of dying. She left a large picture of herself to be hung on the wall. Her love and caring were evident.

EMOTIONAL CARE OF THE CHILD AND HIS FAMILY

A plan for meeting the child's emotional needs can be developed once the assessment has been made. The scope of this chapter precludes dealing with care related to specific behaviors. There are, however, aspects of care that are applicable to all children. Knowledge of growth and development is a must and can be incorporated into a plan of care from the beginning.

Emotional care of the hospitalized child ideally should begin before the fact occurs.

Preparation for anticipated admissions can be individualized and specific as nurses in ambulatory settings assist parents in this task. The informed parent whose own anxieties are adequately controlled may well take the major role in preparing the child. Young children who are not ill may become acquainted with hospitals through stories, play experience at nursery school and visits to the hospital.

For the hospital nurse, the time of admission generally marks the first contact with the child and his family. Regardless of the presenting circumstances it is a time of stress. What transpires during the admission procedure sets the stage for the coming experience. The young child, particularly, is benefited by the presence of his parents. Both child and parents need to know what is being done and why. Orientation to the room and unit as well as to the routines helps to allay anxieties associated with a strange environment. It is helpful at this time to learn of the habits and interests of the child. This is essential if a parent will not be staying with the child. Standard forms routinely ask for data on eating, sleeping, play and toileting. Equally important is information on the child's patterns of coping with new and stressful situations. When six-year-old Kathy was hospitalized the staff was alerted to that fact that her usual coping strategies involved standing back and looking and listening. As a result she was given time to observe before new situations were thrust upon her with the result that she was able to better manage her anxieties.

From the beginning of their child's hospitalization, parents need to feel accepted and needed on the unit. The nurse in essence aids in meeting the emotional needs of the patient as parents are supported to care for their child. Often the verbal expression of welcome is doubted when the nurse does not look up from the desk when a parent arrives on the ward, when mothers are unrecognized as they wait to ask questions, and when parents are told that their child behaves "better" when they are not there. When circumstances prevent parents from staying with a young child or make frequent visits impossible, they must be assured that the needs of their child will be met by those to whom they have entrusted him.

Play is one of the major sources of support for the hospitalized child. Play not only relieves monotony and boredom but stimulates growth and development, relieves tensions, provides an avenue for self-expression and prepares a child for hospital experiences. Often by playing doctor or nurse, anxieties are relieved. For the young child, the old familiar toy from home gives the most comfort. For the adolescent, play as such does not exist. He needs instead a telephone to keep in touch with peers, a radio with ear phones and the support of others his own age. Adolescents more than any other age group benefit from being together. On the other hand, when an age blend occurs on a pediatric unit older children may be greatly benefited as they meet the needs of a young child. Four adolescent boys hospitalized together in one room formed a close relationship that excluded other patients and most staff. When all space generally reserved for toddlers was used, the boys were asked if a 2-year-old child could be placed in their room. Following a conference the four agreed. They were aware that the young patient was refusing to take fluids. Getting him to drink became a project. He was told if he did not drink he could not watch television. The strategy, which might be questioned by some, proved effective. The boys took great pride in achieving where the nursing staff had failed.

If the emotional needs of a hospitalized child are to be fully considered, a plan must include preparation for discharge. For the long term patient, dependence on the hospital may be difficult to terminate. Parents of a young child must be told that clinging behaviors and disturbances in eating, sleeping and toileting may well be expected as the child is working through his response to the recent hospital experience.

The nurse, regardless of the setting, is in a unique position to meet the emotional needs of the hospitalized child and his family. In the home, clinic or pediatric office, focus is on preparation for a specific experience and follow-up care. In the day care setting or school, nurses can become involved in a more general preparation for any hospital experience. The nurse on the pediatric unit, while having the most direct input at the point of maximum stress, is only one member of a team whose energies are directed toward helping children and parents cope with the hospital experience.

BIBLIOGRAPHY

Bergman, T., and Freud, A. *Children in the Hospital.* New York: International Universities Press, Inc., 1965.

Johnson, J. E., Kirchhoff, K. T., and Endress, M. P. Easing children's fright during health care procedures. *MCN: Am. J. Mat. Child Nurs.* 1: 206–10, 1976.

Lindheim, R., Glaser, H., and Coffin, C. *Changing Hospital Environments for Children.* Cambridge, Mass.: Harvard University Press, 1972.

Maier, H. W. *Three Theories of Child Development.* New York: Harper and Row, Publishers, 1965.

Oremland, E. K., and Oremland, J. D. *The Effects of Hospitalization on Children.* Springfield, Ill.: Charles C Thomas, Publisher, 1973.

Petrillo, M., and Sanger, S. *Emotional Care of Hospitalized Children.* Philadelphia: J. B. Lippincott Co., 1972.

Plank, E. N. *Working with Children in Hospitals.* Cleveland: Western Reserve Press, 1962.

Robertson, J. *Young Children in Hospitals.* New York: Basic Books, 1958.

Vernon, D. T. A., Foley, J. M., Sipwicz, R. R., and Schulman, J. L. *The Psychological Responses of Children to Hospitalization.* Springfield, Ill.: Charles C Thomas, Publisher, 1965.

Chapter **28**

treatment of patients with organic brain disease

HARVEY J. WIDROE

Until recently the diagnosis of inoperable organic brain disease has implied that a patient had a poor prognosis. Consequently, psychiatrists and psychiatric nursing staffs have tended to despair at their relative inability to alter the level of cerebral functioning of brain-damaged patients. This attitude of hopelessness often was conveyed directly or indirectly to both patients and their families.

In reality, prospects for improvement in functioning for many brain-damaged patients have existed for some time. The prospects for improvement depend on 1) the etiology of the damage; 2) the location of the damage; 3) the extent of the damage; 4) the duration of the impairment; 5) the age of the patient; 6) the motivation of the patient and 7) the skills of the treatment team. The impressive results of the speech training and motor training programs for patients recovering from cerebrovascular accidents exemplify what can be achieved as a result of skilled therapeutic intervention. Apart from training programs the use of new psychopharmacological agents has substantially improved the prognosis for many brain-damaged patients. Psychophar-

macological agents may alter the operation of the damaged brain to respond positively to the training programs provided by nursing staff, patient activities staff, speech teachers, classroom teachers, etc. (Widroe, 1975).

Current attempts at increasing the level of functioning of damaged brains are based on the following four principles:

1. Nonfunctioning neurons may be sick rather than dead, and sick neurons can improve. Medications which decrease edema, contribute to increased oxygen or blood supply, or the improvement of cellular nutrition may enable a sick neuron to return to normal functioning.

2. Synaptic events can be influenced by psychopharmacological agents. Amphetamines, tricyclic antidepressants and monoamine oxidase inhibitors have significant effects upon the release and re-uptake of norepinephrine. Phenothiazines profoundly affect behavior through blockade of dopaminergic synapses. Lithium affects the stability of postsynaptic membranes, while diphenylhydantoin increases the efficiency of axonal conduction (Jarvik, 1970).

3. Psychoactive agents affect areas of the

brain in a differential fashion. Thus, some areas are more profoundly affected than other areas. If these areas exist in a balance of subsystems, each regulating the electrical outflow of several others, then psychopathology may appear when this functional equilibrium is disturbed. By affecting this equilibrium, psychopharmacological agents can have a substantial effect on both normal and psychopathological behavior. For example, the effect of chlorpromazine in reducing electrical activity in the reticular activating system may decrease the state of hyperarousal of the cortex which has occurred secondary to excessive reticular activating system activity. This diminution of reticular activating system hyperactivity by the use of the chlorpromazine is the mechanism by which chlorpromazine acts to decrease hyperalertness and agitated behavior (Smythies, 1970).

4. Neurons can develop new axonal or dendritic connections as a function of development or regeneration after trauma. Cut axones have been found to sprout new axones that enter and supply nerves to structures in the brain not previously innervated by this group of axones. Nerve cells near damaged cells move in to fill the vacancies. It is possible that training programs for brain damaged patients may be effective in producing experiential events which enhance the proliferation of dendritic connections or axonal regeneration so as to produce "rewiring" of a previously damaged functional system.

These four principles enable us to make more sensible judgements about which medications may effect an increase in a given patient's level of cerebral functioning. In general, if a brain-damaged patient demonstrates affective instability or agitation, then phenothiazines and possibly lithium may be useful. If the patient suffers from an attention-span deficit, then amphetamines or L-dopa may be indicated. If a patient demonstrates seizures, then an appropriate anticonvulsant regimen must be employed. Except for their anticonvulsant effects, cortical acting sedatives such as phenobarbital, chlordiazepoxide and diazepam are of little value toward increasing human brain function. Cortical acting sedatives are to be avoided because they lead to decreased effective control and impairment of judgement and concentration.

HYPERKINETIC ADOLESCENTS

Methylphenidate and the amphetamines are effective in the treatment of hyperkinetic adolescents because they act to increase attention span. This increase in attention span leads to a decrease in distractability, agitation, and drive-related behavior (Wender, 1973). Hyperkinetic adolescents, in contrast to hyperkinetic latency age children, may need a maximally sedating phenothiazine, such as chlorpromazine or thioridazine in addition to amphetamines in order to help check impulse flooding of the cortex via the limbic system. In some instances the inclusion of diphenylhydantoin or lithium carbonate in the psychopharmacological regimen may produce dramatic results in improving the behavior of the disturbed adolescent.

PATIENTS WITH CEREBROVASCULAR ACCIDENTS

Any increase in blood supply to an area affected by but not destroyed by a cerebrovascular accident can greatly increase the level of functioning of the damaged area. The use of cerebral vasodilators may lead to an increase in cerebral functioning at the motor, affective and intellective levels. Papaverine and ergot alkaloids are examples of cerebral vasodilators acting in somewhat different modes which may increase the blood supply to neurons adjacent to an infarcted area of the brain to the extent that a return of functioning is possible.

Dextroamphetamine or methylphenidate aid in the organization of thought processes and in increasing attention span. Consequently, these drugs may be useful in patients whose intellective functions are impaired after a cerebrovascular accident.

Nonsedating phenothiazines such as triflupromazine serve to decrease agitation by limbic system suppression. Moderately sedating phenothiazines such as prochlorperazine or perphenazine may be more effective if a patient's agitation continues. Maximally sedating phenothiazines may be required;

however, the clinician must be aware that maximally sedating phenothiazines such as thioridazine or chlorpromazine may produce or augment an acute brain syndrome and thereby increase intellective impairment.

Diphenylhydantoin increases the efficiency of neuronal conduction and as a consequence should always be given a trial in a patient's post-CVA therapeutic regimen (even in the absence of seizures). For patients who are depressed post-CVA, monoamine oxidase inhibitors such as isocarboxazid or phenylcypramine are preferable to the use of tricyclic antidepressants. Monoamine oxidase inhibitors are less likely to produce an acute brain syndrome when used in combination with other psychoactive medications. In contrast tricyclic antidepressants when combined with other psychoactive agents commonly produce a recent memory defect, poor judgement and confusion.

PATIENTS WITH AMPHETAMINE ADDICTION

Amphetamine abuse by an intravenous route of administration commonly results in brain damage demonstrable as widespread multiple miniscule cerebral cortical infarcts secondary to vasospasm of cortical arterioles.

Former amphetamine addicts demonstrate symptoms of cortical impairment months after they have desisted from amphetamine abuse. The acute withdrawal from amphetamines is no more severe than 48 to 72 hours of sleepiness, depression, hyperirritability and lethargy. But it may take months for the amphetamine addict to become capable of thinking coherently. Nonsedating phenothiazines control the paranoia commonly encountered and aid in reducing the torrent of grossly scattered thinking.

PATIENTS WITH PARKINSONISM

Parkinsonian symptoms and the depression commonly encountered in parkinsonism are both related to monoamine deficits, especially a lack of dopamine in the extrapyramidyl system. L-dopa is metabolized to dopamine in the brain and produces both symptomatic improvement in parkinsonian symptoms and a general improvement of mood. Excess dopamine in the limbic system may lead to an acute brain syndrome or an affective psychosis. Other antiparkinsonian medications, such as trihexyphenidyl hydrochloride, benztropine mesylate, diphenhydramine hydrochloride, all diminish parkinsonian symptoms through their effect on the cholinergic systems. The anticholinergic effects of these medications bring the cholinergic system back into a balance with the dopaminergic systems with a subsequent reduction of pathological symptoms.

PATIENTS WITH IDIOPATHIC TEMPORAL LOBE DAMAGE

Idiopathic temporal lobe damage may be manifest as psychosis, petit mal seizures, psychomotor seizures, dyscontrol syndrome, or borderline character behavior. Once a diagnosis is substantiated by electroencephalogram (especially with nasopharyngeal leads), proper psychopharmacological treatment may be initiated. Idiopathic temporal lobe disturbances may respond well to diphenylhydantoin, phenobarbital, diazepam, or primidone. If these medications are ineffective or if the behavioral pathology becomes more pronounced when these medications are used, then in all likelihood the patient is suffering from temporal lobe dysfunction as a result of electrical overflow from the subcortical amygdaloid nucleus. In such instances medications which suppress the electrical activity of the amygdaloid nucleus, such as fluphenazine, trifluoperazine, or haloperidol should be used instead of or in conjunction with the usual anticonvulsants.

ALCOHOL- OR BARBITURATE-RELATED DEGENERATIVE BRAIN DAMAGE

Withdrawal of alcohol or any other cortical acting sedative to which tolerance has been acquired will result in severe withdrawal symptoms secondary to generalized hyperactivity of the nervous system. In almost all instances substituting another cortical acting sedative which is gradually reduced in dosage enables the patient to withdraw in a safe and relatively comfortable fashion. Diazepam and chlordiazepoxide are the drugs of choice for alcohol withdrawal. Vitamin deficiency may contribute to the acute brain syndrome of withdrawal, and large dosages of vitamins should be part of any alcohol or barbiturate withdrawal regimen.

Chronic brain damage resulting from alcohol or other cortical acting sedatives usually includes frontal lobe damage. This impairment is manifest as poor judgement, a defect of fine nuance of affect, and affective volatility in the face of minimal stress. Improved cortical function can result from treatment with amphetamines, nonsedating phenothiazines and diphenylhydantoin.

PATIENTS WITH LSD-RELATED DAMAGE

The acute brain syndrome secondary to the use of LSD is best treated with moderately or maximally sedating phenothiazines, such as prochlorperazine, chlorpromazine, or thioridazine. In the treatment of symptoms secondary to multiple LSD exposures, flashback can be eliminated by prochlorperazine, diazepam, or a combination of the two. The intellective and affective deficits secondary to chronic LSD abuse persist over a period of many months and may respond to a regimen of amphetamines plus nonsedating or moderately sedating phenothiazines (Widroe, 1968).

PATIENTS WITH HEROIN ADDICTION

Patients who have used heroin may have transient or permanent damage of the median forebrain bundle pleasure centers to the extent that only heroin or methadone can set off the experience of pleasure. An increasing number of psychiatrists have expressed disillusion with methadone as a treatment tool. Instead, acute heroin withdrawal can be achieved most comfortably for the patient by the administration of massive doses of maximally sedating phenothiazines such as thioridizine and chlorpromazine along with large amounts of chlordiazepoxide. Thioridizine is preferable to chlorpromazine because it has less of a hypotensive effect. The hyperactivity of both cortical and limbic systems secondary to heroin withdrawal is diminished by the administration of the two agents, the chlor-

diazepoxide acting at the cortical level, while the phenothiazines act at the limbic system level. Patients under treatment with this regimen are relatively comfortable and are less likely to flee the treatment environment than under a methadone administration program.

After the acute withdrawal period of 7 to 14 days, the dosage of medication can be lowered approximately 50%. It is imperative that the medication regimen not be discontinued. Patients who continue this regimen report a diminution in intensity of the cravings which commonly return the addict to heroin after he has completed acute withdrawal. This regimen must be continued over a number of months until the patient shows substantial improvement in his level of intellectual and social functioning along with the absence of cravings.

Not enough can be said for the constant repetition by nursing and patient activities staff of particular experiences or exercises which literally retrain the brain damaged patient to return to areas of previous competence or to develop new skills. The scope of these exercises is vast and varies with the ingenuity and determination of each treatment team. Areas of functioning commonly affected by training include motor skills (both strength and fine movement), speech, memory, calculation, orientation and sequential reality testing. An individualized program should be devised to meet each patient's needs and the program should be modified as a function of his improvement or lack thereof.

In summary, patients with organic brain damage, regardless of etiology, can now be approached in a thoughtful manner combining both psychopharmacological agents plus an environment that provides a carefully designed, highly individualized training program. Prospects for improvement of cerebral functioning have improved substantially.

BIBLIOGRAPHY

Jarvik, M. Drugs used in the treatment of psychiatric disorders. In Goodman, L. S., and Gilman, A. (Eds.) *The Pharmacological Basis of Therapeutics*, New York: Macmillan, 1970, pp. 151–203.

Smythies, J. *Brain Mechanism and Behavior*. New York: Academic Press, 1970, pp. 113–115.

Wender, P. Some speculations concerning a possible biochemical basis of minimal brain dysfunction. In de la Cruz, et al. (Eds.), *Minimal Brain Dysfunction*. New York: N.Y. Academy of Sciences Pubns., 1973, pp. 18–28.

Widroe, H. A treatment-oriented schema of LSD-induced psychopathology. *Clin. Toxicol.* 1: 179–185, 1968.

Widroe, H. Increasing cerebral function in brain-damaged patients. In Widroe, H. (Ed.), *Human Behavior and Brain Function*. Springfield: Charles C Thomas, 1975, pp. 97–105.

Chapter 29

the "difficult" patient on the burn unit

CAROL FINK

For the past 2 years the author has served as psychiatric liaison to a large metropolitan general hospital burn unit. Twenty-five per cent of the admissions to this unit have a history of alcohol abuse, drug dependence, or other definable psychiatric disorder. Most commonly found are persons with passive-dependent personalities, schizoid "street people" and those who had attempted suicide. These "difficult" patients pose unique and often frustrating problems for the staff. The "normal" patient in the burn situation is extremely demanding of the staff, both physically and psychologically. The "difficult" patient, posing even greater needs for psychological support, can add inordinate pressure to the already overburdened staff.

This discussion attempts to define an expanded role for the psychiatric consultant, a role which goes beyond traditional diagnostic assessment and recommendations for management. This role includes intensive work with patients and their families as well as the crucial task of liaison with the staff. It further provides formal conferences for in-service education, a sharing of ideas and feelings, and mediating conflicts between staff members as well as informal interchanges with staff members which can be invaluable. Pertinent examples of the more common problems are included, and approaches to treatment and management are suggested. A multidisciplinary team model is used. Time and again we are impressed that our "street people" not only survive even the most devastating injuries, but emerge as witty, delightful people, who have found a first real "home."

Including the psychiatric consultant on the burn team can help decrease the anxiety and frustration these patients understandably induce in the staff. This facilitates improved care of *all* patients on the unit, as well as improved staff morale and stability.

In the beginning, I responded hesitatingly to a consultation request from our newly formed burn unit, recalling an earlier meeting with the nursing staff, rife with horror stories of their nightmares of patients' screams, fights with spouses after an arduous day, concern about pain management and feelings of being torturers, as well as questions about management of "difficult" patients. I remember leaving the meeting grateful that I had no responsibility to the unit, but now was fortunate in finding a bright, young staff most eager to discuss its concerns about *all* of the patients, reaching out for any *new* suggestions and approaches and mostly needing support for the *already* quality care being given. It was in response to *this need*, for a listener to explore treatment plans and difficulties, to offer outside *approval* as well as provide patients on the unit with a listening ear and reassurance from one not associated with painful treatment, that I found myself spending more and more time there.

I feel now much as I did then; that there is no simple formula for dealing with specific problems, other than through trial and error, with the staff working as a team, much as a *family*, open to talking out issues and working at solutions. This has been the most challenging part of my role as psychiatric liaison to our six-bed burn unit at San Francisco General Hospital.

The Andreasen group (1972) at the University of Iowa have addressed themselves effectively to the emotional issues involving burn patients in general, the initial emotional shock, the larger issue of pain management, fears of deformity and mutilation, depression and marked regression.

Our population, drawing from a large metropolitan area, seems to fit the epidemiological pattern described by MacArthur and Moore (1975) with alcohol, drug abuse and chronic psychiatric disease as predisposing factors in more than 25% of admissions (frequently *all* patients in the unit).

These alienated, lonely, isolated "street people" pose unique and most frustrating problems for the already overburdened staff; and because of the intense involvement over a lengthy period, unlike other areas of the hospital where acute care predominates, the staff here must come to grips with feelings these patients engender. There can be little question that the patients whom the staff finds "likeable" do indeed heal more quickly, probably getting better nursing care. From the time of admission, meeting with families, with the unit social worker, or more often, attempting to seek out history from hotel clerks, prior medical records, and social service case workers, give the staff a better picture of how and perhaps why, the patient has arrived at the place from which he comes to us. Frequently, the story is not pleasant—broken homes during childhood, early acting out,

seeking parental guidance with none found, dependence upon alcohol or drugs to blot out unpleasant realities, failed attempts at interpersonal relationships where no positive patterns had been formed earlier. Now the staff must deal with massive unmet dependency needs and marked regression in patients who for the most part have no support system. The ward becomes not only a place for treatment of the burn injury, but a new home for people who may have been seeking such warmth and caring, but have not the social skills to interact in such a way as to allow closeness and trust to develop.

J. S., a 22-year-old heroin addict was admitted with 50% 2nd and 3rd degree burns to both hands, arms, shoulders, back, chest and soles of feet—her right hand burned to the bone. Her parents had been divorced when J. S. was 2 years old. The mother had remarried, when the patient was 15, an alcoholic who frequently beat both her and the patient. Frequent moves followed and the patient developed ulcerative colitis, severe enough to necessitate total colectomy and iliostomy. At the time of her thermal injury, the patient was "loaded" and fell asleep while her boyfriend was working. Her hospital course was complicated by the boyfriend frequently being "high" and belligerent while visiting and the entire family, as is frequently the case, became "patients." Her despondency at the need for an above elbow amputation, and further distortion of this lovely young woman coupled with the family's anger toward the boyfriend, as well as guilt, were dealt with by frequent family meetings as well as by a psychology student volunteer, who in thrice weekly visits with her, attempted to provide much needed ego support. Limits around pain medication were set firmly to avoid power struggles, with Methadone used for its longer action. While the goal was to treat her thermal injury, we did attempt to help her to change her characterological patterns without removing defenses, i.e., drug dependence, until replacing them with much needed support over a long period of time.

The staff can decrease its frustration and anger with such patients if it does not feel the need to *change* them into "solid citizens" but rather to attempt to accept them as they are, as individuals with differing needs, treating the presenting injury and offering aids in finding new ways of coping with old problems. We can tend to become somewhat punitive in withholding analgesics from "so-called addictive personalities," often in the name of fear of turning patients into addicts. In this case, the patient had succeeded at transferring her dependency from drugs to other *people* while on the unit, and has maintained her drug-free lifestyle—resulting in a much more satisfactory living situation.

With the alcohol-abusing patient, initially the withdrawal phase can be most frustrating, with the need to restrain frequently, both physically and chemically in order to maintain lines and allow treatment to proceed. We use Valium p.o. or IV as needed until the patient is sedated while also closely observing vital signs, as well as usual nursing approaches to delirium, i.e., keeping lights on at night. The paranoia of the withdrawal state deserves mention in that more suicides from hospital wards occur secondary to the need to escape from imaginary pursuers and the terror of feeling "unsafe" in the strange ward setting, especially the typical burn unit/intensive care setting with so much equipment in view, auditory stimuli and the perceptions of which can be easily distorted. Once over this acute phase, the marked dependency/independency struggle of the alcoholic can become a monumental problem, with the *denial* for needed care which so frustrates our needs as "helpers". Eventually these patients tend to do well while on the unit, feeling "right at home" with their dependency needs being met even in the presence of pain-infliction, and the intense caring by the staff seems to increase their feelings of self-worth. The conflict occurs when, at the time of discharge, one attempts to offer and urge alternative living style, generally with encouragement toward treatment to stop drinking, i.e., AA. Weaning these patient from the unit is a formidable task. We attempt this by sending them to the less acute wards prior to discharge but meet *much* resistance to leaving. We find these patients returning to the unit when intoxicated and in trouble. This group could well benefit from some halfway house setting with limited supervision, where perhaps some drinking could be tolerated. Another option, probably more feasible, would be self-help groups for burn victims, preferably meeting in the inner-city area of the cheap hotels, where when in "trouble" there could be a turning to each other rather than to the bottle.

Another large group which taxes the patience of the staff are the passive-dependent personalities, who are not addicted. These patients exhibit demanding behavior, low frustration tolerance and lack of motivation requiring day-to-day planning. These patients may stir up our own unacceptable desires to be cared for in a dependent manner, resulting in anger and subsequent guilt. Alienated rather schizoid street people, tend to give very little and demand much, making it difficult for the staff to interact with them, except on a treatment-providing level. Consistency in approach, as with all patients seems most helpful, giving choices when possible but taking charge aggressively when necessary. Careful recording of approaches coupled with shift-to-shift reporting is crucial and decreases patients' playing one against the other. The psychiatric consultant in the expanded role may provide instant "on ward" consultation for the staff when the "difficult" patient acts out, particularly during debridement or in other instances requiring sedation or pain management.

With the luxury of time, to sit and listen as a friend and counselor, we can slowly help these people begin to develop trust. Here, being a nurse, not a psychiatrist, can be a real advantage. One is seen as less threatening and more available than the awesome group of doctors who are frequently seen as unapproachable during rounds, and not available at other times. Often patients will express amazement that a doctor "took the time" to sit and talk which frequently can be *most* meaningful. Frequently threats of suicide or signing out are made as attempts to take control of a situation in which one feels helpless, hurting or afraid. I generally interpret these as attempts to be heard, to get attention rather than as genuine intent. We occasionally resort to Valium to help these patients better cope with their anxiety, but using *people* rather than medication is ideal.

Often, what is most needed is a skilled listener. This person need not be a psychiatrist. The physical therapist is in an ideal position to listen, during exercise time, when talk of concerns and dreaded fears about the future may be verbalized. He may be the first to hear the patient's anxiety about disfigurement, disability or limits, and in sharing these comments with the staff, he can offer vital input to total management planning. Also, patients may be reluctant to be critical toward the nursing staff for fear of painful reprisal with the next injection or dressing change, much as they may be reluctant to share their anxiety with the physician, feeling they may "owe him much" for saving their lives, that he is "too busy to be bothered with something trivial." Our comments about "how good" the wounds look may tend to make the patient feel he is being unappreciative if he complains or questions. However, inability to express these "trivial" concerns may be increasing the patient's need for pain medication, keeping his appetite poor, actually impeding his healing process.

The occupational therapist can be most useful with these patients in helping to assess needs and providing impetus to try new things. Typically, patients may resist attempts to become involved in projects; yet, psychologically as well as physically, mastery of new skills as well as the socialization that can occur when several patients are brought together for an activity is crucial. We find that most patients are so involved in "self" during much of their care that they need much added encouragement to interact and we have tried to utilize patients transferred to other wards to spend time with more acute patients on the unit. Again, follow-up care is vital, as dependency on the ward decreases. We do not use antidepressant drugs during the transient situational despondency which so many of these patients experience, preferring to again, use people to listen and offer support.

The psychotic patient who makes a suicide attempt by immolation creates other difficult problems.

S. B, a 23-year-old male, was admitted with 30% burns to head, neck, chest, back and perineum sustained when he poured gasoline on himself in the yard of a Zen Buddhist Center. He had been drifting about the country and had not seen family for years; he first saw a psychiatrist at age 4, with brief psychiatric hospitalizations. Like so many psychotic patients he described no feelings of pain on admission, but was uncooperative, refusing to allow admitting treatment, and was delusional about staff, with homosexual and religious delusions and preoccupation. In this instance, the use of phenothiazines was indicated immediately as treatment of his injury could not be adequately done while the patient was acutely agitated. Working with the staff on allaying anxiety about dosages larger than P.D.R. recommendations, the plan for management and treatment of side-effects was immediately begun. The female staff did all of his care to decrease homosexual anxiety and a special diet was arranged that did not challenge his religious concerns.

The psychotic patient in an intensive care setting creates much anxiety and here the psychiatric consultant can play a more active role. First, suicide potential must be assessed. Our experience has been that once the attempt has been made (necessitating admission) there is a reduction of anxiety, and patients although requiring observation, will *not* make another attempt, while on the ward. At the time of discharge, however, the suicide potential may rise as despondency and anxiety become overwhelming. Careful discharge planning should be begun as early as possible to minimize this risk. The psychiatric consultant may be able to arrange for placement in halfway houses, day treatment centers, etc., so that a sheltered environment can be provided.

Other patients on the unit may require added support while the psychotic patient is acutely disturbed. Fear of going to sleep with that "crazy patient" awake would be very understandable. With reality testing impaired, explanations must frequently be repeated simply, and treatment may have to be completed quickly and efficiently without offering the patient choices in light of his ambivalence. The distorted body image of the schizophrenic may present problems, especially since his psychotic distortions may now become reality. He needs to be able to check things out. Much reassurance and support in frequent doses is necessary. Often these patients are very uncomfortable with being touched, with closeness, and if they become more trusting of certain staff members it is ideal if their care can be done with added consistency. Many of these patients are very creative and can better express themselves with art supplies or notebooks, especially as the acute phase of care is completed. We have found that as the psychosis improves, these patients may do *very* well in the womb-like sheltered environment of the ward, again, making the need for careful discharge planning imperative.

A word about the organic versus functional psychotic state is appropriate. While phenothiazines are the treatment of choice in a functional psychosis, the organic brain syndrome we frequently see secondary to sepsis, hypoxia, or metabolic disturbances, is only made worse by the addition of phenothiazines. Sensorium becomes more clouded, confusion increases, and ability to function is lessened. I have become less comfortable with the term "ICU psychosis" as I see it more as a diagnosis of exclusion. Generally, the acute psychotic picture, characterized by disorientation, confusion, visual hallucinations, fluctuating mental status and frequently paranoid ideation, may be an early symptom of sepsis or prolonged alcohol withdrawal—again the need for a history becomes important. Patients experiencing these acute changes need much reassurance as well as protection from themselves. If chemical controls are necessary, small doses of Valium (5 mg. q./3 to 4 hr.) along with chloral hydrate, Dalmane or Benadryl for sleep appear to be most helpful, using as little medication as possible to avoid distorting the clinical picture.

Other "difficult" problems that have been discussed either informally or in weekly staff meetings have been the frustration of working with the elderly patient, where depression, loneliness and isolation, coupled with increased fatigue and decreased ability to "bounce back" or fight back, make care a challenge. These patients, too may not give back very much, although

when one attempts to use "reminiscent" therapy their often fascinating pasts can make for delightful listening.

Even our population of children tend to be more disturbed and require added psychological support; to this end, we have included liaison with the child-abuse counsel, as well as schools and usual pediatric resources. Having children on the ward has at times created conflicts, both among the physicians as to *where* the child can best be treated (burn unit versus pediatrics ward) and among the nursing staff as to who are the better "mommies." They do, however, do wonders for staff morale.

The *death* of a patient, especially after a lengthy stay, can be devastating to both staff and other patients and is frequently discussed for months. In my observation, intense conflict arises around the issue of how aggressively to treat the severely burned individual with little potential for survival: the dilemma in philosophical approach of the teaching setting utilizing all known technology in order to preserve life versus allowing the patient to die with dignity; arrival at a decision all can feel comfortable with may not be possible, in light of differing philosophies of life and death. My role has been to help the staff accept the decision without "acting out" around it. Anticipatory grief work with family as well as patient can be begun; here again, the consultant may have more flexible time available to deal with this most difficult and necessary task.

This brings me to the most difficult issue of all—how, with patients who are incredibly demanding, both physically and psychologically, can one remain caring and empathetic?

Administration is not always aware of the special needs of the Burn Unit so that staffing problems may not be remedied and indeed are intensified. The intensity of relationships formed by lengthy stays with the need to tolerate patients one feels negatively about—all these create a need for much added support. The staff tends to look to the unit chief and their head nurse for leadership, enthusiasm and approval, which *do indeed* improve the quality of care. The "goodies" tend to come from working together, from sharing goals and accomplishments. As a consultant, I have attempted to be available, to be a sounding board for frustration and anger, which hopefully leaves more energy for patient care. We have had varying degrees of success with formal meetings, the interest peaking and dropping off. More seems to happen on an informal basis. It becomes clear to me that working on a burn unit must be time-limited, that either periodic breaks with more frequent vacations or floating to other areas, perhaps outpatient or community burn clinics might increase one's tolerance. The staff *must* work together, as a team, with open, clear communication between themselves, and provide adequate orientation of newcomers. Only then, when mutual goals for quality care are shared and the pride of success with some of the most difficult patients in the hospital setting can be felt, does the burn unit function as the exciting, challenging area it well can be.

BIBLIOGRAPHY

Andreasen, N. J. C., Noyes, R., Jr., Hartford, C. E., Brodland, G., and Proctor, S. Management of emotional reactions in seriously burned adults. N. Engl. J. Med. 236: 65–69, 1972.

Artz, C. T., and Moncrief, J. A. *The Treatment of Burns*. Philadelphia: W. B. Saunders Co., 1969.

MacArthur, J., and Moore F. Epidemiology of burns. *J.A.M.A.* 231(3): 259, 1975.

Quinby, S. V., and Bernstein, N. R. Identity problems and the adaptation of nurses to severely burned children. *Am. J. Psychiatry* 128: 58–63, 1971.

Sagerhaugh, W. V. Pain expression and control on a burn-care unit. *Nurs. Outlook* 22: 645–650, 1974.

INDEX